Bellevue Hospital Medical College

CITY OF NEW YORK.

SESSION 18

Admit ....

LECTURES

ON

THE PRINCIPLES AND PRACTICE OF MEDICINE.

Austin Flint, M. D., Professor.

Bellevue Hospital Medical College.

CITY OF NEW YORK.

SESSION 1874–'75.

.... *is entitled*

To all the Privileges of the Department of

PRACTICAL ANATOMY,

Until March 1, 1875.

A. Flint jr — M. D., Sec'y of the Faculty.

☞ This Ticket is not an evidence that the holder of it has actually dissected, unless certified by the Professor of Practical Anatomy. [OVER.]

The Education of American Physicians

THE EDUCATION OF AMERICAN PHYSICIANS

Historical Essays

Edited by Ronald L. Numbers

UNIVERSITY OF CALIFORNIA PRESS
Berkeley / Los Angeles / London

This book was published with the assistance of a grant from the Alumni Association of the Loma Linda University School of Medicine.

The endpapers for this book show tickets admitting students to lectures at the Bellevue Hospital Medical College, New York. Courtesy of the Richard W. Schwarz Collection.

University of California Press
Berkeley and Los Angeles, California

University of California Press, Ltd.
London, England

ISBN 0-520-03611-5
Library of Congress Catalog Card Number: 77-20326
Printed in the United States of America

1   2   3   4   5   6   7   8   9

FOR WILLIAM FREDERICK NORWOOD

Contents

Preface

Few topics in the history of American medicine have attracted greater interest than medical education. But because attention has usually focused on institutions rather than on curricula, we know much more about the organization and administration of medical schools than about their methods of instruction and the content of their courses. To correct this imbalance, these previously unpublished essays on the education of American physicians look specifically at the history of subjects taught in medical schools.

Following a brief overview of formal medical training in America since 1765, the chapters first take up the most basic of the preclinical sciences: anatomy, physiology, chemistry, pharmacology, and pathology. Next come essays devoted to the three primary branches of clinical medicine: internal medicine, surgery, and obstetrics. Finally, there are four essays on disciplines—arbitrarily selected—that have fought with mixed success for a place in the medical curriculum: neurology and psychiatry, preventive medicine, medical ethics and jurisprudence, and, of course, the history of medicine.

Perhaps the most important pattern revealed by these disciplinary histories is the gradual shift from what Edward Atwater calls passive to active learning. In the decades following the founding of America's first medical school in 1765, formal medical training consisted almost exclusively of didactic lectures that seldom went beyond the standard texts or notes the instructor himself had copied as a student. During the first half of the nineteenth century medical educators often added demonstrations to their lectures, giving students an opportunity to witness—if not to participate in—activities like anatomical dissections and surgical operations. By the 1890s a number of medical schools had taken the additional step of requiring students themselves to perform laboratory and clinical exercises, a pedagogic revolution that rivals in importance the better-known improvements of that period involving admission requirements, length of terms, and graded curricula. At the same time that preclinical students were entering the laboratory, their more advanced associates were beginning to diagnose real patients, assist with actual deliveries, and aid in surgical procedures.

This was not true, however, of all medical schools in America. As Abraham Flexner discovered in 1909, the better institutions already were emphasizing laboratory and clinical instruction, whereas the worst ones scarcely knew what the terms meant. In harmony with Flexner's recommendations, medical education during the first half of the twentieth century grew increasingly science oriented. As professors with Ph.D.'s displaced the physicians who had traditionally taught the basic sciences, preclinical and clinical training became so estranged that by mid-century many physicians were wondering whether medical schools had forgotten their primary mission of educating medical practitioners.

The twentieth-century medical curriculum, though reasonably stable, also changed in more subtle ways. As the academic calendar grew more and more crowded in response to the appearance of new specialties and accumulating scientific discoveries, medical educators responded by lengthening the school year and requiring additional premedical work at the college level, thus allowing medical schools to drop subjects like botany and inorganic chemistry. Yet by mid-century increased specialization and sophistication had made it impossible to continue providing comprehensive clinical training in the customary two years. Many young physicians found it necessary to continue their education in postgraduate residency programs, which, though beyond the scope of this book, represent one of the most significant recent developments in the history of American medical education.

This volume originated as a festschrift for William Frederick Norwood, America's premier historian of medical education. However, the emergence of common themes in this collection of essays takes it, I believe, far beyond the ordinary honorary volume and celebrates Norwood by carrying his work forward.

Fred Norwood was born in Kansas City, Kansas, on April 20, 1904, the second of twin boys whose father pastored the local Seventh-day Adventist church.[1] From first grade through college Norwood attended Adventist schools, graduating from Walla Walla College in Washington in 1927 with a major in history. Three years later, while teaching at the church's Los Angeles Academy, he enrolled part time in the University of Southern California to continue his historical training in that school's fledgling graduate program. The decision was not without risk for a young Adven-

---

1. Unless otherwise noted, the biographical information that follows is based on a taped interview with William Frederick Norwood, October 27, 1974, a transcript of which is deposited in the Loma Linda University Library, Loma Linda, California.

tist, whose church still viewed secular education as a spiritually hazardous experience.

Norwood received his M.A. degree in history in 1931. Two years later, while continuing his graduate studies, he became registrar of the College of Medical Evangelists, an accredited Adventist medical school with campuses in Los Angeles and Loma Linda. When Dr. Newton G. Evans, the college's former president, urged his junior colleague to focus his doctoral studies on the history of medical education, the suggestion immediately appealed to Norwood, as well as to his professors at USC, particularly Gilbert Giddings Benjamin and Erik McKinley Eriksson. Eriksson's enthusiasm for the idea may have stemmed from his previous work at the University of Iowa with Arthur M. Schlesinger, who personally inspired many of the early studies in the history of American science and medicine.[2]

When, with Eriksson's blessing, Norwood began his dissertation on the history of American medical education before the Civil War, the topic was hardly virgin territory. As early as 1851 Nathan Smith Davis had published a *History of Medical Education and Institutions in the United States,* and various other nineteenth-century writers had produced local medical school histories. Twentieth-century scholars such as Francis R. Packard, Henry E. Sigerist, and Henry B. Shafer had also dealt with the subject. Yet no one had paid much attention to the host of ephemeral medical schools in antebellum America, and no historian had based his conclusions on a thorough search of the available evidence. This Norwood determined to do.

Completed in 1939, his dissertation was one of the first ever written on the history of American medicine, apparently preceded only by the theses of Courtney Robert Hall, Helen E. Marshall, and Henry Burnell Shafer.[3] Norwood's veritable encyclopedia of antebellum medical schools contained historical sketches of eighty-eight different institutions ranging (in the published version) from a twenty-three-page account of the University of Pennsylvania School of Medicine to a one-paragraph note on the College of Physicians and Surgeons of the Upper Mississippi. The picture

2. A. Hunter Dupree, "The History of American Science—A Field Finds Itself," *Am. Hist. Rev.* 71 (1968): 867.

3. See Richard H. Shryock, "The Historian Looks at Medicine," *Bull. Hist. Med.* 5 (1937): 889. Hall and Shafer both studied with Dixon Ryan Fox at Columbia University. In 1934 Hall published *A Scientist in the Early Republic: Samuel Latham Mitchill, 1764–1831* (New York: Columbia University Press), and two years later Shafer brought out *The American Medical Profession, 1783 to 1850* (New York: Columbia University Press). Marshall, who worked with Shryock at Duke University, completed her dissertation in 1934 and later published it under the title *Dorothea Dix: Forgotten Samaritan* (Chapel Hill: University of North Carolina Press, 1937).

that emerged from these sketches was not a pretty one: proliferating schools, low standards, poor instruction, quarreling faculties, and professors interested mainly in the number of lecture tickets they could sell. But in spite of its obvious imperfections, the "American system of medical education," combining an apprenticeship with two identical courses of formal lectures, produced several institutions of relatively high quality and provided an expanding nation with an adequate supply of medical practitioners.

Five years after Norwood finished his dissertation, the University of Pennsylvania Press, assisted financially by sympathetic CME alumni and other private sources, published *Medical Education in the United States before the Civil War*. Wartime restrictions on paper permitted a printing of only five hundred copies, but the response to the book was gratifying. One after another, the leading historians of medicine, from Henry Sigerist to Richard Shryock, praised Norwood for his invaluable contribution to the field.[4] *Medical Education in the United States before the Civil War* quickly became a classic. When a reprinted edition appeared in 1971, it elicited a second round of acclaim for its author. Chester R. Burns, observing that no recent study of American medical education had displayed "the same quality of detailed analysis exhibited by Norwood," suggested that perhaps Norwood's high standards had "inhibited further scholarship."[5] Gert H. Brieger offered similar praise, noting that "all of the work done since 1944 merely adds to and extends Norwood, it doesn't materially change his interpretations."[6]

By the time his book first came out, Norwood had risen to the associate deanship of CME, and he continued, except for two short intervals, to work for the school (which in 1961 became Loma Linda University) until his official retirement in 1974, serving as dean, vice-president, and chairman of the department of cultural medicine. From the late 1930s until 1969 he also taught the history of medicine in one of the few such programs in the country. His first leave of absence from CME came in the early 1950s, when the American Medical Association recruited him for a year to serve as staff associate on a mid-century survey of American medical schools, and the W. K. Kellogg Foundation retained him for a second year to evaluate its program of financing continuing medical education. In

4. One of the few criticisms came from Erwin H. Ackerknecht, who felt that Norwood had focussed too exclusively on "the non-medical aspects of school life." Although Ackerknecht regarded the book as "a valuable and reliable survey," he did not think that it dealt with "the history of medicine proper, that is, the history of diseases and their treatment" (*Quart. Rev. Bio.* 20 [1945]: 96; and *Psychosomatic Medicine* 7 [1945]: 193).

5. Chester R. Burns, *J. AMA* 220 (1972): 1621–22.

6. Gert H. Brieger, *Bull. Hist. Med.* 48 (1974): 300–301.

1960/61 he returned to the AMA for eighteen months as staff director of a special committee investigating the financial problems of medical students and interns. Although these administrative responsibilities frequently took Norwood away from the history of medicine, he continued to write historical articles and book reviews; and in 1979, after a decade and a half of work, he completed the final chapter of a volume entitled *American Medicine and the Civil War*.

This collection of essays on the changing education of American physicians complements Norwood's institutional history of American medical schools. It honors a man who chose never to teach at one of the nation's great universities, who never directed a doctoral dissertation, yet who won the love and respect of all who knew him. It is a monument to a wonderful white-haired gentleman who pioneered in the writing of American medical history, who persevered in the teaching of the history of medicine, and who enriched the lives of countless students and friends. In editing this collection I have incurred many debts of gratitude. First, I would like to thank Lloyd G. Stevenson and my thirteen collaborators, who good naturedly put up with my editorial idiosyncrasies and—in some cases—with interminable delays in publication. If this book is a success, they deserve the credit. Vern Carner, a former associate of mine at Loma Linda University, initially suggested that I edit a volume in honor of our friend Fred Norwood. Anna Bresnahan and Ada Turner assisted in preparing the biographical material. Judith Walzer Leavitt, John L. Parascandola, Guenter B. Risse, and Patricia Spain Ward—all colleagues at the University of Wisconsin—each offered to read one or more chapters. Gert H. Brieger generously read the entire manuscript. Marilyn Schwartz, of the University of California Press, performed the herculean task of editing the manuscript, appreciably improving its clarity, precision, and style. William J. Orr, Jr., checked copy and proofread, and Barbara Ingle prepared the index.

Finally, I am indebted to the Alumni Association of the Loma Linda University School of Medicine for financially supporting the publication of this volume. Fittingly, this same association a quarter-century ago contributed to the cost of printing Norwood's *Medical Education in the United States before the Civil War*. I particularly appreciate the cooperation of Walter E. Macpherson, M.D., chairman of the publications board; Alma O. Johnson, office manager; and Harvey A. Elder, M.D., who lent his support at a crucial time.

RONALD L. NUMBERS
Madison, Wisconsin
April 1978

Introduction

LLOYD G. STEVENSON

LESS than a century ago the learned and indefatigable Theodor Puschmann wrote, without collaborators, a comprehensive history of medical
education.[1] The nearest recent counterpart of this study, a panoramic
history edited by the late Professor C. D. O'Malley and published in
1970, involved a large number of scholars, who contributed essays on
medical instruction ranging from classical antiquity to the modern era and
covering both eastern and western hemispheres.[2] The majority of historians of medical education have been less ambitious, often limiting their
work to national histories, organized in a variety of ways. The most recent
example of a short, one-man job is Martin Kaufman's *American Medical
Education: The Formative Years, 1765–1910* (1976), which begins not
long after the beginning and goes as far as the Flexner Report. William
Frederick Norwood's classic *Medical Education in the United States be-*

1. Theodor Puschmann, *A History of Medical Education from the Most Remote to the
Most Recent Times*, trans. and ed. Evan H. Hare (London: H. K. Lewis, 1891).
2. Charles Donald O'Malley, *The History of Medical Education: An International Symposium Held February 5–9, 1968* (Berkeley and Los Angeles: University of California Press,
1970).

1

fore the Civil War (1944) focused on an even briefer period. Norwood's book devoted little attention to the maturation of the medical sciences and the development of clinical specialties, much of which took place after 1865. But now comes a study which does just that. Ignoring the subspecialties, which split the physician's employment into hematology, cardiology, rheumatology, and the like, it separates the training of doctors into the broad categories that have long characterized research and practice. It narrows the focus and in doing so sharpens it. Although each contributor to this volume restricts his survey, the totality of the work has a very wide purview.

In one sense the present book complements *Medical Education in the United States before the Civil War;* in another sense it is antithetical to Norwood's pioneering work. Its coverage extends into the twentieth century, and it looks at medical education in America from a totally different viewpoint. In his foreword to Norwood's book Henry Sigerist quoted with approval a statement by Richard Shryock that had just appeared in *Isis:* "The value of studies in the history of American science is not to be found primarily in contributions to the history of science as such, but rather to the history of the United States." This assertion Sigerist thought could be extended: "Shryock's statement fully applies to the history of medicine. . . . Medical education as it was practised in the United States before the Civil War had certainly nothing to give to the world, and yet it was undoubtedly an important factor in the life of the nation."[3]

Were science and medical education in antebellum America so puerile? Or had Shryock and Sigerist shorn history of its beams? Even Norwood, in his laboriously researched and well-considered survey, found little to praise, reporting not merely frontier hardship but many of the least engaging aspects of "a society that worshiped the principles of unchecked free enterprise and unlimited laissez faire." (The phraseology is obviously Sigerist's and comes from his foreword to Norwood's book.) Disregard of educational standards was only one feature of the soggy prewar medicine exposed by Norwood; American medical education must have picked up considerably in the half century before Abraham Flexner came along to inspect and condemn.

And yet the commanding strength of Nathan Smith and the bombast of Charles Caldwell were a part of American medical education before the Civil War. And Erasmus Darwin Fenner—whose work Norwood handled well, but not so well as the present book—seems to have been right up

3. Foreword by Henry E. Sigerist to William Frederick Norwood, *Medical Education in the United States before the Civil War* (Philadelphia: University of Pennsylvania Press, 1944), p. vii.

with the vanguard of European medical education in the clinical instruction he offered in New Orleans on the very eve of the war.

Edward Atwater can improve upon Norwood's account of clinical instruction largely because the rise, the competition, and the success or fall of medical schools do not (and need not) concern him more than incidentally. He can concentrate on the teaching of medicine, as John Blake can concentrate on the teaching of anatomy and Gert Brieger on the teaching of surgery. After a preliminary overview of American medical education by Martin Kaufman, each of the contributors to this book is free to focus on a single medical science or clinical specialty, unmindful for the most part of economics, politics, or other distractions. (Of course, discussing these external factors can be a strength rather than a distraction, as Atwater demonstrates in his chapter on internal medicine.) Because of the organizational pattern of this book and because of Norwood's prior work, his successors can now largely ignore the organizations and disorganizations, the strikes and lockouts and sieges, the rivalries and pitched battles (a term both figurative and literal), and the dreadful fusillades of rhetoric that characterized medical education in an apparent rehearsal for the Civil War. They can train their sights on targets that are clearly defined and well within range. They can tell us where, when, and how the various disciplines of medical education took their form and place in the medical curriculum and show us how the changes (and also the absence of change) in American medicine found representation in the course of study. They can show us how medical educators of the past taught their young students to dissect, to auscultate, to prescribe. Whereas Norwood's attention centered on the schools and their quarrelsome faculties, the attention of the contributors to this volume focuses on the relations between teacher and student and, above all, on the content and method of teaching. To this extent the book contributes not just to American history, the stated theme of the volume, but to the history of medicine generally—a subject that makes a few historians unaccountably shy and causes them to flee back as quickly as possible to the shelter of their traditional fields. The essayists in this volume are, by and large, brave enough to insist on the point.

There was a time, of course, when not a few teachers of medicine were, or thought themselves, extremely versatile. There was no more presumption in a preceptor undertaking to teach his apprentice virtually everything than in his undertaking general and indeed total practice. Probably the majority welcomed the opportunity, when it came, to pass along to other hands certain duties, especially surgical procedures, certain difficult and dangerous cases, and certain demands for teaching. And yet medical philosophers of vast expertise were not unknown. Dr. John Delamater, apparently regarded everywhere as a man of lofty talent, was known in half a dozen medical colleges in New England and New York and in four situated in what was then the great Northwest (Ohio and Illinois). He held chairs in nine or ten medical schools, and for nearly forty years (1823–1860) he delivered lectures "in almost every branch of medical science."[4] But after the Civil War it became a mark of sophistication for teachers to restrict their teaching, like their medical practice, to one or two areas, no longer taking the world for a parish. The broad fields of medicine, like the wide plains of America, were ultimately subdivided, cultivated, fenced. And if medical teachers lacked the splendid versatility of a Delamater, many of them lacked very little of his superb self-confidence.

This narrowing of areas of competence staked out by practitioners and teachers came rather late, the date varying from field to field. Each of our authors deals to some degree with this dating. Several are quite precise, but they have been luckier than others in the nature and amount of data available to them. All the contributors to this book find ample evidence of change in what was taught, if not evidence of improvement or change in the manner of teaching. And toward the end of the nineteenth century and the beginning of the twentieth they all discover signs—indeed sometimes flags and banners—of a move toward a new era in medical education. Thus Sigerist's apologetic attitude toward what he plainly regarded as little more than mediocrity (of value to American history only) can be replaced by a mixture of damning criticism and dawning pride, a singular combination that recalls the not altogether unwelcome Flexner Report. True, the measure of mediocrity in medical instruction at the turn of the century remained large; but just as Norwood found in the antebellum period, described in his splendid book, it is a mediocrity illumined by shafts of the most varied and interesting light, gleams that occasionally light up not only the history of the United States but also the history of medical education in broader realms. This is not to imply that American history can shed light on the European experience only by having something "to give to the world." Both goodness and badness (and bad medical education has not been unknown in Europe) can be revealing. Whether seen from this broader perspective or from the viewpoint of having something to give to the world, American medical education grows increasingly worthy of historical attention. Bad and good, it grows, in these pages, more interesting.

From every angle, then, the international as well as the national, the

---

4. Norwood, *Medical Education*, p. 153. "As a builder of western medicine Delamater ranks with Daniel Drake."

post–Civil War history of American medical education is here seen, for all its grave (and not infrequently ludicrous) defects, as a matter of slowly increasing importance and interest. American medicine ultimately assumed major, and generally recognized, significance toward the end of the nineteenth century. But into the first quarter of the twentieth century American medical education retained defects so serious that it could give only limited promise of the real distinction to come; and when the distinction was at last apparent, not all of the shortcomings had disappeared. Some of the less exhilarated scholars, the more reproachful, even believe that as the old defects vanished new ones replaced them.

It was the Civil War that turned the attention of American medical schools to the teaching of public health, as Judith Leavitt shows in her essay. More surprising, perhaps, is the part played by women's medical colleges in bringing about this change. Even if readers know that medical ethics and jurisprudence found a place in the medical curriculum at an early date, a number of those who read the essay by Chester Burns will learn with some surprise of the comprehensive lectures on the legal responsibilities of doctors delivered in New York a century ago; for there presently exists a widespread erroneous impression that malpractice suits are comparatively novel.

That the transformation of medicine, growing ever more scientific as the nineteenth century advanced, should have brought with it extensive changes in the substance of teaching we can to some extent take for granted. How inorganic and pharmaceutical chemistry gave way to medical chemistry and how medical chemistry grew into biochemistry demonstrate, according to James Whorton, a rough but not inexact parallel between the evolution of science and evolution of teaching. In other disciplines, however, such an equivalence has not always proved easily traceable.

What many will learn from these pages is that changes did not always solve problems but occasionally caused them. What was to be the proper relationship between research and teaching? Would the concept of anatomy sustained by Franklin P. Mall and Ross Harrison satisfy the surgeons? Would it satisfy the students? Pondering such questions with knowledge and insight, John Blake illumines both past and present. Another element in the story of the teaching of anatomy is its relationship with physiology on the one hand and pathology on the other, an issue approached from different perspectives by John Warner and Russell Maulitz, who have written key chapters dealing with the structure of nineteenth-century medicine and hence of medical education. Both sciences, of course, were intimately linked with the clinic, although pathology at that time better served the needs of clinicians and better integrated with their teaching. The changing relationship between neighboring disciplines is further exemplified, with its implications for teaching, in Jeanne Brand's essay on neurology and psychiatry, an essay which also reveals, as not all of the others do, the impact of government aid and intervention in the period since World War II.

Another area in which neighborhood relationships are shown undergoing change is that of materia medica and pharmacology, the subject of David Cowen's essay. Here again the status of chemistry is relevant, and also that of physiology. Conceding some truth to Carleton Chapman's statement that materia medica was "more Pharmacy than Pharmacology" in the mid-nineteenth century, Cowen nevertheless insists on the continuance of the close relationship with therapeutics. Pharmacology itself gradually becomes the principal concern; but, as some readers will learn with surprise, the separation of departments of physiology and pharmacology in the major medical schools became virtually complete only at the beginning of the present decade.

The historians of clinical teaching, especially Edward Atwater and Gert Brieger, are concerned with student opportunities to observe, to take active part, and to assume responsibility. Lawrence Longo informs us that the introduction of demonstrative teaching of obstetrics dates for practical purposes only from 1850. The findings of J. Whitridge Williams's survey of the teaching of obstetrics and gynecology, published soon after the appearance of the Flexner Report, are less well known than Flexner's findings but hardly less startling.

Other kinds of teachers have surveyed their pedagogic fields earnestly and even anxiously, but none, perhaps, have done so as keenly in recent years as medical historians; and none, as Genevieve Miller (I think) indicates, have had more reason for anxiety. And yet the work progresses. Not all of it can be as clearly and solidly relevant as the history of medical education. But the present book comes triumphantly home to our bosoms and businesses in a way that can leave little doubt of the use of medical history. Would that every carpenter of a new curriculum could be counted on to read and ponder it.

American Medical Education

MARTIN KAUFMAN

U NTIL well into the nineteenth century the vast majority of American physicians were trained through apprenticeship. That was fully in line with the European methods of educating surgeons, apothecaries, and other tradesmen. In colonial days boys were often apprenticed before they reached their sixteenth birthday, and the apprenticeship often lasted from five to seven years. In return for financial compensation and the labor of the boy, the preceptor would prepare his apprentice for the "successful" practice of medicine. The student would act as a body servant, tending the horse, cleaning the office, and sometimes trying to collect bills. During the term of apprenticeship, the student would "read medicine" in the preceptor's library and join the master on his rounds. In addition, some students would learn anatomy through dissection, although that often caused problems with the local citizenry, who were not enthusiastic about having their cemeteries raided for subjects.[1]

1. See Genevieve Miller, "Medical Apprenticeship in the American Colonies," *Ciba Symposia* 8 (January 1947): 502–10; Genevieve Miller, "Medical Education in the American Colonies," *J. Med. Educ.* 31 (February 1956): 82–94. For more complete substantiation of

7

Martin Kaufman

Some physicians were excellent preceptors, with a genuine interest in their students, a library of the leading medical works of the day, and an intense desire to improve the quality of medical care in the region. The evidence indicates, however, that most physicians had only a few books and were too busy to devote much time to the needs of their apprentices. In addition, because only a few physicians were willing to take the chance of teaching anatomy through dissection, most students had to learn anatomy by reading anatomy textbooks.[2] On the other hand, it was necessary to have trained physicians, and apprenticeship served that purpose without forcing students to attend medical school in Europe, which was out of the reach of all but upper-class students. With all its faults, apprenticeship did assure that practicing physicians had clinical experience, even if that simply meant watching a preceptor tend to his patients, and it assured that practitioners were not totally unschooled.

A few students who could afford to do so would serve their apprenticeship and then complete their education by attending lectures at the University of Edinburgh or some other European school. After receiving their medical degrees, they would often make the grand tour of the Continent, attending clinical lectures at leading hospitals and enrolling in private courses taught by the most famous physicians and surgeons of the time. It has been estimated that of the three thousand physicians who practiced medicine during the colonial period, only about four hundred were medical graduates, and most of those had graduated from European institutions.[3]

The first medical college in America was established in 1765 by John Morgan and William Shippen, Jr., young Philadelphians who had recently returned from Europe, where they had received medical degrees from Edinburgh and taken the grand tour of the day. Morgan, Shippen, and other American students at Edinburgh had discussed the need for medical colleges in the colonies and had resolved to establish one when

---

the generalizations in the first half of this essay, see Martin Kaufman, *American Medical Education: The Formative Years, 1765–1910* (Westport: Greenwood Press, 1976). For a systematic survey of the antebellum medical schools, see William F. Norwood, *Medical Education in the United States before the Civil War* (Philadelphia: University of Pennsylvania Press, 1944).

2. For specific examples of the benefits and the problems of apprenticeship, see Kaufman, *American Medical Education*, ch. 1.

3. For information on the European medical training given to American students, see Whitfield J. Bell, Jr., "Medical Students and Their Examiners in Eighteenth Century America," *Trans. & Stud. Coll. Phys. Phila.*, 4th ser., 21 (June 1953): 14–24; Genevieve Miller, "European Influences in Colonial Medicine," *Ciba Symposia* 8 (January 1947): 511–21. See also Whitfield J. Bell, Jr., "A Portrait of the Colonial Physician," *Bull. Hist. Med.* 44 (November–December 1970): 497–517.

they returned to Philadelphia. Morgan, who had the support and encouragement of Dr. John Fothergill, a leading physician and scientist, managed to convince the trustees of the College of Philadelphia to establish a medical college modeled after the University of Edinburgh.[4]

Morgan's intention was to enable students who had completed their apprenticeship to review the various branches of medical science, "concentrated into as small a part of the year as possible." In effect, the medical college would combine the work of several preceptors, each of whom would theoretically be an expert in a specific field of medical science. The student would review anatomy through dissection, medicine and materia medica through practical lectures, and surgery, medicine, and midwifery by observing a variety of cases at a local hospital. It was virtually impossible for all of that to be obtained in a single preceptor's office.[5]

When the college opened in 1765, it had a two-man faculty, with Morgan as professor of the theory and practice of medicine, and Shippen as professor of anatomy and surgery. It was not until 1767 that the trustees decided to confer degrees, the bachelor's degree in "physic" and the doctor's degree in "physic," the latter to be awarded to students who had received their bachelor's degree at least three years earlier and who presented and defended a thesis. On June 21, 1768, America's first medical commencement was held, with ten young men receiving bachelor's degrees. The students had sat through lectures given by the two fledgling professors, and they had heard Thomas Bond's clinical lectures at the Pennsylvania Hospital. Within the next two years the faculty grew. Adam Kuhn, a student of Linnaeus, was appointed professor of botany and materia medica, and Benjamin Rush, a member of that first graduating class in 1768 who went on to complete his education at Edinburgh, was named professor of chemistry.[6]

In 1767 the second medical school was established in the colonies, this time in New York City. Like the one in Philadelphia, it was organized by a young graduate of Edinburgh, Samuel Bard. The governors of King's College appointed Bard and five others as professors, including three of

4. Whitfield J. Bell, Jr., *John Morgan: Continental Doctor* (Philadelphia: University of Pennsylvania Press, 1965), pp. 72–73. For a complete description of the development of the University of Pennsylvania Medical School, see George W. Corner, *Two Centuries of Medicine: A History of the School of Medicine, University of Pennsylvania* (Philadelphia: J. B. Lippincott, 1965).

5. N. S. Davis, *Contributions to the History of Medical Education and Medical Institutions in the United States of America, 1776–1876* (Washington, D.C.: Government Printing Office, 1877), p. 11.

6. Bell, *John Morgan*, pp. 143–44. See also Elizabeth H. Thomson, "Thomas Bond, 1713–84," *J. Med. Educ.* 33 (1958): 614–24.

the best-known and most experienced men in the colony: Samuel Clossy, Peter Middleton, and John Jones. On May 3, 1769, ten months after the first commencement at Philadelphia, King's College graduated its first class.[7]

In 1782 Harvard established a medical college, and fifteen years later Nathan Smith, a Harvard graduate who had recently returned from Edinburgh, helped establish the fourth American school, which was affiliated with Dartmouth College in New Hampshire. At Transylvania University in Kentucky at the turn of the century, a fifth institution was organized, but it did not graduate its first class until 1802. Thus by the beginning of the nineteenth century there were five medical colleges in the United States, all connected with colleges of arts and sciences.

Soon several new colleges appeared, including the College of Physicians and Surgeons in New York City, the University of Maryland, Yale University, and the College of Physicians and Surgeons of the Western District of New York. Until the War of 1812, America's medical schools were either branches of colleges and universities or affiliates of medical societies. After the war, however, most new schools were proprietary, generally established by local physicians who wanted to add to their prestige by being professors at a local medical school, to supplement their income by dividing the student fees, and to achieve a competitive advantage by being able to advertise a college connection.[8] Local citizens were generally enthusiastic about the establishment of medical colleges as long as their cemeteries were not ransacked for cadavers. The development of a local college gave residents a sense of pride; after all, they then lived in a "seat of learning," like Paris, Rome, London, or Philadelphia. No longer were they frontiersmen—they lived in the midst of a civilized society.[9]

Since the primary impetus for establishing proprietary colleges was financial, the schools tried to improve their competitive advantage over other institutions. Because students had to take two courses of lectures for their degrees, the schools tried to schedule their sessions so it was possible for students to transfer after having attended one course elsewhere; students who did so would be able to graduate in less than one year of study. Indeed, as schools proliferated, they began to compete for students

7. See Byron Stookey, *A History of Colonial Medical Education in the Province of New York, with Its Subsequent Development* (Springfield, Ill.: Charles C. Thomas, 1962).

8. See Frederick Waite, "Birth of the First Independent Proprietary Medical School in New England, at Castleton, Vermont, in 1818," *Ann. Med. Hist.*, n.s., 7 (May 1935): 242–52. Waite provides an interesting analysis of the reasons for the development of proprietary institutions.

9. Daniel J. Boorstin, *The Americans: The National Experience* (New York: Random House, 1965), pp. 152–61.

by reducing requirements, cutting fees, and offering "scholarships" to students who otherwise would have filled the benches of competing institutions.[10] The curriculum was ungraded, having no sequence of basic and advanced courses. Students at one college would hear the same professors giving the same lectures in two different terms. The system tended to encourage students to transfer so they would benefit from the lectures of a different set of professors.

Although the proprietary school has traditionally been blamed for lowering standards of medical education in the early nineteenth century, there is evidence that the problem began earlier. In 1792, for instance, the University of Pennsylvania abolished the bachelor's degree in medicine and reduced its requirements for the doctor's degree. Since it was possible to practice medicine without having attended college (before the advent of medical license laws), and as it was "both tedious and expensive" to attend medical school, many young men attended only long enough to receive the bachelor's degree in medicine, or they practiced without attending any lectures. It was simply not worthwhile financially for students to attend classes if they could not then advertise themselves as "doctors." And the requirements for the doctorate were so stringent that only a handful of graduates ever returned for that degree. The response of the professors was natural: they eliminated the bachelor's degree altogether and offered doctor's degrees for less than what previously had been required for the bachelor's, at the same time reducing the length of the medical course from seven or nine months to a more appealing four or five months.[11] Students flocked to the schools which offered degrees in the shortest period of time.

Throughout the nineteenth century medical colleges proliferated, and the number of colleges was further increased by the development of competing medical sects. Twenty-six new schools were established between 1810 and 1840, and forty-seven more were organized between 1840 and 1877. By 1876, the nation's centennial, eighty medical colleges had been established and sixty-four were still in operation.[12] It was a very volatile period in the history of medical education. Indeed, some of the new schools developed not because of any real need for more or better

10. Frederick Waite, *The First Medical College in Vermont: Castleton, 1818–1862* (Montpelier: Vermont Historical Society, 1949), pp. 83–84.
11. Frederick Waite, "Medical Degrees Conferred in the American Colonies and in the United States in the Eighteenth Century," *Ann. Med. Hist.*, n.s., 9 (July 1937): 315–20; N. S. Davis, *History of Medical Education and Institutions in the United States, from the First Settlement of the British Colonies to the Year 1850* (Chicago: S. C. Griggs, 1851), pp. 50–55.
12. Davis, *Contributions to the History of Medical Education*, p. 41.

medical colleges, but rather as a result of intrafaculty disputes. An argument over who should hold the prestigious chair in medicine, for instance, could easily result in the organization of a competing institution committed to the destruction of the original school.[13]

Friction between schools often led to pamphlet warfare and, on occasion, even to open strife. In at least one case, involving the Eclectic Medical Institute of Cincinnati, violence erupted between factions competing for control of the college. Opposing armies of students and professors faced each other with knives, pistols, bludgeons, and blunderbusses, and the faction defending the college building eventually brought in a six-pound cannon. At that point the besieging forces dispersed, to continue their war in a court of law.[14]

Prior to the Civil War the typical medical school had five or six professors, most of whom were general practitioners teaching in their spare time. A few instructors, however, were professional medical educators who taught at two or more institutions during the same year. They would teach during the winter, spring, and summer terms, often travelling great distances. Nathan Smith, for instance, taught in the same years at Yale, Vermont, and Bowdoin, travelling from Connecticut to Vermont and then to Maine. Other educators went from Michigan to New York City, and so on. As long as the colleges had four-month courses—and it was possible to teach an intensive course in less than that—a number of these professional medical teachers supported themselves from student fees at several institutions.

Until specialization began in the decades after the Civil War, professors taught what they preferred, or in the case of newcomers to the faculty, what was left after the veteran professors selected their courses. There were usually nine specific courses—anatomy, botany, chemistry, diseases of women and children, materia medica, obstetrics, physiology, principles and practice of medicine, principles and practice of surgery. Because the typical school had only five or six professors, some instructors had to teach more than one subject. For instance, in 1822 New York's College of Physicians and Surgeons had seven professors and a demonstrator of anatomy (who was responsible for procuring subjects and assisting students who chose to learn anatomy through dissection). Anatomy and physiology, botany and materia medica, and obstetrics and the diseases of women and children were each taught by one professor.[15] The chair of

13. See examples in Kaufman, *American Medical Education*, ch. 3.
14. Harvey W. Felter, *History of the Eclectic Medical Institute* (Cincinnati: Alumni Association of Eclectic Medical Institute, 1902), pp. 41–42. See also Ronald L. Numbers, "The Making of an Eclectic Physician," *Bull. Hist. Med.* 47 (March-April 1973): 155–66.
15. College of Physicians and Surgeons, *Catalogue, 1822* (New York, 1822).

clinical medicine at the College of Physicians and Surgeons was unique for its day, as only a few schools had access to hospitals, and teaching was almost exclusively by the lecture method. Indeed, until the twentieth century it was possible to graduate from medical school without ever setting foot in a hospital.

It is difficult to assess the quality of the various institutions; until the late 1840s virtually all the historian has to work with are college announcements, editorials and articles in medical journals, and student notebooks and diaries. In addition, the announcements often exaggerated the facilities in an attempt to attract more students, who were the lifeblood of the colleges. One New York physician and author, Edward H. Dixon, asserted that "no tribe of wandering gipsies or rope dancers can surpass their show-bills, announcing the enticing facilities with which their college abounds." In an essay entitled "Medical Lying, as illustrated in our College Circulars," Dixon declared that "lying like a college catalogue" was the epitome of that art. He insisted that the catalogues claimed "pretensions" which could not be read in faculty meetings without the professors "laughing at one another." As a result of the misrepresentations, students complained about the "hospital" which consisted of two beds in an attic, or the "extensive course" which consisted of two lectures with no apparatus or demonstrations.[16]

Late in 1846 or early in 1847 a committee of the convention which developed into the American Medical Association sent questionnaires to determine conditions in the colleges. Nineteen institutions replied, representing slightly more than half the schools. The survey indicated great variations. The term extended from three months in some schools to eight in others; the faculty numbered from three to eight; clinical instruction was required in twelve colleges but not in seven; and dissection was required in only five of the schools.[17]

The committee recommended that the term be standardized at six months, that graduates be required to take two courses of lectures and to present evidence of having served an apprenticeship with a qualified preceptor. Finally, the committee suggested that each school have seven professors, providing instruction in seven branches of medical science: theory and practice of medicine, principles and practice of surgery, general and special anatomy, physiology and pathology, materia medica,

---

16. *The Scalpel* 3 (November 1850): 59–60, and 5 (February 1853): 104–7. For more evidence of misrepresentation and exaggeration in announcements, see Andrew Boardman, *Essay on the Means of Improving Medical Education and Elevating Medical Character* (Philadelphia, 1840), pp. 5–7.

17. *Proceedings of the National Medical Conventions, Held in New York, May, 1846, and in Philadelphia, May, 1847* (Philadelphia, 1847), p. 70.

therapeutics and pharmacy, chemistry and medical jurisprudence, and midwifery and the diseases of women and children. In addition, the committee recommended that each student be required to devote three full months to anatomical dissection, and that the colleges require hospital work.[18]

Two schools, the University of Pennsylvania and New York's College of Physicians and Surgeons, lengthened their courses in response to the AMA recommendations, and for both it was disastrous. In 1847 the schools announced six-month courses of lectures. When the Jefferson Medical College of Philadelphia and New York University continued to advertise four-month courses, the inevitable result was an increase in enrollment at Jefferson and NYU and a decrease at Pennsylvania and the College of Physicians and Surgeons. It did not take long for the two reforming institutions to return to the traditional four-month program. In 1849 a more complete survey demonstrated that although twenty-two of the twenty-eight colleges had seven or more professors, only seventeen schools required dissection and only seven required hospital attendance.[19]

During the Gilded Age of American history, when material success took precedence over moral or ethical considerations, proprietary colleges continued to proliferate. In 1880 there were 90 colleges; ten years later the number had increased to 116, and by 1900 there were 151.[20] During this period many large cities had three, four, or even more competing colleges, and the weakest ones often attracted the largest classes because of their low standards.

Significantly, the proliferation of colleges came at precisely the time when medical and scientific knowledge was advancing at a rapid pace. The bacteriological revolution increased the importance of chemistry, pathology, bacteriology, and physiology, all of which required laboratory facilities and trained instructors. In order to provide an adequate education, medical colleges needed laboratories with costly equipment and more teachers than ever before. It was becoming more expensive to provide the modern scientific medical education. A college that depended solely upon student fees for support could not possibly remain in existence. Those schools that were branches of universities were in the best position to survive; after all, the universities had laboratories that medical

18. Ibid., pp. 73–74.
19. *Trans. AMA* 2 (1849): 281–99; *St. Louis Medical and Surgical Journal* 12 (August 1854): 471; William Pepper, *Higher Medical Education* (Philadelphia: J. B. Lippincott, 1894), pp. 24–25.
20. *Medical Schools of the United States, 1906* (Chicago: AMA Council on Medical Education, 1906), p. 46.

students could utilize. In addition, the new scientific emphasis meant that medical students had to be better prepared than ever before; without a firm foundation in physics, chemistry, and biology they would find it impossible to keep up with the professors during their first year of medical college.[21]

With the scientific revolution came a tremendous increase in the amount of medical knowledge to be acquired. It became more difficult for professors to cover their areas in the short time allocated, whether four, five, or even six mmnths. in addition, as medicine became more firmly based on scientific knowledge, the traditional ungraded curriculum no longer served its purpose. In the past the medical course had provided a rapid review for students who already had several years of informal clinical experience as apprentices. Now the apprenticeship was disappearing and the colleges had to provide students with their entire medical training.

The professors were in a difficult position. They recognized that they needed more time to educate their students, and they knew that more money was required to provide laboratories and to pay laboratory instructors. Moreover, they knew that the preliminary education of students had to be improved to insure that they could benefit from ths course. Yet if they lengthened the lecture term, required higher standards, or increased fees, they would drive students to schools with lower standards.

The colleges responded to this dilemma in a number of ways. A few institutions adopted reform in spite of the difficulties of competing with schools having less rigorous standards. The Chicago Medical College is a case in point. Nathan Smith Davis, a founder of the AMA and a leader in the continuing fight to improve medical education, was the most influential member of the faculty. He insisted that the school maintain high standards even if that tended to increase enrollment at the competing Rush Medical College. While other institutions continued to admit all who applied and provided them with an ungraded four-month course of lectures, the Chicago Medical College only admitted college graduates or those who could pass entrance examinations. In addition, the students had to take a graded five-month course. From 1859 to 1870 the Chicago Medical College was alone in its attempt to provide a medical education of exceptional quality. In 1870 Harvard joined the crusade. Charles Eliot, the president of Harvard University, decided that Harvard's medical edu-

---

21. N. P. Colwell, "Medical Education," in U.S. Commissioner of Education, *Report, 1915* (Washington, D.C.: Government Printing Office, 1915), 1:185–220. For a detailed description of the scientific and bacteriological developments, see Richard H. Shryock, *Development of Modern Medicine* (New York: Alfred A. Knopf, 1947), pp. 336–55.

cation had to be improved, and he convinced the members of the corporation, which determined university policy, to make changes: a three-year graded curriculum, a nine-month term, oral and written examinations, and faculty salaries subsidized by the university. Harvard's enrollment decreased substantially after 1870, but the college did reform. Then, in 1877, the University of Pennsylvania developed a three-year graded curriculum, and Syracuse and Michigan followed in short order.[22]

Schools that could not pay salaries to the professors had to find other ways of solving the problem. Some retained the two-year ungraded curriculum but offered an optional three-year graded course for students who wanted a more coordinated and a more rational program. The third year included practical work in medicine, surgery, and obstetrics. New York's College of Physicians and Surgeons developed an optional course in 1879, and the Jefferson Medical College eventually followed in the early 1880s.[23]

Jefferson had earlier developed a third way to solve the problem, but only for those students who wanted a more complete medical education. In the early 1870s the professors at Jefferson had recognized the need to lengthen the course, but they had been reluctant to do so because it would have reduced their competitive advantage over the University of Pennsylvania. As a result, in 1872 they had established a "supplemental" course, offered in April, May, June, and September for only a five-dollar fee. The course consisted of a series of lectures on the so-called special subjects, for which there was insufficient time in the regular program. Samuel Gross discussed aspects of surgery that were apparently omitted in the regular course. John Biddle lectured on materia medica and therapeutics, Charles Meigs on paralysis, J. Solis-Cohen on the throat and chest, and Isaac Ray on insanity. In addition, students could attend lectures on eye and ear surgery and venereal diseases.[24] Other schools found time for the special subjects during the regular program by filling the students' free time with additional lectures. In 1876, to take one example, the Bellevue Hospital Medical College had nine professors of special subjects teaching such subjects as orthopedic surgery, diseases of children, dermatology, and psychological medicine.[25]

22. N. S. Davis, "The Earlier History of the Medical School," in Arthur H. Wilde, *Northwestern University: A History* (New York: University Publishing Society, 1905), 3:298–308; Thomas F. Harrington, *The Harvard Medical School* (Chicago and New York: Lewis, 1905), 3:1020–43, 1057; Fred B. Rogers, "William Pepper, 1843–1898," *J. Med. Educ.* 34 (September 1959): 885–89.
23. From an examination of college announcements.
24. Jefferson Medical College, *Catalogue, 1872* (Philadelphia, 1872).
25. Bellevue Hospital Medical College, *Catalogue, 1876–77* (New York, 1876).

Country medical schools like the University of Vermont quickly recognized the potential of such arrangements, which allowed them to bring in specialists from the cities and have them lecture to the students and hold clinics without any financial burden on the college. Indeed, at Vermont the professors of special subjects supported themselves on fees from patients happy to have an opportunity to be treated by a specialist from Boston, New York, or Philadelphia.[26]

In the 1870s and 1880s, when Koch, Lister, Pasteur, and others were revolutionizing medical science, the public attitude towards physicians began to change. Earlier, when thousands of poorly trained "doctors" had been annually graduated "to cure or to kill," and when physicians had practiced bloodletting and had administered harsh drugs, the doctor had been considered a tradesman, one to be avoided. During the Jacksonian period, when it was insisted that the common man had the right to become a physician without worrying about restrictive legislation, and when the practices of the orthodox physicians made it difficult for them to counter the claims of the competing medical sects, state after state repealed their medical licensing laws. As a result, from the 1840s to the early 1870s there was little protection against practice by unschooled quacks. By the early 1870s some states began to pass licensing laws, but these provided for the automatic licensing of medical graduates. With schools frantically competing to reduce standards, the new laws were hardly better than no laws at all. By placing a premium on the possession of a diploma, such laws actually encouraged the growth of diploma mills in the 1870s and early 1880s. When it became obvious that the laws contained an immense loophole, the states began amending their statutes to provide for the examination of all applicants. In 1888 only five states required such examination; by 1896 twenty-three did.[27]

As the years passed, state examining boards began to insist that all applicants meet certain standards. In order to qualify for examination, students had to present evidence of having completed high school or its equivalent and having graduated from colleges that maintained high standards of medical education. This forced schools to reform or face the prospect that their graduates might not be able to practice in some states. Illinois led this move in 1877, and others soon followed. These states insisted that acceptable colleges have a minimum number of professors,

26. University of Vermont Medical Faculty Minutes (May 22 and June 3, 1875), University of Vermont Medical Archives, Burlington, Vermont; John Brooks Wheeler, *Memoirs of a Small-Town Surgeon* (New York: Frederick A. Stokes, 1935), pp. 164–65.

27. For information on the history of medical licensing, see Richard H. Shryock, *Medical Licensing in America* (Baltimore: Johns Hopkins Press, 1967). See also John H. Rauch, "Address on State Medicine," *J. AMA* 6 (June 12, 1886): 645–52.

provide laboratory and hospital experience for their students, and prepare them for rigid examinations in the various fields of study. By the 1890s it was necessary for the colleges to increase their terms to the six months required by the licensing agencies, to develop a three-year and then a four-year graded curriculum, to teach the special subjects as part of the regular program, to require dissection, and to assure that their students had an adequate preliminary education.

Toward the end of the nineteenth century, Baltimore provided the nation with an example of the ideal medical school: the Johns Hopkins Medical School. The university's endowment assured complete independence from student fees and student demands, which made it possible to institute far-reaching reforms patterned after the German system of medical education. The school began with a four-year graded curriculum, with an emphasis on laboratory and clinical training and with full-time professors of the preclinical sciences. As the years passed, licensing agencies began to insist that every acceptable school have a specific number of full-time professors. No longer could the schools be staffed by general practitioners who taught medicine in their spare time. By the early years of the twentieth century, at least in laboratory courses, full-time trained scientists would provide their expertise to the students.[28]

Beginning in the 1820s, representatives of medical schools and societies had met in a number of futile attempts to improve medical education. Until the 1890s they had been almost certain to fail in their efforts because it would have been suicidal for a handful of colleges to raise standards and increase requirements. Medical professors profited directly from high enrollments, and they were hesitant to accept any change which might drive students to other institutions. In addition, as long as it was possible to practice medicine without having to demonstrate proficiency, attendance at medical school was not necessary. For the schools to survive, they had to provide some attraction, and a long and difficult course and stringent examinations hardly constituted attractions.

By the last decade of the nineteenth century the situation had dramatically changed. The state licensing boards required a certain level of preliminary education (and a constantly higher one), and the colleges were expected to provide a specified medical training. If the schools could not regulate their own affairs and maintain acceptably high standards, the state agencies threatened to do so. That threat encouraged the colleges to unite. In 1890 a number of medical teachers met just prior to the annual

28. Richard H. Shryock, "The Influence of the Johns Hopkins University on American Education," *J. Med. Educ.* 31 (April 1956): 228–29.

AMA convention to discuss "Medical Education in this Country and Measures for Its Improvement."[29]

The meeting resulted in the establishment of the Association of American Medical Colleges, which soon was setting standards to be enforced by the state licensing agencies. While in 1880 only 26.8 percent of the schools required three years of study, by 1894, 96.3 percent did so. Four schools—Pennsylvania, Harvard, Michigan, and the Chicago Medical College—had four-year courses.[30] Moreover, the advantages of attending the better schools were becoming obvious. Statistics indicated that one-quarter of the graduates of the inferior schools were unable to pass licensing examinations, compared with only 1.5 percent of those from the better colleges.[31] Soon virtually every school had a graded four-year course, taught the required subjects, and at least advertised that they offered laboratory and hospital instruction and admitted only qualified students.

In 1903 the AMA established a committee on education, soon to be known as the Council on Medical Education, which inspected and evaluated the colleges.[32] In 1907 the council found that many of them were "absolutely worthless, without any equipment for laboratory teaching, without any dispensaries, without any hospital facilities." Indeed, the report indicated that some schools were "no better equipped to teach medicine than is a Turkish-bath establishment or a barbershop."[33] With Arthur Dean Bevan and Nathan P. Colwell leading the way, the council invited Henry S. Pritchett, the president of the Carnegie Foundation, to examine the results of the recent survey of medical schools. Bevan and Colwell obviously hoped to encourage the foundation to undertake an independent examination that could be publicized.[34] An aroused American people would then presumably demand reform. Pritchett agreed to sponsor such a survey and invited Abraham Flexner, a professional educator with no medical training, to make the investigation. After acquainting himself with the literature in the field, visiting Johns Hopkins to learn about the ideal medical college, and speaking with leading medical educators at the better schools, Flexner began his inspection. He tried to

29. Dean F. Smiley, "History of the Association of American Medical Colleges, 1876–1956," *J. Med. Educ.* 32 (July 1957): 512–25; William J. Means, "The History, Aims, and Objects of the Association of American Medical Colleges," *Proc. AAMC* (1919): 5–12; *J. AMA* 20 (January 7, 1893): 24; 22 (March 17, 1894): 393–94.

30. *J. AMA* 22 (March 17, 1894): 393–94.

31. *J. AMA* 20 (January 7, 1893): 24.

32. See Kaufman, *American Medical Education*, ch. 10.

33. *Report of the Third Annual Conference, 1907* (Chicago: AMA Council on Medical Education, 1907), p. 10.

34. Abraham Flexner, *Henry S. Pritchett: A Biography* (New York: Columbia University Press, 1943), p. 108.

determine whether the colleges were capable of financing a modern medical education without depending solely on student fees. He inspected the
laboratories to determine if they were sufficient for the required scientific
work of the preclinical years. He inspected the hospital to see if the
college could provide sufficient clinical experience for the students. He
studied the size of the faculty and the training of the various professors to
assess whether there were enough teachers to provide good instruction in
the various fields of medical science. Then he examined the entrance
requirements and admission records to determine whether the requirements were being enforced.[35]

   After gathering an immense amount of information and personally inspecting all the schools, Flexner submitted his report, published in 1910.
His findings shocked the nation. Flexner had found that only a handful of
the schools were capable of providing an adequate medical education. He
revealed that a large number of schools had violated their own admission
requirements in order to fill empty seats and to add to the income of the
professors. He disclosed that many colleges had inadequate laboratory
and clinical facilities. He showed that almost all medical professors were
practicing physicians who taught in their spare time.[36] His conclusion was
inescapable—the colleges were turning out "physicians" in name only,
men and women whose preliminary education was inadequate, whose
medical education was limited, and who would threaten the health and
welfare of the American people when they began to practice medicine.

   Following the Flexner Report, the Association of American Medical
Colleges and the AMA Council on Medical Education continued periodically to examine and rate the colleges. By the second decade of the
century, state licensing agencies were insisting that candidates graduate
from schools acceptable to the Council on Medical Education. The proprietary schools, unable to provide the laboratory facilities, the clinical
material, and the additional staff required for a modern medical education, were consequently forced either to close their doors or to merge
with more viable institutions. The result was a substantial decrease in the
number of schools, from 155 in 1910 to 85 in 1920, and finally to a low of
77 in 1941/42. The schools that remained in existence were not always

    35. See Abraham Flexner, *Abraham Flexner: An Autobiography* (New York: Simon and
Schuster, 1960), for information on how he developed his plan to survey the colleges. For a
brief analysis of the role of Flexner, see Robert P. Hudson, "Abraham Flexner in Perspective," *Bull. Hist. Med.* 46 (November-December 1972): 545–61.
    36. Abraham Flexner, *Medical Education in the United States and Canada* (New
York: Carnegie Foundation for the Advancement of Teaching, 1910). The Flexner Papers,
in the Library of Congress, are a gold mine of information, and they demonstrate the
tremendous amount of work that went into the 1910 report.

equal to Johns Hopkins, but they maintained certain minimum standards and requirements that were constantly being raised.

A substantial improvement in the quality of medical education resulted. After the reforms of the early twentieth century, medical graduates received clinical instruction and experience in municipal or affiliated hospitals, were taught by full-time scientists in the preclinical fields, and were given a modern (scientific) medical education. Unfortunately, one by-product was a drastic reduction in the number of physicians, a problem which still plagues America in the 1970s. The shortage of physicians was especially severe in rural areas, as almost all of the country medical schools were forced to close in the aftermath of the Flexner Report. Those schools had been educating general practitioners for rural and small-town America, and their disappearance was especially crucial for those areas. In addition, the increased standards coupled with a decrease in the total number of colleges and students enabled medical educators to establish stringent quotas for Negroes, Jews, and other minorities.

As executive secretary of the General Education Board, John D. Rockefeller's charitable foundation, Abraham Flexner exerted a profound and lasting influence on American medical education. He channeled funds into Yale, the University of Chicago, and other promising institutions, enabling them to improve to such an extent that soon they were rivalling Johns Hopkins, Harvard, and Pennsylvania as the nation's leading schools.[37] In 1913, as a result of Flexner's suggestion that one million dollars be given to Johns Hopkins to place the clinical professors on full-time salary, the General Education Board initiated a movement towards full-time professors of medicine, surgery, obstetrics, and pediatrics.[38] In 1914 the AMA established a committee to investigate the need for a "thorough reorganization of clinical teaching," which reported in favor of full-time clinicians, following the example set by Johns Hopkins.[39]

The experiment at Johns Hopkins was an attempt to reform medical education from the top, with the university compensating full professors to free them from private practice. Most colleges, however, could not possibly afford to pay the salaries of their leading clinicians. At most schools reform had to start at the bottom, with recent graduates agreeing to be full-time teachers. As these men had not yet developed extensive practices, academic medicine seemed reasonably attractive to them. In

37. Flexner, *Autobiography*, pp. 161–74, 196–98.
38. Donald Fleming, "The Full-Time Controversy," *J. Med. Educ.* 30 (July 1955): 398–406.
39. *Report to the House of Delegates, 1914* (Chicago: AMA Council on Medical Education, 1914), p. 17; *Bull. AMA* 10 (March 15, 1915): 244–68.

1920 the University of Michigan developed another alternative allowing professors to practice in a university clinic. Fees received from the patients went directly to the departments of the medical college to pay the clinicians' salaries. This seemed to be a perfect solution; the college gained full-time professors without adding to its financial burden. Unfortunately, the "Michigan Plan" led to a great deal of trouble.

First, the members of the preclinical staff and other university professors were outraged by the difference in salary levels at the college. To prevent a wholesale defection to private practice, the university had to pay professors of clinical medicine considerably more than those teaching the basic sciences. In addition to the "divided faculty engaged in a pitched battle . . . marked by incriminations and imputations," there was opposition from private physicians throughout the state, who believed that the clinic at Ann Arbor, supported by state funds, would steal their patients.[40]

A more workable system was the so-called geographic full-time. Under this plan professors were allowed to maintain a limited private practice as long as most of their time was devoted to teaching, research, or administrative duties at the college. Although the specifics differed from school to school, teachers generally received a base salary and a portion of what they earned in private practice. This supplemental income allowed medical schools to retain professors who otherwise would have left for a more lucrative private practice. The colleges and affiliated hospitals were compensated for the facilities provided to the professors, and any surplus supported departmental and research budgets.[41]

During the decade from 1910 to 1920, while medical educators were debating the merits of the full-time concept, several other developments were accepted almost without question. First, virtually every school became affiliated with a university, which enabled it to increase both the length and value of the preclinical years. Moreover, an increasing number of the professors of preclinical subjects held Ph.D. degrees in their specialties rather than M.D. degrees, which had been the case in the past. Unfortunately, the influence of the university was usually limited to improving the teaching of science. The humanistic values of the liberal arts seldom affected either medical educators or their students. As the schools began to require one, two, and then three years of college preparatory

40. G. Canby Robinson, "The Use of Full-Time Teachers in Clinical Medicine," *South. Med. J.* 15 (December 1922): 1009–13; George Dock, "Full-Time Clinical Departments," *South. Med. J.* 15 (December 1922): 1013–25. See also A. C. Furstenberg, "A Consideration of Full Time and Part Time Faculty Services," *J. AAMC* 20 (November 1945): 339–48. Furstenberg describes and analyzes four different systems of supporting clinical faculty.

41. Saul Jarcho, "Medical Education in the United States, 1910–1956," *J. Mt. Sinai Hosp.* 26 (1959): 363–64; *Proceedings of the Annual Congress on Medical Education, Medical Licensure, and Hospitals, 1930* (Chicago: AMA, 1930), pp. 47–55.

work prior to enrollment in medical school, the situation did not improve. Premedical students spent their time in the laboratory, either avoiding or paying little attention to the humanities and social sciences. According to one historian, Saul Jarcho, the result was that medical graduates "lacked the wide ranging cultural interests which are expected in educated men," and they "were consequently incompetent to fill their proper roles in American society."[42]

In addition to developing a university affiliation and hiring a scientifically trained preclinical staff, every medical college by 1921 had an affiliation agreement with a local hospital, which was either owned or controlled by the faculty. This was an important step towards clinical excellence, because, to a large extent, the hospital *was* the medical college. Only through extensive clinical observation and experience could students develop the practical skills needed for successful medical practice.[43]

Also by the 1920s, some schools began to work towards greater correlation of preclinical and clinical work. Previously, professors of the preclinical sciences had taught their subjects without specific reference to practice, while teachers of clinical subjects taught without relating medical practice to the sciences. By the mid-1920s a number of schools had successfully experimented with interdepartmental correlation, and a few institutions like the Universities of Pennsylvania and Illinois developed medical clinics for first-year or second-year students.[44] Since the twenties the colleges have continued to work towards the integration of clinical and preclinical work. A study of the literature seems to indicate, however, that medical school deans and the members of the various curriculum committees were working without any knowledge of earlier developments elsewhere. A large number of articles appeared pleading for more correlation between the laboratory and practical years or describing some revolutionary new experimental program—programs which often were strikingly similar to the ones developed earlier at Pennsylvania and Illinois.[45] Indeed, such ignorance of the past seems to be a continuing phenomenon.[46]

42. Jarcho, "Medical Education, 1910–1956," pp. 345–47, 369.
43. Ibid., p. 356. See also N. P. Colwell, "The Hospital's Function in Medical Education," *J. AMA* 88 (March 12, 1927): 781–84.
44. Jarcho, "Medical Education, 1910–1956," p. 360. See also articles in *J. AMA* 66 (February 26, 1916): 629–35; 81 (August 18, 1923): 599–601; 82 (May 17, 1924): 1632–34; (June 28, 1924): 2139–40; *South. Med. J.* 10 (March 1, 1917): 187–91, and 19 (September 1926): 704–5.
45. Hugh Cabot, "A Plea for the Further Extension of Clinical Opportunity into the Earlier Years of the Medical Course," *Bull. AAMC* 2 (April 1927): 105–15; G. S. Eadie, "Integration of the Curriculum of the Pre-Clinical Years," *J. AAMC* 12 (March 1937): 65–68.
46. George E. Miller, "Bedside Teaching for First-Year Students," *J. Med. Educ.* 29

At about the same time that schools began to improve clinical instruction, especially by providing experience in the early years, the "first modern preceptorships made their appearances."[47] In 1927 N. S. Davis III, of Northwestern University, wrote about the problem of teaching the art and business of medicine. The modern physician, he said, knew "much of the science of medicine," but "because nothing has been substituted" for the preceptorships of the past, he was unprepared for the realities of medical practice. Just prior to his analysis, however, some colleges had begun to develop experimental programs in the hope of solving the problem. Harvard organized a tutorial system, with students assigned to professors of clinical medicine in their third and fourth years, while Stanford required all students to spend some time as assistants to general practitioners.[48]

Wisconsin and Michigan established similar programs, as did the University of Vermont. At Wisconsin Dean C. R. Bardeen developed a preceptor system, which was really an organized extern system in the fourth year. The "Wisconsin Plan" gave students experience in hospitals and clinics throughout the state. At Michigan Dean Hugh Cabot followed the Stanford example by emphasizing work with general practitioners. At Michigan and Vermont the intention was to teach the art of medicine as well as to encourage students to become general practitioners, it was hoped, in rural areas of the state.[49]

By the mid-1920s, however, the systematic development of standards in medical education tended to prevent experimentation or change in the curriculum. The schools were in "a strait jacket composed of specific and detailed requirements" of the state examining boards. Moreover, as medical specialism developed on a large scale in the twentieth century, colleges responded by increasing the number of hours in the curriculum and by developing short courses on every new specialty. In 1925 the Association of American Medical Colleges tried to respond to the problem by establishing the Commission on Medical Education, with Dr. Willard C. Rappleye as director. Rappleye followed the example of Abraham Flexner, comparing medical education in Europe and America and developing intricate statistical studies to determine the need for physicians and the problems of medical education.

(January 1954): 28–32. See also I. Davidsohn, "Integration of Clinical and Preclinical Studies," *J. Med. Educ.* 30 (November 1955): 637–40.

47. Jarcho, "Medical Education, 1910–1956," p. 360.

48. N. S. Davis III, "Preceptorships," *J. AMA* 89 (August 20, 1927): 578–79.

49. C. R. Bardeen, "The Preceptor System at Wisconsin," *Bull. AAMC* 3 (January 1928): 31–37; Hugh Cabot, "The Preceptor System at Michigan," ibid., pp. 37–39.

Perhaps in its most important move the commission called for a truce between the Federation of State Medical Examining Boards and the members of the Association of American Medical Colleges, so member schools could experiment in curriculum development without penalty to the graduates. In 1929 and 1930 the federation voted to continue the truce, which had the effect of giving the schools "a permanent charter of liberty with respect to curriculum and educational requirements." Then, in keeping with its basic premise, the commission decided against recommending any specific changes in the curriculum. Thus, the medical curriculum was able to evolve continually, and the colleges were released from the "strait jacket" of the immediate post-Flexner period.[50] The leading medical schools responded almost immediately to the truce by developing innovative programs, including the preceptorships already described. Yale, Johns Hopkins, and Harvard all developed new programs that basically included a reduction in the number of required courses and lectures and an earlier introduction to clinical medicine.[51]

In spite of the experimentation of the late twenties and early thirties, curriculum development remained a problem. By the 1940s the colleges had increased the number of hours in response to the growth of specialism. For instance, Stanford added nine hundred hours to its program between 1940 and 1955. The options and free time which once existed were disappearing, and the medical student was more burdened than ever.[52] In the past the student had been trained to be a general practitioner. He had listened to a few lectures in the special subjects so he would know when to summon a specialist and which kind to call. By the late forties and early fifties, students were required to take courses in virtually all the specialties, many irrelevant to their future plans. At the same time, the curriculum was scientifically oriented to the exclusion of the humanities and the social sciences related to medical practice.[53]

Some medical educators recognized the problem and complained in medical journals of curricular difficulties. They noted that the curriculum was too detailed, that it was growing too large to be manageable. It made little provision for individual differences. Regardless of whether a student

50. Samuel P. Capen, "Results of the Work of the Commission on Medical Education," *J. AMA* 100 (April 22, 1937): 1217–19; *Final Report of the Commission on Medical Education* (New York: Office of the Director of the Study, 1932).
51. G. Canby Robinson, "A Study of Several Experiments in Medical Education," *J. AAMC* 6 (May 1931): 129–45.
52. John Field, "Medical Education in the United States: Late Nineteenth and Twentieth Centuries," in C. D. O'Malley, ed., *The History of Medical Education* (Berkeley and Los Angeles: University of California Press, 1970), p. 519.
53. Jarcho, "Medical Education, 1910–1956," p. 374.

intended to practice obstetrics or neurosurgery, he would take the same courses, even though much of the program would be meaningless to his later practice.[54]

A handful of schools continued to experiment with the curriculum, the most important being Western Reserve. When Joseph T. Wearn became dean in 1945, he initiated discussions on the problems of the modern medical program. Over the next seven years, eleven of the thirteen departments appointed new heads, all of whom expressed a desire to re-evaluate the curriculum. In 1950 the Commonwealth Fund granted $435,000 for a five-year program of curriculum planning and revision, and the task was started. With the general faculty overseeing the entire process and demonstrating that democratic decision making could bring about needed change, Western Reserve reduced the common core, allowed more time for electives, and let students develop their own major programs. The new plan also provided for a more complete integration of studies through the use of "multi-discipline laboratories."[55]

In 1953 Dean George Packer Berry of Harvard suggested the need to analyze the curriculum critically, to make it relevant to the changing medical world of the twentieth century. He insisted, quite correctly, that the "whole system of medical education urgently needs restructuring," and he called for the use of teaching institutes of the Association of American Medical Colleges to be the "effective device" to that end. Berry wanted to eliminate unnecessary material and to add the social and behavioral sciences which were relevant to medical life and practice.[56] The teaching institutes suggested by Berry were subsequently held, bringing together medical college administrators and teachers to discuss curricular modification in general and specific terms.

During the 1950s and early 1960s discussion turned into action. A number of colleges began to make significant changes in their programs, following the example set earlier by Western Reserve.[57] In general, they modified the post-Flexner approach, creating more programs relevant to individuals' future plans and including courses in medical history, medical sociology, medical economics, and medical ethics.

54. Langley Porter, "The Present Curriculum and the Aims of Medical Education: Are They Compatible?" in *Proceedings of the Annual Congress on Medical Education, Medical Licensure, and Hospitals, 1936* (Chicago: AMA, 1936), pp. 35–38; W. T. Sanger and A. W. Hurd, "What the Educator Thinks the Ideal Medical Curriculum Should Be," *J. AAMC* 21 (January 1946): 8–18.

55. *Proceedings of the Annual Congress on Medical Education and Licensure, 1953* (Chicago: AMA, 1953), pp. 21ff.

56. George Packer Berry, "Medical Education in Transition," *J. Med. Educ.* 28 (March 1953): 17–42. Quotes on pp. 41–42.

57. P. V. Lee, *Medical Schools and the Changing Times* (Evanston: Association of American Medical Colleges, 1962).

At the same time some institutions began to develop ways to produce well-trained physicians in less time than it had previously taken. This seemed necessary in view of the severe shortage of physicians in some areas. Curriculum committees questioned the sanctity of the traditional four-year program and investigated the possibility of streamlining the program to provide adequate training in shorter periods of time. Johns Hopkins, Northwestern, and Boston University all experimented in this direction. Soon other colleges were developing combined six-year pre-medical and medical programs, while others were operating twelve months a year and eliminating an entire year from the program of instruction in the process.

In 1964 the Council on Medical Education found that eighteen of the eighty-eight accredited medical schools had significantly modified their curricula. The trend was clearly towards more elective time and greater integration of the basic and clinical courses.[58] The new programs allowed students to select courses in line with their own interests and career goals, and in many cases the common core included basic courses in medical economics, ethics, history, and sociology. Also during the fifties and sixties the number of medical schools increased dramatically through increased federal and state funding to help eliminate the shortage of physicians. The newer schools were in the best position to experiment; they were not committed to any traditional programs and thus could develop entirely new and innovative curricula. Significantly, some of the newer institutions were the leading experimenters.[59]

In a relatively short essay covering several hundred years, it is impossible to do more than trace in bold strokes the major developments in the history of American medical education. In sum, it can be said that medical education has changed greatly over the years, but the attempt to develop perfection has failed in every period. Indeed, although a change in the focus of medical education itself may have appeared at the time to have been a revolutionary improvement, in retrospect that great advance often brought with it a new set of problems. For instance, although the modern medical student is trained in more ideal physical surroundings and by better trained professors than his eighteenth-century or nineteenth-century counterpart, he has little of the personal contact that typified the apprenticeship.

Similarly, in bygone days the high school (or academy) graduate was liberally educated; he had read the classics, disciplined himself on lan-

58. Field, "Medical Education in the United States," p. 521; *J. AMA* 194 (1965): 731–823.
59. Vernon W. Lippard and Elizabeth Purcell, *Case Histories of Ten New Medical Schools* (New York: Josiah Macy, Jr., Foundation, 1972).

guages, developed a multiplicity of interests, learned to debate and to think. The student was able to become an integral part of the society in which he lived. Over the years, however, as medical science proliferated and the colleges tried to impart the new knowledge to the undergraduate medical student, the science of medicine eclipsed the humanities and social sciences. In earlier times the student had obtained more clinical experience than he was capable of understanding. In the twentieth century the situation was reversed. He received too much science and too little bedside experience. The ideal situation would produce a scientifically trained physician who had clinical experience and an awareness of his role in society. Over the course of time all the schools have tried to find that delicate balance. Undoubtedly that search will continue into the future.

Anatomy

JOHN B. BLAKE

WHEREAS anatomy is allowed on all hands, to be the foundation both of physick and surgery. . . ." So begins the first known public announcement of a course of lectures in anatomy in what is now the United States. The advertisement was placed by Thomas Wood, surgeon, of New Brunswick, New Jersey, in a New York newspaper on January 27, 1752. Whether the course was given is not known.[1] Long before then, however, transplanted Englishmen in the North American colonies had recognized the importance of anatomy. Indeed, the earliest effort to promote medical instruction in the colonies was in this field, long since accepted as an essential part of medical education.

Soon after their arrival in the New World the Massachusetts leaders saw the necessity of training their own doctors as well as their own ministers for the future. John Eliot, the apostle to the Indians, wrote in 1647 of his hope that a school might be established "wherein there should be

---

1. E. B. Krumbhaar, "The Early History of Anatomy in the United States," *Ann. Med. Hist.* 4 (1922): 274.

Anatomies and other instructions that way" for "our young Students in Physick," who now had "onely theoreticall knowledge, and are forced to fall to practise before ever they saw an Anatomy made." There had been "one Anatomy . . . which Mr. *Giles Firman* . . . did make and read upon very well," but none since, and Firman had returned to England. Also in 1647 the Massachusetts legislature agreed, upon the petition of the president of Harvard, that "such as studies phisick or chirurgery may have liberty . . . to anotomize once in foure yeares some malefactor, in case there be such as the Courte shall alow of." In 1676 Judge Samuel Sewall recorded his attendance at the dissection of an Indian executed the previous day, but such occasions must have been rare and we have no record of any formal anatomical instruction, other than Firman's lecture and demonstration, until well into the eighteenth century.[2]

In the evolution of American medical education, the first stage was the immigration of physicians trained in Europe. These were soon supplemented by Americans trained at home through apprenticeship. Eventually an increasing number, dissatisfied with this system, travelled to Great Britain or the Continent for additional formal education. They returned to America eager in many cases to impart their new knowledge gained at the centers of medical learning and thus instituted the third phase, formal courses in medical subjects. Teaching in anatomy came first. Thomas Cadwalader of Philadelphia, after studying with William Cheselden in London, is said to have given lectures in anatomy with demonstrations on a cadaver to a number of Philadelphia physicians about 1730, and Sylvester Gardiner has been credited with giving private lectures illustrated with imported anatomical preparations in Boston somewhat later. In 1750 John Bard and Peter Middleton of New York dissected the body of an executed criminal for the instruction of students. Two years later, as noted above, Thomas Wood proposed giving a lecture course. In 1755 a Scottish physician, William Hunter, who had arrived in Newport, Rhode Island, about three years earlier, presented a series of lectures on anatomy which were apparently well attended and probably repeated in 1756. To date, they are the first systematic, advertised public lectures known to have been delivered in the United States, but they did not lead to any permanent institution.[3]

2. Ibid., p. 271; J. B. Blake, *Public Health in the Town of Boston, 1630–1822* (Cambridge: Harvard University Press, 1959), pp. 7–8.

3. Krumbhaar, "Early History of Anatomy," pp. 272–73; James Thacher, *American Medical Biography*, 2 vols. (New York: Da Capo Press, 1967), 1:52, 271; H. Montgomery, "Prescholastic Anatomical Instruction as a Factor in Medical Professionalization in British

The honor of establishing the first permanent teaching program in anatomy must be accorded to William Shippen. Born in Philadelphia in 1736, Shippen served an apprenticeship with his father and then studied with William and John Hunter in London, took his M.D. at Edinburgh in 1761, and returned to Philadelphia in 1762. In March of that year he presented a course of lectures on midwifery. In November he began his first course of lectures on anatomy, also including surgery, bandaging, and midwifery. Ten students attended. Those who wished to learn the art of dissecting by seeing the subject prepared for the lecture could do so by coming early and paying extra. There is no indication that the students might themselves dissect. Shippen continued giving the lectures in subsequent years. With the establishment of a medical school at the College of Philadelphia in 1765, he became the country's first professor of anatomy. His lectures were largely didactic, and, at least in the early years, based largely on those he had attended under the Hunters in London. [4]

Soon comparable facilities began to emerge in other cities. In New York Samuel Clossy, who had received his M.D. in Dublin in 1755, emigrated from Ireland in 1763. That fall he offered a course of anatomical lectures in which he proposed to demonstrate the parts and to explain as well their "Uses, Motions, and Diseases." He lectured forty-four nights, but could not complete the third part of the course because, as more people learned what he was doing, he could not get a third cadaver for his demonstrations. In 1765 Clossy was elected professor of natural history at King's College with the expectation that he would also teach anatomy, and in 1767 he received an additional appointment as professor of anatomy in the newly organized medical school. The announcement for his first course indicated that those who wished to witness "Dissections and Preparations" might do so for an extra fee. Clossy lectured until the outbreak of the Revolution, when, as a Loyalist, he fled New York. He returned during the British occupation and lectured again at the New York Hospital but went to England in 1780. [5]

North America," in K. Lanzinger, ed., *Americana-Austriaca* (rpt. Vienna: W. Braumüller, [n. d.]), p. 155; William Frederick Norwood, *Medical Education in the United States before the Civil War* (Philadelphia: University of Pennsylvania Press, 1944), p. 39; E. B. Krumbhaar, "Doctor William Hunter of Newport," *Ann. Surg.* 101 (1935): 506–28.

4. F. R. Packard, *History of Medicine in the United States*, 2 vols. (New York: Hafner, 1963), 1:306–22; J. B. Blake, "The Anatomical Lectures of William Shippen, 1766," *Trans. & Stud. Coll. Phys. Phila.*, 4th ser., 42 (1974): 61–66.

5. B. Stookey, "Samuel Clossy, A.B., M.D., F.R.C.P. of Ireland, First Professor of Anatomy, King's College (Columbia), New York," *Bull. Hist. Med.* 38 (1964): 153–67.

In Baltimore Charles Frederick Wiesenthal, who was born in Prussia in 1726 and settled in Maryland in 1755, soon became a leading practitioner and preceptor. In time—probably in 1769—he developed a teaching program sufficiently extensive to lead him to build a substantial schoolhouse (still standing in 1900) with ample space for dissection. The importance he placed on this may readily be seen in a letter written in 1781 to his son, then a student in Philadelphia: "We received your letters . . . in which I see your beginning to dissect yourself which pleases me and I insist that you continue to do the same manually in *propria persona*, and not being content with merely demonstrations after the Subject is prepard, as I want the practical part. It will lead you towards Operations and will make that part of Surgery more intelligible." After Wiesenthal died in 1789, his son Andrew continued to lecture on anatomy and surgery to classes of private students until his death in 1798.[6]

In Boston, leadership in anatomy came from John Warren, the younger brother of the patriot-physician Joseph Warren. Interested in anatomy since his college days, John Warren took advantage of his appointment as supervising surgeon of the military hospital in Boston in 1777 to further his studies. In 1780 he presented a private course of lectures and demonstrations at the hospital. The following year he gave a public course that so impressed the authorities of Harvard that they appointed him professor of anatomy and surgery in 1782 and established the Harvard medical school. In 1797, when sufficient funds had accumulated, Warren was appointed Hersey Professor, the first, and for a long time the only, endowed chair in anatomy in the country.[7]

After the Revolution new medical schools joined those already established at Philadelphia, New York, and Boston. Anatomy was invariably an accepted part of the curriculum, often combined with physiology as well as with surgery. The formal teaching consisted of lectures by the professor, often illustrated with anatomical demonstrations prepared by prosectors. Although students were sometimes allowed to undertake some dissecting, it was not required for graduation. Hence we find in the medical college building constructed in Baltimore in 1812 only four small dissecting rooms, chiefly for prosectors, surrounding the much larger anatomical theater.

6. E. F. Cordell, "Charles Frederick Wiesenthal, Medicinae Practicus, the Father of the Medical Profession of Baltimore," *Bull. Johns Hopkins Hosp.* 11 (1900): 170–74; idem, *The Medical Annals of Maryland, 1799–1899* (Baltimore: Medical and Chirurgical Faculty of the State of Maryland, 1903), pp. 15–17; G. H. Callcott, *A History of the University of Maryland* (Baltimore: Maryland Historical Society, 1966), pp. 17–18.

7. T. E. Moore, Jr., "The Early Years of the Harvard Medical School: Its Founding and Curriculum, 1782–1810," *Bull. Hist. Med.* 27 (1953): 530–61.

One result was that the stature of a professor was often determined by his brilliance as a lecturer. Thus James Thacher describes Caspar Wistar, Shippen's successor as professor of anatomy at Pennsylvania from 1808 to 1818, in glowing terms:

> Dr. Wistar as a public teacher . . . appeared in all the fulness of his intellectual powers. He brought to the anatomical theater his deep and various learning, his habitual feelings, and even something of his colloquial vivacity. Although he was strikingly fluent, and truly learned, still there was something in his eloquence peculiarly his own. Not that he was lofty in his manner and imposing by his voice, for he was neither. His was the eloquence of sentiment, rather than of manner; and his persuasiveness owed almost as much to his disposition, as to the great importance of the truths which he unfolded. . . . An unrivalled fluency and simplicity attended him through every step of the demonstration, however complicated; and he knew, of all men we have ever heard, the best how to be interesting, and at the same time rigorously minute. A broad and clear light shone steadily around him. He seemed to have identified anatomy with his common thoughts; and the language in which he expressed himself on this subject, seemed like the appropriate expressions of his familiar conversation.[8]

By contrast with his reputation as a lecturer and author of the first American textbook of anatomy, Wistar as a practical anatomist is remembered chiefly for "the elucidation of the correct anatomical relations between the ethmoid and sphenoid bones."[9]

Later in the century Oliver Wendell Holmes attained an even more enviable reputation in the lecture hall. As his erstwhile demonstrator, David W. Cheever, recalled:

> He enters [the amphitheatre], and is greeted with a mighty shout and stamp of applause. Then silence, and there begins a charming hour of description, analysis, simile, anecdote, harmless pun, which clothes the dry bones with poetic imagery, enlivens a hard and fatiguing day with humor, and brightens to the tired listener the details of a difficult though interesting study. . . . The student is now listening to his *fifth* consecutive lecture that day, beginning at nine o'clock and ending at two; no pause, no rest, no recovery for the dazed senses. . . . One o'clock was always assigned to Dr.

8. Thacher, *American Medical Biography*, 2:219.
9. F. R. Packard, "Caspar Wistar," in *Dictionary of American Biography*, reprint ed., vol. 10, pt. 2 (New York: Scribner's, 1936), p. 433.

Holmes because he alone could hold his exhausted audience's attention.

Holmes's successor, Thomas Dwight, reinforced Cheever's description: "No one but Dr. Holmes could have been endured under the circumstances." Dwight also reported another aspect of Holmes's teaching that may have added to his popularity. Holmes, wrote Dwight, lectured to the "lower half of the class. . . . He felt a sympathy for the struggling lad preparing to practise where work is hard and money scarce. 'I do not give the best lectures that I can give, . . . I should shoot over their heads. I try to teach them a little and to teach it well.' "[10]

By the time Holmes had reached these peaks of oratorical distinction, dissection in most schools was at least ostensibly required. At Maryland the trustees in 1833 required all students to take at least one "ticket" from the demonstrator. However, this was dropped six years later and not reinstituted until 1848. Daniel Drake at Cincinnati began requiring all students to take the dissection course in 1835; how much actual dissection each student carried out is difficult to say. Many students no doubt were eager to do and learn as much as they could. Yet as late as 1849 the University of Pennsylvania, Jefferson Medical College, the College of Physicians and Surgeons in New York, and Yale still did not require dissection.[11]

It has often been suggested that American medical education, notoriously faulty as it was in the nineteenth century, was better than its system. Certainly this was true of anatomy for many students. Denied an opportunity for careful or extensive dissection in the medical school curriculum, many students sought other means to learn what they knew they must before practicing surgery. Apprenticeship was still an important part of medical education in the first part of the century. Though no doubt they were often perfunctory, practical instruction and guidance in the study of anatomy by dissection must have been obtained by many students under some preceptors. Since it was necessary to obtain cadavers by stealth, one learns of these cases largely by indirection. Thus an aspiring physician in 1819 explained to his brother why he had returned home to Leominster precipitately:

> The students of Dr. [James] Thacher, four in number including myself, animated with a *laudable* desire of obtaining useful knowl-

10. J. T. Morse, Jr., *Life and Letters of Oliver Wendell Holmes*, 2 vols. (Boston: Houghton Mifflin, 1896), 1:176, 178, 182.
11. Norwood, *Medical Education*, p. 239; G. W. Corner, "The Role of Anatomy in Medical Education," *J. Med. Educ.* 33 (1958): 2; Callcott, *History of the University of Maryland*, pp. 113–14.

edge, particularly anatomy, a branch essential to the well-bred physician, & having, as they thought, a good opportunity to effect their wishes, by the death of an old worthless fellow in Plymouth, did, on a certain night, about three weeks since, take up the body of said fellow with the view carefully to dissect the same, & obtain the skeleton.

Unfortunately the resurrection was discovered, and court action appeared imminent.

I had notice of this, & took French leave of P., fled to the Carter Mountain of Leominster for safety, & am now enjoying a "dignified retirement" otium cum dignitate.[12]

Some years later Nathan Smith Davis wrote that as a young practitioner in Binghamton, New York, about 1840, "I occupied every leisure moment in study . . . every winter refreshing my anatomical knowledge by dissecting one or more subjects in the work-room over my office and instructing students (generally had to get the subjects with my own hands). . . ."[13]

Preceptors like Thacher and Davis were no doubt the exception; more common presumably was the "tedious and too often unprofitable course of anatomy" mentioned by Drake. Even as late as 1881 the president of the Maine Medical Society complained that preceptors advised their students not to pay much attention to chemistry or physiology or the microscope because they would not use them in practice. "These students avoid dissection, or try to, altogether," he wrote. "Instead of seeking every opportunity for the study of practical anatomy, they do only so much as they must, to receive the demonstrator's ticket."[14] Yet the number of grave-robbing stories and scandals of nineteenth-century American medicine clearly suggests that self-study of anatomy and teaching by preceptors was by no means uncommon.

In some cases such private teaching took on the character of an unchartered school, like the Wiesenthals' in Baltimore. While most such schools were intended chiefly for the office students of the professor, some offered wider opportunities. Especially notable was the Philadelphia School of Anatomy, started by Jason Valentine O'Brien Lawrance (or Lawrence)

12. C. B. to his brother, Leominster, 4 March 1819, transcript courtesy of Samuel X. Radbill.
13. W. J. Bell, Jr., "Nathan Smith Davis: An Autobiographical Letter, Previously Unpublished," *J. AMA* 224 (1973): 1014–16.
14. Daniel Drake, *Physician to the West: Selected Writings of Daniel Drake on Science and Society*, ed. H. D. Shapiro and Z. L. Miller (Lexington: University of Kentucky Press, 1970), p. 192; W. W. Greene, "President's Address," *Trans. Maine Med. Soc.* 7, pt. 2 (1881): 239–40.

in 1820. He proved to be a popular teacher and opened the school to all medical students. By 1822 he was offering a six-month course in anatomy and surgery which began after the medical school commencement in spring and lasted, except during August, to November. At the same time Lawrance was actively engaged in dissections and upon his early death in 1823 left, according to Thacher, some three thousand pages of notes. Unlike most such schools, which ceased operation when the founder quit, the Philadelphia school continued after Lawrance's death under John D. Godman, who also developed an enviable reputation for his work in anatomy and pathology. Others continued the school until its final demise in 1875. Meanwhile it had been the scene of much excellent teaching, extensive opportunities for dissection, and original physiological and anatomical research.

> Within its walls [wrote W. W. Keen], earnest, intelligent, laborious men of science have taught, experimented, and investigated, and published the results of their work in many a book and pamphlet and scientific paper . . . thousands of men . . . have studied and dissected here, and here begun their scientific lives, and are now spread all over the country . . . doing the best of work as practitioners, teachers, writers, and original investigators.[15]

Despite Keen's glowing account, comparable opportunities for learning anatomy elsewhere in the country were scarce, and many of the more eager Americans who could afford to do so continued their studies in Europe. Early in the nineteenth century emphasis shifted from London and Edinburgh to Paris, largely because of the superior opportunities for dissections, especially for training in pathological anatomy and surgery. During the 1850s and later, Americans turned increasingly to some of the German universities and to Vienna, where the anatomical material was said to be inexhaustible.[16] It is quite clear that one of the seriously limiting factors in the teaching of anatomy in America was the difficulty in obtaining cadavers.

As early as 1641 the Massachusetts General Court had already recognized the principle, accepted in English common law, that a judge might sentence the body of a convicted criminal to dissection, and occasionally

15. Thacher, *American Medical Biography*, 1:353–55; W. W. Keen, "The History of the Philadelphia School of Anatomy and Its Relation to Medical Teaching," in his *Addresses and Other Papers* (Philadelphia: Saunders, 1905), pp. 41–67; quotation on p. 41.
16. R. M. Jones, "American Doctors and the Parisian Medical World, 1830–1840," *Bull. Hist. Med.* 47 (1973): 40–65, 177–204; J. I. Waring, "William Middleton Michel in Paris, 1842–1846: A Vignette of Cruveilhier," *J. Hist. Med.* 23 (1968): 349–55; T. N. Bonner, *American Doctors and German Universities* (Lincoln: University of Nebraska Press, 1963), p. 71 and passim.

courts did order bodies turned over to physicians for this purpose. In 1784 Massachusetts passed a law requiring judges to turn over for dissection the body of anyone executed for killing another in a duel (obviously to increase the penalties for duelling!) and in 1805 provided statutory authority for so disposing of other executed criminals. In New York, as a result of the famous "Doctor's Mob" riot in 1788, the legislature in 1789 passed "an Act to prevent the odious practice of digging up and removing for the purpose of dissection dead bodies interred in cemeteries or burial places." While providing penalties for grave-robbing, it also empowered judges (but did not require them) to order the bodies of persons executed for murder, arson, or burglary turned over to a surgeon for dissection; the declared purpose of this provision was to facilitate the study of anatomy. In 1824, following a riot in New Haven against the Yale medical school, the Connecticut legislature went further, providing that unclaimed bodies of persons who died in the state prison, as well as executed criminals, might be used for anatomical study. Such provisions, however, even if they had been routinely administered to the benefit of anatomical teaching, could never have provided an adequate supply, especially as the number of students and the demand for bodies expanded rapidly during the nineteenth century.

In Massachusetts, beginning in 1825, members of the Harvard medical faculty joined leaders of the state medical society in a forceful campaign for an anatomy statute. They lobbied the legislature and sought public support through pamphlets, magazine articles, and other means. They argued that anatomical knowledge was necessary for physicians and surgeons and could be obtained only by the practice of dissection. Under the licensure statutes surgeons had to know anatomy and were subject to malpractice suits if they did not. Thus the law denied them the very means to acquire what the law required them to have. The chief beneficiaries, however, would not be physicians but the public, and especially the poor, who would get better medical care and the assurance that the graves of their loved ones need no longer be violated to satisfy the demands of the dissectors.

As a result of this effort, Massachusetts in 1831 passed the country's first real anatomy act. As amended in 1834, it authorized appropriate public officials to turn over to physicians and surgeons for teaching purposes unclaimed bodies which would otherwise have had to be buried at public expense, provided the person had not during his final illness requested burial. Connecticut passed a similar law in 1833, New Hampshire in 1834, and Michigan in 1844, but all three were repealed less than a decade after passage. Only two states, Massachusetts and New York, where a law was enacted in 1853, retained anatomy acts when the Civil War broke out.

After the war, under increasing pressure from medical schools and societies, a number of states passed anatomy acts, beginning with Pennsylvania in 1867. By 1881 fifteen of the then thirty-eight states authorized the use of unclaimed bodies that must otherwise be buried at public expense for anatomical purposes. Nevertheless, as late as the 1890s, under Maryland's anatomy act of 1882, the Johns Hopkins medical school obtained over half its cadavers from extralegal sources. With the overall improvement of medical education and the rising status of the medical profession in public esteem in the late nineteenth and early twentieth centuries came further improvement in anatomical laws. Many previously permissive laws were made mandatory, requiring the managers of public charitable institutions to turn over unclaimed bodies. Additional states passed laws, so that by 1913 only two of the thirty-nine states with medical schools lacked anatomical laws. In one of these, Tennessee, graverobbing continued into the 1920s. Elsewhere it had long since ceased. Meanwhile, many were the hair-raising encounters faced by professors and students, which must have reinforced the importance of bold, decisive, and rapid action in emergency situations, especially in surgery, rather than the desirability of quiet, studied research. Securing the passage of reasonable anatomy acts was one of the most significant advances in the teaching of anatomy during those years.[17]

Despite the increasing availability of subjects after 1865 and routine dissection requirements, both teaching and learning conditions left much to be desired. Students often came to medical school with less than a high school education and with no background in biology or training in dissection of animals. The result, as a later critic claimed, was in most cases no more than "indecent butchery." It would be much better, he argued, "to let these ill-trained hands learn the difference between muscle and fascia, nerve and vessel—which is about all such bungling teaches them—upon the dead bodies of the lower animals. . . ." Medical students, he thought, should start out on cats.[18]

In most schools until nearly the end of the century anatomy consisted almost exclusively of gross anatomy, taught as a background for surgery.

17. J. B. Blake, "The Development of American Anatomy Acts," *J. Med. Educ.* 30 (1955): 431–39; S. L. Clark, "Medical Education from the Ground Up or Our Late Resurrection Men," *J. Med. Educ.* 37 (1962): 1291–96.

18. J. B. Roberts, "Some Defects in Anatomical Teaching in the Medical Schools of the United States," *Transactions of the First Pan-American Medical Congress Held in the City of Washington, D.C., U.S.A., September 5, 6, 7, and 8, A.D. 1893*, 3 vols. (Washington, D.C.: Government Printing Office, 1895), 2:1147.

Teachers were generally practicing surgeons, and often took an anatomy chair in hope of something better. Indeed, George W. Corner has recorded the story of a surgeon who bought a professorship of anatomy for one thousand dollars as an investment toward a surgical career.[19] Demonstrators often were filling in time until they could build a surgical career. Even when the opportunity to dissect became routine, most medical school teaching still consisted of drill and memory work, and emphasized textbooks, diagrams, models, and examinations rather than principles and methods or independent thought. Despite stated requirements, some students could get by without ever dissecting, and the anatomy halls were often filthy, the bodies ill kept. As one critic reported, "Nerves, arteries, veins, muscles, become to him [the student] streaks of yellow, red, blue and brown color, formed into intricate diagrams to be memorized by constant conning over."[20] Dissections were made, wrote another critic, as a manual exercise, to illustrate the book. "Most men," he wrote, "when asked to describe a bone, visualize—not the bone, but the picture of the bone in 'Gray's Anatomy.' "[21]

The existence of these complaints and a substantial number of articles and addresses on the teaching of anatomy published between 1880 and 1910 indicate the extent of concern during these years.[22] The authors exhibited very general dissatisfaction with the way anatomy was being taught and urged substantial reforms. This outburst was part of the general movement for the reform of medical education initiated by Charles W. Eliot at Harvard in 1871 and later carried further, especially at Johns Hopkins. Certain special considerations, however, applied to anatomy that did not hold equally true for all the basic medical sciences, much less the clinical specialties. Until late in the century, anatomy was traditionally the only laboratory course in medical school. It was, however, generally taught simply for its practical value, chiefly for surgery,

19. G. W. Corner, "The Past of Anatomy in the United States," *Anat. Record* 137 (1960): 180.

20. G. F. Shiels, "A Plea for the Proper Teaching of Anatomy," *J. AMA* 23 (1894): 110–12.

21. W. T. Porter, "The Teaching of Physiology in Medical Schools," *Boston Med. & Surg. J.* 139 (1898): 648. Generally, see G. H. Monks, "The Study of Anatomy: Its Position in Medical Education in England and in America," ibid. 113 (1885): 104–7; Roberts, "Some Defects in Anatomical Teaching," pp. 1147–51; E. W. Holmes, "The Dissecting Room," *Transactions of the First Pan-American Medical Congress*, 2: 1152–54; F. P. Mall, "On Some Points of Importance to Anatomists," *Anat. Record* 1 (1907): 24–29; C. R. Bardeen, *Anatomy in America*, Bulletin of the University of Wisconsin No. 115, Science Series, vol. 3, no. 4 (Madison: University of Wisconsin, 1905), pp. 137–38, 171; E. W. Holmes, "Modern Anatomy," *J. AMA* 32 (1899): 852–55.

22. See bibliography in C. R. Bardeen, "Report of the Sub-committee on Anatomy to the Council on Medical Education of the American Medical Association, April, 1909," *Anat. Record* 3 (1909): 435–37.

and, unlike the other medical sciences, gross human anatomy had very
limited potential for stimulating original research.

While they agreed on the need for change, the reformers did not
necessarily agree on the changes needed. Some took a rather conservative
stance on the purpose of anatomical teaching and the kind of teaching
proper for medical students. George Franklin Shiels of San Francisco, for
example, stressed the need for teaching by training instead of cramming,
the need for continuing, systematic anatomical instruction, emphasizing
dissection, over three years. He thought each student should dissect the
body three times, with the last time devoted to purely medical and surgical anatomy.[23] Edmund W. Holmes, demonstrator of anatomy and lecturer on surgical anatomy at the University of Pennsylvania, wanted more
dissection and less didactic teaching of anatomy. Writing late in the
1890s, when the influence of Franklin P. Mall was already being felt, he
insisted that embryology, histology, and comparative anatomy should be
taught in premedical years. Medical school was the place to train practical
physicians, not scientists. The time for training physicians was too short
anyway, and anatomy was being pushed aside for *ologies* and *isms*.

> Most of the errors in actual practice [he complained] are due to a
> lack of knowledge of practical applied human anatomy. Yet its de-
> tails are despised, and the utmost enthusiasm, the finest museum
> and laboratory facilities, the latest apparatus, the costliest build-
> ings are lavished on the collateral branches, whilst the practical
> knowledge of the human body . . . seems to be more and more lost
> sight of.

Dr. Irving S. Haynes, a professor at the Cornell University Medical
College, commenting on Holmes's presentation to the Association of
American Anatomists in 1898, agreed that the object of a medical school
was to graduate successful practitioners. The teacher of anatomy, he believed, should be actively engaged in the practice of his profession. The
facts of anatomy by themselves were uninteresting to medical students,
but if "clothed . . . with the charm of a practical application" to medicine
or surgery, they became alive and the student would remember them.[24]
Dr. C. A. Hamann of Cleveland, Ohio, expressed similar views at the
annual meeting of the Association of American Medical Colleges in 1901.
Perhaps rich medical schools should have full-time professors to advance
the science, but they were not the right teachers for medical students,

---

23. Shiels, "A Plea for the Proper Teaching of Anatomy," pp. 110–12.
24. Holmes, "Modern Anatomy," pp. 852–55; E. W. Holmes, "The Defects of Our
Present Methods of Teaching Anatomy in Our Medical Schools," *Proc. Assoc. Am. Anat.
1898* 11 (1899): 49–54; I. S. Haynes, comment on Holmes, ibid., p. 59.

who were future practitioners, not embryo scientists. They should be taught what was useful in practice by practitioners, not by those who neither knew nor were interested in anatomy from a medical point of view.[25]

Other reformers in the 1890s and after sought a more fundamental change in the teaching of anatomy. In essence, they wanted anatomy to be taught by active research scientists who pursued the subject for its own sake rather than as a basis for surgery. They sought and found their intellectual colleagues as much among zoologists as among physicians, and they tended to look upon anatomy as a branch of human biology rather than as a branch of medicine.

Among the early exemplars of this new tradition was Charles Sedgwick Minot. After receiving a doctorate of science in natural history from the Harvard graduate school in 1878, Minot joined the Harvard faculty in 1880, first in the dental school, later in the medical school, where he made a major contribution to the development of human embryology. A more influential figure in the reform of anatomical teaching generally was Franklin P. Mall. A graduate of the University of Michigan medical school in 1883, Mall went to Germany intending to take special training in ophthalmology. There he fell under the influence of Wilhelm His and Carl Ludwig, who turned his interests to scientific research in embryology and microscopic anatomy. After returning to the United States in 1886, Mall spent three years as a fellow in William Welch's department of pathology at the Johns Hopkins Hospital, followed by appointments at Clark University and Chicago. In 1893 he returned to Baltimore as the first professor of anatomy in the new Johns Hopkins medical school. There he was to follow a highly productive career of research in histology and embryology.

Mall also set about reforming the teaching of anatomy. He believed strongly that medical schools should train physicians in scientific attitudes and observation. To accomplish this, anatomy had to be taught as a science for its own sake, and not as preparation for surgery. For this kind of teaching it was essential to have teachers who were themselves engaged in scientific research and whose teaching techniques would imbue in students a research spirit of independent observation and judgment. In the long run, he believed, this would actually make better practicing physicians than any amount of supposedly practical drill or instruction.

In line with these views, Mall eliminated the formal lecture as a teaching device and instead set new medical students immediately to work at

---

25. C. A. Hamann, "The Teaching of Anatomy in Medical Schools," *Bull. Am. Acad. Med.* 5 (1901): 511–21.

the dissecting table, with textbooks, atlases, and competent instructors available to help them as needed. For the large dissecting hall common in medical schools at the time he substituted small, scrupulously clean rooms where students might work in the atmosphere of a research laboratory. For demonstrators he brought in persons who showed outstanding promise as future scientists, rather than budding surgeons. The wisdom of his choices was shown by the number of his demonstrators—at least eighteen—who subsequently headed departments of anatomy in other medical schools, not counting those who otherwise contributed to scientific research. In addition, Mall was a strong advocate of a system of concentrated study, in which a student spent full time on one or at most two areas of study. This was the way any scholar worked, he argued, and he saw no reason why medical students should not do the same. Among other advantages, it would allow the more capable students time for electives and independent study. Most of Mall's teaching ideas were instituted at Hopkins and in time were accepted at other schools as well. Of the few that were not adopted, one was his belief that medical students, like graduate students, should write a thesis based on original research.[26]

By the time Minot, Mall, and others were beginning to turn anatomy departments of medical schools into research centers, the traditional primary subject for medical students—gross human anatomy—was no longer a major field for scientific research. Some professors made valiant efforts to turn it into a research subject by emphasizing the observation and recording of variations in the structure of human bodies. This was, wrote C. R. Bardeen, "the salvation of gross anatomy as an object of intellectual interest to teachers and students."[27] In fact, anatomists were able to grow as scientists by bringing into their field such relatively new subjects as microscopic anatomy and embryology, where research opportunities were many. It was this, as George Corner has written, that enabled anatomy to save its "intellectual soul."[28]

In his presidential address to the American Association of Anatomists in 1912, Professor Ross Harrison, head of the department of zoology at Yale

26. For Mall's views on teaching, see especially his "On Some Points of Importance to Anatomists," pp. 24–29; his "On the Teaching of Anatomy," *Anat. Record* 2 (1908): 313–35; F. R. Sabin, *Franklin Paine Mall: The Story of a Mind* (Baltimore: Johns Hopkins Press, 1934). The number of department heads is from Corner, "The Role of Anatomy," p. 4.

27. C. R. Bardeen, C. M. Jackson, and W. R. Keiller, "Report of the Committee on the Teaching of Gross Human Anatomy," *Proc. AAMC* 30 (1920): 20; Bardeen, "Use of the Material of the Dissecting Room for Scientific Purposes," *Bull. Johns Hopkins Hosp.* 12 (1901): 155–58; Bardeen, "Recent Progress in Anatomy," *Wis. Med. J.* 3 (1904–1905): 616; T. Dwight, "Problems of Clinical Anatomy," *Med. Comm. Mass. Med. Soc.* 19 (1903): 429–38.

28. Corner, "The Role of Anatomy," p. 5.

and a former member of Mall's department, expressed the scientists' views. Anatomy, he stated, as a science, was most closely related to zoology; whether one was a zoologist or an anatomist was determined not so much by subject matter or training as by "present fortuitous attachments." While the necessity of teaching medical students the facts of human structure would no doubt keep the distinction alive, anatomists must be alive to the greatest danger to their subject: its practical importance, for this posed the constant threat of making anatomy subservient to practice and turning it into dulling routine drill. The "purely morphological conception of anatomy" had "led us to a barren field where we still are plodding. . . ." Anatomy must return to a concern with all phases of form and development in living organisms and, like other sciences, adopt the experimental method.[29]

The results of this attitude may be seen not only in the great expansion of research undertaken in anatomy departments between 1912 and the 1940s but also in the direction the research took. In a review of these trends in 1942, A. M. Lassek described the previous thirty years as "characterized by free, expanding, unbridled research by investigators interested in anatomy." Analyzing some 3,655 articles from abstracts in the *Anatomical Record*, he found that the research was conducted on rodents in 27 percent of the reports, on submammalian species in 24 percent, and on primates in 21 percent. Some 25 percent of the studies were in embryology, 20 percent in histology, 11 percent in endocrinology, but only 8 percent in gross anatomy. Of the studies on man, embryology ranked first with 34 percent; 21 percent were in gross anatomy. Lassek's general conclusion was that the purpose of anatomical study was to increase the knowledge of the field throughout the animal kingdom; that nearly all the work on man was purely descriptive anatomy; and that probably very little of the research was used by clinicians.[30] A somewhat later survey of fields of research showed no significant change in the trend: research interests of anatomists varied widely, but very few concerned themselves with pure form. Only 9 percent of the papers published between 1956 and 1961 were in gross anatomy; other figures included embryology, 10 percent; neuroanatomy and physiology, 15 percent; histology, 13 percent; histochemistry, 11 percent; endocrinology, 21 percent.[31]

29. R. G. Harrison, "Anatomy: Its Scope, Methods and Relations to Other Biological Sciences," *Anat. Record* 7 (1913): 401–10. See also J. Loeb, "On the Teaching of Anatomy," *Anat. Record* 5 (1911): 306–8.
30. A. M. Lassek, "Anatomical Research in the United States during the Past Thirty Years," *J. AAMC* 7 (1942): 387–90.
31. E. Eldred and L. Gadbois, "Fields of Research of American Anatomists," *Anat. Record* 144 (1962): 165–67.

While anatomy departments were becoming more research oriented, they were also, as Mall predicted, doing a better job of teaching anatomy. The inferior pedagogy (lectures, drills) and execrable facilities still so widespread at the time of Abraham Flexner's survey in 1910 were subsequently replaced in the general reform of medical education that was carried out during the 1910s and 1920s. The dissecting table became the primary locus for teaching gross anatomy, and by 1920, according to a report to the Association of American Medical Colleges, the general standard was for two students to share in the dissection of one cadaver.

At the same time the growth of medical science and the demands of other departments led to a reduction in the amount of time allotted to the teaching of anatomy. From 1902 to 1903 the average total length of the curriculum in forty-one medical colleges with a four-year course was 4,095 hours, of which 768 hours (19 percent) were devoted to anatomy (including 549 for gross anatomy and 219 for embryology and histology). After considerable discussion the Committee on the Medical Curriculum recommended 700 hours (500 for gross anatomy) in a total of 4,100. C. R. Bardeen, reporting to his fellow anatomists, indicated his dissatisfaction, feeling that it should be longer. He admitted, however, "There is undoubtedly at present a desire on the part of those teaching other branches to curtail anatomy so that more time may be given to those branches." Their desires have continued unabated. By 1920 C. R. Stockard of Cornell (probably the first Ph.D. anatomist to head an anatomy department in a medical school) could remark that "the modern anatomical laboratory is covering twice as much ground in half the time. . . ." By about 1955 the average amount of time in required anatomy courses was down to 622 hours with only 330 hours for gross anatomy.[32]

This decrease was no doubt disturbing to some teachers, but not to all. Presumably there were those glad to see their teaching load lightened, especially in a subject that was not their primary interest, so that they could devote more time to research. A nonanatomist and former dean, looking back over the period from 1920 to 1970, recalled that in the earlier decades "the first year was a grueling experience for students who did not possess retentive memories . . . and many young people who showed promise of becoming good physicians fell by the wayside because of their inability to describe . . . the origin and insertion of the gastrocnemius

---

32. Bardeen, *Anatomy in America*, p. 173; Bardeen, "Report of the Sub-committee on Anatomy, 1909," pp. 415–22; Bardeen et al., "Report of the Committee," p. 33; "The Teaching of Anatomy and Anthropology in Medical Education: Report of the Third Teaching Institute, Association of American Medical Colleges," *J. Med. Educ.* 31, no. 10, pt. 2 (Oct. 1956): 14.

muscle."[33] For such students the change was certainly welcome.

Others took a more positive view. In his Terry Lecture of 1939, Lewis H. Weed, professor of anatomy at Johns Hopkins, reminded his audience that the purpose of medical school was to produce the best kind of physician; medical faculties must guard against the danger of producing superb technicians lacking in intellectual curiosity. Teachers must encourage the inquiring mind through "the blending of teaching and research, not only in the classrooms but also in the wards and laboratories. . . ." The specific curriculum, Weed continued, was of secondary importance. Hence, rather than deploring the continuing reduction in required hours for anatomy, one should see this as an opportunity. Whereas once anatomy formed almost the entire basis of preclinical instruction, no longer was there time to teach students details or techniques. Now the teacher could present biological viewpoints and encourage intellectual inquiry. The development of mere technical proficiency might be postponed to postgraduate years. Medicine, said Weed, a worthy exponent of the Mall tradition, was becoming more and more biological, and he applauded the change.[34]

Even when Mall had been urging reform in anatomical teaching, there had been those, as we have seen, who agreed with him on the need for reform but not on teaching anatomy for its own sake. Though the views of Mall predominated from the 1920s, voices were still heard in opposition. Objectors sometimes argued that researchers were not good teachers, at least of anatomy, because they were not interested in teaching or in gross anatomy, but in their own work in some other field. As academic prestige and advancement came to depend increasingly on research production, especially after the influx of federal money in the late 1940s, the objections increased. Critics, chiefly clinicians, also protested that as anatomists (now usually Ph.D.'s rather than M.D.'s) became increasingly specialized, they lost knowledge of or interest in the clinical applications of their subject, which made them increasingly unsatisfactory as teachers of medical students, however much their research might add to fundamental science. Surgeons especially complained that students were not learning enough anatomy.[35]

33. V. W. Lippard, *A Half-Century of American Medical Education: 1920–1970* (New York: Josiah Macy, Jr., Foundation, 1974), p. 8.
34. L. H. Weed, "The Anatomist in Medical Education," *J. AAMC* 14 (1939): 281–91. Similar views are expressed in A. Gregg, "Perspectives on the Teaching of Anatomy," ibid. 17 (1942): 273–82.
35. Corner, "The Past of Anatomy," pp. 181–82; Corner, "The Role of Anatomy," p. 5; Lippard, *Half-Century*, pp. 12–13, 46–48.

Thus in 1932 the Commission on Medical Education, while recommending a decided decrease in the amount of time devoted to gross anatomy in the first year and less emphasis on memorization of detailed facts, argued that steps should be taken to provide opportunities for review and extension of anatomical knowledge later, thus helping to weave together the preclinical sciences and clinical medicine in a closer relationship. Better correlation was needed: students should not be successively students of anatomy, physiology, and biochemistry, but students of medicine.[36]

A decade later William Dock, professor of pathology at the Cornell medical school, noted that the "competent, ingenious and energetic men" who had made American anatomy departments outstanding were mostly students of physiology. Dissection played little or no part in their research. As a result, some of the country's best physiologists were teaching gross human anatomy while those who had greatest need for and interest in the subject—the surgeons—were not. His recommendation was to introduce medical students to medicine through the fast-growing and exciting subjects of physiology and biochemistry. "Anatomy," he noted, "was never thought of as a cultural subject, valuable in weaning the young American student from didactic methods of teaching, until after physiology, biochemistry and bacteriology were part of the curriculum." Return dissection, "a thoroughly utilitarian subject," to a place in the curriculum where it was likely soon to be applied and let it be taught by those who used the knowledge: internists, radiologists, and especially surgeons.[37] What anatomy departments needed, argued a physician-instructor, just as much as research trailblazers, were "anatomical utility men who know by experience what in the vast encyclopedia of anatomy is important clinically. . . ."[38] From students, too, came complaints that instructors too interested in research were not good teachers and failed to relate the preclinical subjects to their application in medicine.[39]

In 1950, subject to ever-increasing pressure from other areas of medical knowledge, the place of anatomy in the traditional sense was still retreat-

36. *Final Report of the Commission on Medical Education* (New York: Office of the Director of the Study, 1932), pp. 182–84, 189.
37. W. Dock, "Anatomical Dissection: Its Place in the Curriculum," *J. AAMC* 17 (1942): 383–86.
38. W. D. Gardner, "The Young Physician Anatomist in Medical Education and Research," *J. AAMC* 24 (1949): 162–65.
39. J. E. Deitrick and R. C. Berson, *Medical Schools in the United States at Mid-Century* (New York: McGraw-Hill, 1953), p. 335; "The Teaching of Anatomy," pp. 70–71.

ing in the medical curriculum (though anatomy generally still had the largest budget among preclinical departments).[40] The viewpoint of Mall, though still dominant, was under increasing attack. Once the premier medical science, anatomy was becoming to a large extent a victim of its own success.

40. Deitrick and Berson, *Medical Schools in the United States*, pp. 165–66.

Physiology

JOHN HARLEY WARNER

P HYSIOLOGY," wrote Abraham Flexner in 1910, is "the central discipline of the medical school."[1] Although few American medical educators before the late nineteenth century would have agreed with Flexner's singular emphasis, nearly all contended that physiological instruction offered the aspiring physician something of value. Whether a student learned physiology by reading a textbook borrowed from his preceptor's library in the eighteenth century, by listening to lectures in a proprietary medical school in the nineteenth century, or by observing physiological phenomena through his own experiments in a twentieth-century laboratory, his efforts reflected the belief that a knowledge of the functioning of the human body enhanced the physician's understanding of both disease and therapeutics. Educators often stressed the medical value of physiological knowledge, yet they seldom defined its clinical value; the meaning of physiology for the practitioner was elusive. Nevertheless, while the structure, content, and specific objectives of physiological instruction for medical students varied widely from the colonial period to the twentieth

1. Abraham Flexner, *Medical Education in the United States and Canada* (New York: Carnegie Foundation for the Advancement of Teaching, 1910), p. 63.

48

century, the belief that physiological knowledge would help the student become a more successful physician consistently underlay the teaching of physiology.

Until the 1760s medical education in America was synonymous with apprenticeship, and at least until the 1830s nearly all American physicians studied medicine under a preceptor before entering a medical school.[2] Educational quality depended as much on the preceptor's knowledge and resources as on the student's diligence. Poorly trained, ill-equipped preceptors gave their students little physiological instruction.[3] The best preceptors, on the other hand, offered a sound education, providing their pupils with books such as Hermann Boerhaave's *Institutiones Medicae* (1708), the favored text for physiology in eighteenth-century America. Benjamin Rush, who studied in the early 1760s with John Redman, the leading preceptor in Philadelphia, described his apprenticeship:

> I read in the intervals of business and at late and early hours all the books in medicine that were put into my hands by my master, or that I could borrow from other students of medicine in the city. I studied Dr. Boerhaave's lectures on Physiology and Pathology with the closest attention.[4]

Before the turn of the century Rush and over two hundred other colonial medical students supplemented their American apprenticeships by attending medical schools in Britain, where they studied physiology with such leading teachers as William Cullen in Edinburgh.[5]

The earliest medical colleges in America formalized physiological instruction in chairs of the theory of medicine or the institutes of medicine. When the College of Philadelphia opened the first medical school in the colonies in 1765, John Morgan became professor of the theory and practice of medicine, modeling his course after the one he had attended at Edinburgh.[6] "THE THEORY OF PHYSIC, more commonly termed Medical

---

2. George W. Corner, "Apprenticed to Aesculapius: The American Medical Student, 1765–1965," *Proc. Am. Phil. Soc.* 109 (1953): 251.

3. Daniel Drake commented on the qualifications of the average preceptor in *Practical Essays on Medical Education and the Medical Profession in the United States* (Cincinnati: Roff and Young, 1832), p. 30.

4. Quoted in Genevieve Miller, "Medical Education in Colonial America," *Ciba Symposia* 8 (1947): 515.

5. Whitfield J. Bell, Jr., "Medical Students and Their Examiners in Eighteenth Century America," *Trans. & Stud. Coll. Phys. Phila.*, 4th ser., 21 (1953): 14–24; idem, "Some American Students of 'That Shining Oracle of Physic,' Dr. William Cullen of Edinburgh, 1755–1766," *Proc. Am. Phil. Soc.* 94 (1950): 275–81; Francis R. Packard, "How London and Edinburgh Influenced Medicine in Philadelphia in the Eighteenth Century," *Ann. Med. Hist.*, n.s., 4 (1932): 219–44.

6. George W. Corner, *Two Centuries of Medicine: A History of the School of Medicine, University of Pennsylvania* (Philadelphia and Montreal: J. B. Lippincott, 1965), p. 40.

Institutions, comprehends under it, the most important doctrines of Physiology and Pathology," Morgan wrote in 1765. "PHYSIOLOGY teaches the uses of the several parts in the human body, it treats all the functions, vital, animal, and natural, in a sound state."[7] At King's College Medical School in New York, founded in 1767, Peter Middleton included physiology in his lectures on the theory of physic.[8]

Courses in anatomy frequently included some physiology as a functional corollary to human structure, and occasionally overlapped considerably with courses in the theory of medicine. At Harvard in the 1780s Benjamin Waterhouse thoroughly surveyed contemporary physiological knowledge in his lectures on the theory and practice of medicine,[9] while his colleague John Warren, professor of anatomy and surgery, stressed function in his anatomical course. Proper study of the parts of the body, Warren maintained, necessarily involved the "deducing of their Functions from their form and situation," and in his course he attempted "to intersperse such physiological observations as obviously occur in the definition" of human anatomy.[10] A similar situation existed at the College of Physicians and Surgeons in New York in the early 1810s. David Hosack, professor of the theory and practice of physic and clinical medicine, began his course with a "compendious view" of the functions of the body in health, while John Augustine Smith, professor of anatomy, surgery, and physiology, endeavored to integrate structure and function and "to present such physiological views of each part as necessarily arise from considering its peculiar nature and functions."[11] Physiological instruction clearly occupied an important but dispersed place in the curricula of early American medical colleges.

The physiological content of courses in the institutes or theory of medicine was relatively standardized before the rapid proliferation of medical schools in the early nineteenth century. The professor usually introduced his subject with a brief survey of the chemical and structural

7. John Morgan, *A Discourse upon the Institution of Medical Schools in America* (Philadelphia: William Bradford, 1765), p. 11.

8. Byron Stookey, *A History of Colonial Medical Education in the Province of New York, with Its Subsequent Development (1767–1830)* (Springfield, Ill.: Charles C. Thomas, 1962), p. 53.

9. Benjamin Waterhouse, *A Synopsis of a Course of Lectures on the Theory and Practice of Medicine* (Boston: Adams and Nourse, 1786).

10. Warren quoted in Thomas Edward Moore, Jr., "The Early Years of the Harvard Medical School: Its Founding and Curriculum, 1782–1810," *Bull. Hist. Med.* 27 (1943): 549; see also p. 554.

11. "Syllabus of the Several Courses of Lectures Delivered in the College of Physicians and Surgeons, New-York," in Daniel D. Tompkins, *An Historical Sketch of the Origin, Progress, and Present State of the College of Physicians and Surgeons of the University of the State of New-York* (New York: C. S. Van Winkle, 1813), p. 28.

composition of the body. He then proceeded to the organic and animal or "vital" properties of the body, like mobility, irritability, vital affinity, and sensibility. The bulk of the lectures treated the functions of the body: nutrition and digestion, respiration, locomotion, excretion, reproduction, and the circulation of the blood. Finally, he considered the "faculties and operations of the mind" and the "moral faculties." A discussion of hygiene—particularly the influences that climate, exercise, food, sleep, clothing, occupation, and atmosphere exerted on the human constitution—served as a transition from the lectures on physiology to those on pathology.[12] Medical students in Philadelphia, Boston, or New York in the 1810s heard, in essence, a diluted version of the lectures on the institutes of medicine given in Edinburgh, modified only by the particular interests or weaknesses of their American professors.

Except for the knowledge an imaginative student may have gained from envisioning in motion the parts of a dissected corpse, physiological training came solely from didactic lectures and textbooks. The instructors in physiology in the eighteenth and nineteenth centuries were almost always practicing physicians, whose knowledge of the subject frequently did not extend beyond the instruction they had received from their preceptors and from physiology lectures. Faculty quality varied considerably, especially toward mid-century, as the number of medical schools increased. Few teachers illustrated their didactic lectures with demonstrations or experiments until after the 1840s, and many read their physiology lectures directly from textbooks or from the notes of courses they had taken as students. Charles Caldwell, who received his M.D. at the College of Philadelphia in 1796, later recalled that his professors

> entered the hall, ascended the platform, seated themselves in their chairs, and calmly read their lectures—some of them without animation or emphasis, and, not infrequently, without abstracting their eyes from their manuscript, from the beginning to the close of their sober exercise—a mode of lecturing as unprofitable to those who, instead of listening, too often slumbered, as it was saturnine and ungraceful in those who practiced it.[13]

12. James Jackson, *A Syllabus of the Lectures Delivered at the Massachusetts Medical College to the Medical Students of Harvard University* (Boston, 1816); Benjamin Rush, *Sixteen Introductory Lectures, to Courses of Lectures upon the Institutes and Practice of Medicine, with a Syllabus of the Latter* (Philadelphia: Bradford and Innskeep, 1811); "Syllabus of the Several Courses of Lectures Delivered in the College of Physicians and Surgeons, New-York," in Tompkins, *An Historical Sketch.*
13. Charles Caldwell, *Thoughts on the Education, Qualifications, and Duties of the Physician of the United States. A Valedictory Address, Delivered on the 5th Day of March, 1849* (Louisville, Kentucky: Currier Job Room, 1849), p. 9.

Although Benjamin Waterhouse claimed in 1786 that "all the knowledge
the Physiologist pretends to, he derives from *Experiment, or the use of
his senses,*"[14] few American medical students before the 1870s learned any
physiology through their own experience.

The physiological knowledge a student acquired in medical school,
however, sometimes went beyond the required lectures and assigned
books. From the 1790s to the 1810s a number of American medical students elected to write theses on such physiological subjects as respiration,
animal heat, and the nature of the living principle.[15] John R. Young, who
graduated from the University of Pennsylvania in 1803, based his thesis,
*An Experimental Inquiry into the Principles of Nutrition and the Diges-
tive Process,* on simple digestive experiments he performed on a frog, a
fellow student, and himself. Young concluded that gastric juice contained
phosphoric acid, which explained the stomach's acidity.[16] Most theses,
however, merely reviewed existing physiological theories and evaluated
their evidential foundations. Still, writing a physiological thesis did encourage the student to go beyond the content of his required lectures,
instructing him in a single branch of physiology through his own evaluation of extracurricular sources.

Instruction in physiology was also available outside the customary institutions. Harvard undergraduates, who later may have studied medicine, took advantage of private physiological instruction as early as the
1690s,[17] and beginning with the early nineteenth century, an increasing
number of "private" schools emerged to supplement the courses offered
by medical colleges.[18] The Philadelphia Anatomical Rooms, later the
Philadelphia School of Anatomy, offered students instruction in anatomy
and surgery from April to November, when the city's medical colleges

14. Waterhouse, *A Synopsis of a Course of Lectures,* p. 16.
15. For examples of student theses see Samuel Martin, *An Inaugural Essay on Respira-
tion* (Baltimore: S. P. Child, 1813); Robert Morrell, *An Inaugural Dissertation on Animal
Heat* (New York: T. and S. Swords, 1810); Matthias E. Sawyer, *An Inaugural Dissertation:
Containing an Inquiry into the Existence of the Living Principle and Causes of Animal Life*
(Philadelphia: T. Dobson, 1793); Lyman Spalding, *An Inaugural Dissertation on the Pro-
duction of Animal Heat* (Walpole, New Hampshire: David Carlisle, 1797); Joseph Youle, *An
Inaugural Dissertation on Respiration: Being an Application of the Principles of the New
Chemistry to that Function* (New York: T. and J. Swords, 1793).
16. John R. Young, *An Experimental Inquiry, into the Principles of Nutrition, and the
Digestive Process* (Philadelphia: Euken and Mecum, 1803).
17. F. Guerra, "Harvey and the Circulation of the Blood in America During the Colonial
Period," *Bull. Hist. Med.* 33 (1959): 214, 228. See also Josiah Bartlett, *A Dissertation on the
Progress of Medical Science in the Commonwealth of Massachusetts* (Boston: T. B. Wait,
1810), pp. 12–13.
18. See, for example, David Hosack, *Plan of Study Adopted in the Private Medical
School, Established by David Hosack* (New York, [ca. 1812]).

were closed.[19] Physiological instruction accompanied dissection, as James M'Clintock, professor of anatomy at the school in 1840, explained:

> In our attempts to obtain an acquaintance with the structure and connections of the different parts forming our bodies, we can hardly fail to obtain some idea of the functions they subserve. The student, even when most closely engaged in examining the bodily organization, imperceptibly becomes a physiologist.[20]

Perhaps the best known private institution was Boston's Tremont Street School, which four Harvard professors established in 1838, and which, like the other private schools, included physiology in its curriculum.[21] Given these sources of physiological instruction—preceptors, medical colleges, and private medical schools—the ambitious American medical student did not need to travel to Europe to gain a sound knowledge of physiology.

The presence of physiological instruction in medical college curricula plainly indicates that the faculties perceived in physiology something of value for the future practitioner. The role of scientific training in providing physicians with a justification of their professional status is obscure, especially before the emergence of "scientific medicine" after the mid-nineteenth century. Much clearer was the assumption, shared by most medical teachers, that physiological knowledge was of practical utility to the physician and surgeon. John Morgan argued in 1765 that "every disease we labor under is a disorder of the vital, animal, or natural functions"; therefore, "a thorough acquaintance with these in the sound state is implied before we can pretend to understand their morbid affections, or how to remedy them." For therapeutics, he added, "PHYSIOLOGY gives us the clearest light in the cure of diseases, which is the grandest object of all our inquiries in medicine."[22] Daniel Drake over fifty years later defended the medical relevance of physiology in similar terms:

> Without a knowledge of Anatomy and Physiology, no pupil can prosecute the study of the profession; for diseases consist either in alterations of structure, or in disordered and irregular movements in the functions of that structure; and in both cases, without an ac-

19. William Williams Keen, "The History of the Philadelphia School of Anatomy and Its Relations to Medical Teaching," in idem, *Addresses and Other Papers* (Philadelphia and London: W. B. Saunders, 1905), pp. 42–43.

20. James M'Clintock, *Annual Lecture: Introductory Lecture to the Winter Course of Anatomy, in the Philadelphia School of Anatomy, Delivered on Monday Evening, November 2d, 1840* (Philadelphia: Charles A. Elliott, 1840), p. 7.

21. James Bordley III and A. McGehee Harvey, *Two Centuries of American Medicine, 1776–1976* (Philadelphia, London and Toronto: W. B. Saunders, 1976), p. 23.

22. Morgan, *A Discourse Upon the Institution of Medical Schools*, p. 12.

quaintance with the *healthy* condition, no degree of genius can enable us to understand the morbid.[23]

Physiology, or a knowledge of the normal functions of the body, prepared the student to understand how disease altered these functions and how to remedy these morbid alterations through therapeutics.

As the number and variety of medical schools increased in the nineteenth century, particularly in the southern and western states, physiological instruction became less uniform in both quality and focus. When a country medical school hired a poorly trained practitioner to teach physiology, instruction of a high caliber could not be expected. A well-educated and conscientious professor with access to a good library, on the other hand, could offer his students a comprehensive view of the most current physiological knowledge. The focus of physiological teaching was equally variable, depending on the school and interests of its instructor. Before Samuel Gregory founded the Boston Female Medical College in 1848, for example, he gave popular lectures on physiology and personal hygiene, emphasizing the value of these subjects in preserving health. This emphasis continued in the lectures given at the Female Medical College, which, in deference to the particular needs of its students, also stressed the physiology of pregnancy and parturition.[24]

William G. Rothstein has argued that the scientific content of nineteenth-century medical education differed little among regular, homeopathic, and eclectic schools.[25] The focus of physiological teaching, however, varied substantially. The eclectics generally stressed the value of physiology as a guide to health and a guard against empiricism. At the Eclectic Medical Institute of Cincinnati, which in the mid-1850s claimed the greatest enrollment of any medical college outside Philadelphia and New York,[26] students read the same physiology textbooks used by their counterparts in regular schools,[27] but the lectures they heard placed an

23. Daniel Drake, *An Inaugural Discourse on Medical Education; Delivered at the Opening of the Medical College of Ohio, in Cincinnati, November 11th, 1820* (Cincinnati: Looker, Palmer and Reynolds, 1820), p. 5. See also John D. Godman, *Introductory Lecture to the Course of Anatomy and Physiology, in the Rutgers Medical College, New York, Delivered, December 11, 1826* (New York: H. Stevenson, 1826), p. 5.

24. Frederick C. Waite, *History of the New England Female Medical College* (Brattleboro, Vermont: Vermont Publishing Co., 1950), pp. 12–19.

25. William G. Rothstein, *American Physicians in the Nineteenth Century: From Sects to Science* (Baltimore and London: Johns Hopkins University Press, 1972), pp. 166, 228, 238–39.

26. Ronald L. Numbers, "The Making of an Eclectic Physician: Joseph M. McElhinney and the Eclectic Medical Institute of Cincinnati," *Bull. Hist. Med.* 47 (1973): 157–58.

27. "Annual Announcement of Lectures of the Eclectic Medical Institute of Cincinnati, Session 1852–3," *Eclectic Med. J.* 11 (1852): 426.

unusual emphasis on theories of brain function and neurophysiology. The school's *Annual Circular* for 1849 stated that

> in physiology and medical philosophy, the instructions of the Institute are essentially different from those of any other school in Europe or America. This is the only school in which the facts of Phrenology and Animal Magnetism have been properly recognized and explained as a portion of medical science. It is the only school in which the functions of the brain, as a physiological organ, have been taught.[28]

This emphasis reflects both the school's eclectic philosophy and the particular interests of Joseph R. Buchanan, its professor of physiology and institutes of medicine, who was particularly intrigued by the functions of the brain and its "mental and physiological powers."[29] The Eclectic Medical Institute highlighted its emphasis on neurophysiology in 1850 by separating the professorships of physiology and "cerebral physiology."[30] Knowledge of the physiology of the brain and nervous system, the faculty hoped, would "give the pupil a philosophical understanding of the mysterious operations of the human consitution, its varieties, temperaments, and pathological conditions, by the exhibition of vital laws, facts and principles heretofore unknown."[31] Clearly, by the mid-1850s the content of physiological instruction—particularly the attention paid to different branches of physiology—was not constant in American medical schools.

Nor was the amount of physiological instruction the same in all regular medical schools. The first annual announcement (1849) of the Medical College of Evansville made it clear that Charles S. Weever's course in anatomy and physiology would be primarily anatomical, and that Weever would devote only "as much time to the science of Physiology, as may be consistent with giving a full and complete course of lectures on Anatomy."[32] Robley Dunglison, on the other hand, emphasized physiology at the expense of anatomy in his lectures at the University of Virginia. When the department of medicine opened at Charlottesville in 1825, Dunglison became the the first full-time medical instructor in America. His chief interest was physiology, and he assisted William Beaumont with his experiments on gastric juice in the early 1830s. Dunglison considered him-

    28. "Eclectic Medical Institute, Fifth Annual Circular," *Eclectic Med. J.* 8 (1849): 327–28.
    29. Ibid., p. 328.
    30. "Eclectic Medical Institute of Cincinnati," *Eclectic Med. J.* 9 (1850): 385.
    31. "Annual Announcement of the Eclectic Medical Institute of Cincinnati, for the Session of 1853–4," *Eclectic Med. J.* 12 (1853–54): 338.
    32. Burton D. Meyers, *The History of Medical Education in Indiana* (Bloomington: Indiana University Press, 1956), p. 31.

self a pioneer in the teaching of physiology in America, commenting in his lectures that "this interesting department of science has of late years acquired a value which it did not previously possess."[33] The five thousand or more medical students whose diplomas bore Dunglison's signature[34] obviously received substantially more instruction in physiology than did Weever's students at Evansville. Dunglison's most important contribution to the teaching of physiology, however, was his textbook *Human Physiology* (1832),[35] the first comprehensive textbook in the field by an American author.

Until Dunglison's textbook appeared, the paucity of good, available treatises on physiology seriously hindered successful teaching of the subject. One physician who studied in Philadelphia in the 1790s later recalled the ineptness of his physiology instructors and the lack of good books to compensate for poor teaching:

> Nor did the English language afford books, by the study of which the defect could be remedied. As far as I was then, or am yet informed, the libraries of Philadelphia did not contain, on physiological science, in the English tongue, more than four small volumes, amounting, in the aggregate, to less than twelve hundred octavo pages. And, to say the least of them, their quality was in no degree superior to their bulk. So scanty and unprofitable were the resources of physiology, in the school of Philadelphia, in the fortieth year of the institution's existence.[36]

He added that the translation from Latin of Johann Friedrich Blumenbach's *Elements of Physiology* in 1795 improved the situation somewhat.[37] But until 1815 most Harvard students used only Albrecht von Haller's *First Lines of Physiology*,[38] and as late as 1833 Oliver Wendell Holmes supplemented the lectures he attended at Harvard only with Haller's treatise and Anthelme Richerand's *Elements of Physiology*.[39]

33. Dunglison quoted in Samuel X. Radbill, "Robley Dunglison, M.D., 1798–1869, American Medical Educator," *J. Med. Educ.* 34 (1959): 90.

34. Samuel X. Radbill, "Robley Dunglison," *D. S. B.* (1970–1976), 4:252.

35. Robley Dunglison, *Human Physiology, Illustrated by Engravings*, 3rd ed., 2 vols. (Philadelphia: Carey Lea and Blanchard, 1838).

36. Caldwell, *Thoughts on the Education, Qualifications, and Duties of the Physicians of the United States*, p. 10.

37. Johann Friedrich Blumenbach, *Elements of Physiology*, trans. Charles Caldwell, 2 vols. (Philadelphia: Thomas Dobson, 1795).

38. Walter J. Meek, "The Beginnings of American Physiology," *Ann. Med. Hist.* 10 (1928): 112; Albert von Haller, *First Lines of Physiology* (Troy, New York: Obadiah Penniman, 1803).

39. Meek, "The Beginnings of American Physiology," p. 112; Anthelme Balthasar Richerand, *The Elements of Physiology: Containing an Explanation of the Functions of the Human Body; in Which the Modern Improvements in Chemistry, Galvanism, and Other*

Shortly after the publication of Dunglison's book, Nathaniel Potter wrote the author. "While the physiologist will find himself pleased and instructed," he commented, "the pupil will perceive, that he has, at last, found a safe and easy guide to the fundamental principles of his profession. As a *textbook*, it will take precedence of all other systems."[40] Potter's prediction was largely realized, and by 1858 more than ninety-five thousand copies of Dunglison's book had been sold. Samuel D. Gross later remarked that "what Haller's great work accomplished for surgery in the eighteenth century, Dunglison accomplished for physiology in America in the nineteenth."[41] After the mid-1840s several other texts appeared, providing comprehensive and accessible sources of physiological knowledge and greatly facilitating the teaching of physiology.[42] For the interested medical student, this increased availability of good textbooks was perhaps the most important advance in American physiological education in the prelaboratory period.

During the 1840s some instructors in medical schools began to illustrate their didactic lectures on physiology with demonstrations. At the University of Pennsylvania in 1841, drawings constituted the only illustrations used in the physiology course.[43] But during the same decade the Rock Island Medical School, a third-rate midwestern proprietary institution, was illustrating its physiology lectures "by plates and diagrams" as well as by demonstrations using the microscope.[44] And in 1846 Jeffries

Sciences, Are Applied to Explain the Actions of the Animal Economy, trans. Robert Kerrison (Philadelphia: Hopkins and Earle, Fry and Kammerer, 1808).

40. Nathaniel Potter to Robley Dunglison, 29 April 1833, in Samuel X. Radbill, "The Autobiographical Ana of Robley Dunglison, M.D.," *Trans. Am. Phil. Soc.*, n.s., 53, pt. 8 (1963): 57.

41. Gross quoted in Meek, "The Beginnings of American Physiology," p. 118.

42. John C. Dalton, *A Treatise on Human Physiology; Designed for the Use of Students and Practitioners of Medicine* (Philadelphia: Henry C. Lea, 1871); John William Draper, *Human Physiology, Statical and Dynamical; or, the Conditions and Course of the Life of Man* (New York: Harper and Brothers, 1856); Austin Flint, *A Text-Book of Human Physiology; Designed for the Use of Practitioners and Students of Medicine* (New York: D. Appleton, 1876). Textbooks by English authors which were popular in America included William B. Carpenter, *Elements of Physiology, Including Physiological Anatomy, for the Use of the Medical Student* (Philadelphia: Lea and Blanchard, 1846), and Robert Bentley Todd and William Bowmann, *The Physiological Anatomy and Physiology of Man*, 2 vols. (London: John W. Parker, 1845). On textbooks used see John S. Billings, "Literature and Institutions," in *A Century of American Medicine, 1776–1876* (1876; reprint ed., New York: Burt Franklin, 1971), p. 301; Jonathan Forman, "The Worthington School and Thomsonianism," *Bull. Hist. Med.* 21 (1947): 777; *Catalogue of the Officers and Students of Harvard University for the Academical Year 1862–63* (Cambridge, Mass.: Sever and Francis, 1862), p. 91.

43. The Medical Faculty of the University of Pennsylvania, *Medical Department of the University of Pennsylvania* (Philadelphia, 1841), pp. 26–27.

44. *Prospectus of the Rock Island Medical School, to be Opened on the First Monday of*

Wyman proposed to demonstrate his physiology lectures at Hampden-Sidney Medical College with experiments "illustrating the chemistry of Digestion Respiration &c."[45] On the whole, however, physiological demonstrations as teaching aids in the 1840s were infrequent and nowhere systematic.

Demonstrations illustrating physiology lectures became more common in the 1850s. John C. Dalton, whom S. Weir Mitchell called America's "first professional physiologist,"[46] returned from studying experimental physiology with Claude Bernard to take up the chair in physiology and morbid anatomy at the University of Buffalo. To illustrate a lecture in physiology in 1854, Dalton experimentally created a gastric fistula in a dog in order to reproduce some of Beaumont's classic experiments with Alexis St. Martin's stomach.[47] This was apparently the first instance of teaching physiology with illustrations by vivisection in an American medical school.[48] The following year Dalton became professor of pathology and physiology at the Vermont Medical College at Woodstock, which announced that "in the department of Physiology the lectures will be illustrated by a series of highly interesting and valuable experiments upon living animals, particularly in the action of the gastric juice, and other elements of the process of digestion."[49]

S. Weir Mitchell described one physiology lecture in the 1850s as being "a more or less well stated resume of the best foreign books, without experiments or striking illustrations. It was like hearing about a foreign land into which we were forbidden to enter."[50] But some physiology instructors were already incorporating Dalton's methods into their own courses. James Aitken Meigs, professor of the institutes of medicine in the medical department of Pennsylvania College, illustrated his lectures on physiology "with an extensive series of vivisectional demonstrations."[51] And William Thompson Lusk at Harvard systematically employed vivi-

November Next, at Rock Island Illinois (Chicago: J. Campbell, 1848), p. 11.

45. Jeffries Wyman to David Humphreys Storer, 29 November 1846, in George E. Gifford, Jr., "Twelve Letters from Jeffries Wyman, M.D., Hampden-Sydney Medical College, Richmond, Virginia, 1843–1848," J. Hist. Med. 20 (1965): 326.

46. S. W. Mitchell, "Biographical Memoir of John Call Dalton," Biogr. Mem. Nat. Acad. Sci. 3 (1895): 179.

47. Frederick Clayton Waite, The Story of a Country Medical College: A History of the Clinical School of Medicine and the Vermont Medical College, Woodstock, Vermont, 1827–1856 (Montpelier: Vermont Historical Society, 1945), p. 115.

48. William B. Atkinson, The Physicians and Surgeons of the United States (Philadelphia: Charles Robson, 1878), p. 658.

49. Waite, The Story of a Country Medical College, p. 115.

50. Mitchell, "Biographical Memoir of John Call Dalton," p. 179.

51. Atkinson, The Physicians and Surgeons of the United States, p. 158.

sectional experiments in 1870. Such experimentation on living animals for educational purposes inevitably attracted public criticism, but Lusk defended the practice, arguing in his introductory lecture that "the destruction of life which this may involve can hardly be objected to by those who constantly acquiesce in the sacrifice of animals for a much lower purpose viz.: the gratification of the palate."[52]

The medical students enrolled in Dalton's or Meigs's courses in physiology in the 1850s, or even Lusk's course in the 1870s, merely observed demonstrations; they did not perform experiments. No medical school in America taught physiology—with the single exception of microscopic physiology—in the laboratory until the 1870s.[53] Although one medical educator dismissed the microscope as "one of those new-fangled European notions,"[54] American physicians began to recognize the medical value of microscopy by the 1840s, and a few medical schools began offering students practical training in microscopic anatomy and physiology.[55] At the Vermont Medical College students used the microscope to become "practically familiar with many of the important facts of Minute Anatomy and Physiology." According to the school's *Announcement*, microscopes "are extensively used, and all the students will be enabled to become familiar with most of the leading physiological phenomena."[56] Similarly, the Berkshire Medical Institution organized a department of surgical pathology and microscopy in 1854, holding classes "on stated evenings for practical and personal instruction with the Microscope, that all the students may become familiar with the elementary structures, and interesting physiological phenomena."[57] Other schools soon began providing students with the opportunity to study histophysiology by experiment and personal observation.[58] Most instruction in microscopy emphasized anatomy rather than physiology; nevertheless, microscopy was the one part of the medical curriculum where the student before the 1870s could pursue practical laboratory study of physiological phenomena.

52. Graham Lusk, "Physiology at the Harvard Medical School, 1870–1871: A Part of the Introductory Lecture and Synopsis of the Experimental Demonstrations Given by William Thompson Lusk," *Boston Med. & Surg. J.* 167 (1912): 922.

53. Keen, however, claimed that in 1856 S. Weir Mitchell gave a "purely experimental course on Physiology" at the Philadelphia School of Anatomy (Keen, "The Philadelphia School of Anatomy," p. 60).

54. Waite, *History of the New England Female Medical College*, p. 29.

55. James H. Cassedy, "The Microscope in American Medical Science, 1840–1860," *Isis* 67 (1976): 76–97.

56. Waite, *The Story of a Country Medical College*, p. 114.

57. Peter D. Gibbons, "The Berkshire Medical Institution," *Bull. Hist. Med.* 38 (1964): 58.

58. C. I. Reed, "Development of the Teaching of Physiology in Ohio," *Ohio St. Arch. & Hist. Q.* 60 (1951): 360; Corner, *Two Centuries of Medicine*, p. 156.

Attempts to elevate the status of physiology in American medical schools after the Civil War often elicited an apathetic response and sometimes encountered strong resistance. When curricular reforms at Harvard in the early 1870s introduced the laboratory method of teaching physiology, one faculty member objected to having students "while away" their time "in the labyrinths of Chemistry and Physiology."[59] Even the American Medical Association's Committee on Medical Education, which recommended in 1867 that "the curriculum of instruction should be materially, if not completely, reformed," called for a reduction in the teaching of physiology, chemistry, obstetrics, and materia medica to provide more time for lectures on pathological anatomy, toxicology, medical jurisprudence, medical ethics, and medical history.[60] Nevertheless, the early postbellum period saw a reconstruction of medical school curricula encompassing both reforms in the methods of teaching the subject and a more rigorous defense of the value of physiological training for the future practitioner. As a result of these changes, physiology came to occupy a leading position in the programs of the better schools.

One of the most influential attempts to upgrade the teaching of physiology took place at Harvard during the 1870s. Charles William Eliot, who became president of Harvard in 1869,[61] wrote in his annual report for 1871 that "the whole system of medical education in this country needs thorough reform,"[62] introducing a three-year graded curriculum and the laboratory method of instruction. In physiology and the other basic sciences, "laboratory work is substituted for, or added to, the usual didactic lectures, and laboratory work is as much required of every student as attendance at lectures and recitations."[63] In recognition of the subject's importance in the new curriculum, the reorganized school created an independent department of physiology, appointing Henry Pickering Bowditch as its head.[64]

Since his graduation from the Harvard Medical School in 1868, Bow-

59. Donald Fleming, *William H. Welch and the Rise of Modern Medicine* (Boston: Little, Brown, 1954), p. 5.

60. S. D. Gross, "Report of the Committee on Medical Education," *Trans. AMA* 18 (1867): 365.

61. Frederick Rudolph, *The American College and University: A History* (New York: Knopf, Vintage Books, 1962), pp. 290–95.

62. Eliot quoted in Hebbel E. Hoff, "Medical Progress a Century Ago: A New Medical Curriculum in America," *Conn. Med.* 36 (1972): 58. See also *A Catalogue of the Officers and Students of Harvard University for the Academic Year 1871–72* (Cambridge, Mass.: Riverside Press, 1871), p. 89.

63. *Ninetieth Annual Catalogue of the Medical School (Boston) of Harvard University, 1872–73* (Cambridge, Mass.: Charles W. Sever, 1873), p. 3.

64. [Harold C. Ernst, ed.], *The Harvard University Medical School, 1782–1906* (Boston: Harvard University, 1906), p. 90.

ditch had studied experimental physiology in France and Germany. He brought with him to Harvard in 1871 not only laboratory apparatus, which he had purchased in Germany, but also an approach to physiological research and teaching that he had learned from his mentor Carl Ludwig at the Physiological Institute in Leipzig.[65] Under Bowditch's tutelage, first-year students at Harvard learned physiology from lectures, recitations, and practical laboratory demonstrations, while third-year students could elect to undertake original physiological research in the laboratory.[66] For the first time in America the laboratory had joined the lecture hall as a locus of physiological instruction for medical students.

Although first-year medical students at Harvard entered the physiological laboratory in 1871, for over a decade they did not undertake experiments but merely observed demonstrations executed by instructors. More advanced students pursued their own original research in increasingly sophisticated and well-equipped laboratories (see illustration). Between the time Bowditch created his physiological laboratory and the turn of the century, however, the methods of laboratory teaching in physiology changed markedly. Educators at Harvard and elsewhere came to believe that student experimentation was a more constructive use of laboratory facilities than faculty demonstrations. William Townsend Porter, assistant professor of physiology in 1898, decried the use at many schools of physiological demonstrations performed in the lecture hall simply to illustrate required textbooks and lectures: "Never was the pedagogical cart more squarely before the horse!"[67] By the 1890s first-year students at Harvard were learning much of their physiology by doing, rather than merely observing, physiological experiments.

In 1898 Harvard required its first-year medical students to take a laboratory course in experimental physiology in which each pupil carried out more than one hundred experiments, thereby "emancipating the student from the textbook and accustoming him to form independent judgements."[68] Instruction in physiology included 118 hours of lectures, 64 hours of laboratory work, and 32 hours of recitations. In addition, about 15 percent of the class elected to write theses on physiological topics.[69] Experiments, designed to give the future physician "the point of view of

65. Everett Mendelsohn, "Henry Pickering Bowditch," *D. S. B. (1970–1976)*, 2:365–68.
66. *Ninetieth Annual Catalogue of the Medical School (Boston) of Harvard University, 1872–73*, p. 9.
67. W. T. Porter, "The Teaching of Physiology in Medical Schools," *Boston Med. & Surg. J.* 139 (1898): 647–48.
68. *Announcement of the Medical School (Boston) of Harvard University for 1898–99* (Cambridge, Mass.: Harvard University, 1898), p. 14.
69. Porter, "The Teaching of Physiology in Medical Schools," p. 647.

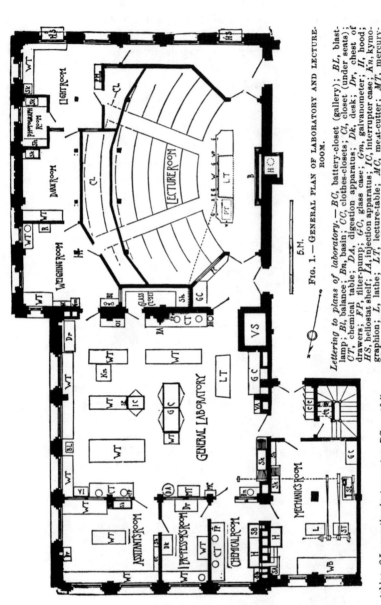

5.M.

FIG. 1. — GENERAL PLAN OF LABORATORY AND LECTURE-
ROOM.

Lettering to plans of laboratory. — *BC*, battery-closet (gallery); *BL*, blast-
lamp; *Bl*, balance; *Bn*, basin; *CC*, clothes-closets; *Cl*, closet (under seats);
CT, chemical table; *DA*, digestion apparatus; *Dk*, desk; *Dr*, chest of
drawers; *FP*, filter-pump; *GC*, glass case; *Gm*, galvanometer; *H*, hood;
HS, heliostat shelf; *IA*, injection apparatus; *IC*, interrupter case; *Kn*, kymo-
graphion; *L*, lathe; *LT*, lecture-table; *MC*, meat-cutter; *MT*, mercury-
table; *OI*, operating instruments; *PC*, portfolio-case; *PM*, pendulum myograph; *R*, refrigerator; *RA*, respiration apparatus; *SA*,
soldering apparatus; *SB*, steam-bath; *SE*, steam-engine; *Sh*, shelves; *Sk*, sink; *SP*, seconds pendulum; *ST*, saw-table; *TU*, tele-
scope; *VA*, varnishing apparatus; *VS*, ventilating shaft; *WB*, work-bench; *WT*, working-table. *Lecture-room.* — *A*, air-blast;
B, blackboards; *E*, electricity; *G*, gas; *PT*, pneumatic trough; *W*, water; *WP*, waste-pipe.

The Harvard Physiological Laboratory in 1884. First-year medical students witnessed demonstrations in this
laboratory while advanced students used its extensive apparatus in original physiological research ("The Harvard
Physiological Laboratory," *Science* 4 [1884]: 128).

the physiologist,"[70] became the focus of the teaching of physiology. Porter commented that "instructors saturated with the *ancien régime* . . . will exclaim, 'Why! you have made the lectures merely explanatory of the experiments,' " adding emphatically: "Precisely, that is the chief excellence of this plan of instruction."[71] A decade later first-year students were spending 200 hours in the physiological laboratory, listening to lectures for 90 hours, and writing a required thesis in physiology.[72] The laboratory had thus become the principal setting of instruction in physiology at Harvard. Experiments no longer merely illustrated lectures; lectures explained experiments.

Laboratory instruction in physiology, following Bowditch's efforts at Harvard, soon appeared in the educational programs of other leading medical schools. The University of Pennsylvania opened a physiology laboratory in 1874, and the University of Michigan organized a physiology and histology laboratory three years later.[73] Courses in experimental physiology, optional at first, became integral parts of the curricula of America's foremost medical schools in the 1880s and 1890s.

As physiology won recognition as an autonomous science in the last third of the nineteenth century, it also gave rise to several new subdisciplines. Looking back at the 1870s and 1880s, the physiologist Henry Sewall could write in 1911 that

> whereas physiology was then the dependent runt of the medical family it is today the eldest son in a stable system of primogeniture. As with a noble jewel whose beauty depends on the cutting, we may name one facet Pathology, another Pharmacology, another Biochemistry, another Psychology, and so on, the jewel itself remains and ever will be Physiology.[74]

As early as 1875, for example, Yale's Russell Henry Chittenden, who established the first physiological chemistry laboratory for teaching purposes in America, was advocating the incorporation of his subject into the curriculum of every medical school.[75] Thus, besides their laboratory work

70. *Announcement of the Medical School (688 Boylston Street, Boston, Mass.) of Harvard University for 1900–01* (Cambridge, Mass.: Harvard University, 1900); W. T. Porter, "The Laboratory Teaching of Physiology," *Science*, n.s., 14 (1901): 567–71.

71. Porter, "The Teaching of Physiology in Medical Schools," p. 651.

72. *Announcement of the Medical School, Longwood Avenue, Boston, Mass., of Harvard University for 1909–10*, 2nd ed. ([Cambridge, Mass.]: Harvard University, 1909), p. 27.

73. Corner, *Two Centuries of Medicine*, p. 156; Wilfred B. Shaw, ed., *The University of Michigan: An Encyclopedic Survey, in Nine Parts* (Ann Arbor: University of Michigan Press, 1942–1958), pt. 5, *The Medical School, the University Hospital, the Law School, 1850–1940*, pp. 917–19.

74. Henry Sewall, "Henry Newell Martin, Professor of Biology in Johns Hopkins University, 1876–1893," *Bull. Johns Hopkins Hosp.* 22 (1911): 328.

75. Frederick A. Fuhrman, "Development of Laboratories for Teaching the Medical

in general physiology so named, some medical students received additional physiology instruction in laboratory courses in physiological chemistry, pharmacology, and pathological physiology.[76]

The rapid advance of physiological knowledge in the second half of the nineteenth century clearly fostered certain changes in American medical education, yet the stimulus of this increasing body of knowledge does not in itself explain the growth of the laboratory teaching of physiology in medical schools from the early 1870s through the turn of the century. This growth rested largely on a complex of other factors external to physiology as a science. As long as medical colleges offered only ungraded courses with terms lasting only a few months, there simply was not room in the crowded curriculum for time-consuming laboratory work. The advent of the graded curriculum and the progressive lengthening of terms after the Civil War obviated this problem in many schools.[77]

Moreover, most practicing physicians who made up the faculties of antebellum medical schools had neither the laboratory experience nor the time required for laboratory teaching. After the 1870s the marked increase in the number of American nonmedical graduate students, coupled with the large number of American physicians who gained practical experience in German physiology laboratories, provided the educated manpower to fill these new faculty positions.[78] At the same time, the increasing number of full-time chairs in physiology enabled professors to devote more time to teaching.[79] Laboratory instruction was also expensive, demanding both faculty time and specialized apparatus.[80] Most proprietary schools could not afford to teach physiology in the laboratory. But as the best medical colleges strengthened their university affiliations and became increasingly dependent on philanthropy, they freed themselves

Sciences," in idem, *Multidiscipline Laboratories for Teaching the Medical Sciences* (Palo Alto, Calif.: Stanford University School of Medicine, 1968), p. 20.

76. See, for example, W. G. MacCallum, "On the Teaching of Pathological Physiology," *Bull. Johns Hopkins Hosp.* 18 (1907): 327–30.

77. Frederick C. Waite, "Advent of the Graded Curriculum in American Medical Colleges," *J. AAMC* 25 (1950): 315–22; Robert P. Hudson, "Abraham Flexner in Perspective: American Medical Education, 1865–1910," *Bull. Hist. Med.* 46 (1972): 551.

78. Richard Hofstadter and C. DeWitt Hardey, *The Development and Scope of Higher Education in the United States* (New York: Columbia University Press, 1952), p. 64; Thomas Nelville Bonner, *American Doctors and German Universities: A Chapter in International Intellectual Relations, 1870–1914* (Lincoln: University of Nebraska Press, 1963), p. 23.

79. John A. D. Cooper, "Undergraduate Medical Education," in John Z. Bowers and Elizabeth F. Purcell, eds., *Advances in American Medicine: Essays at the Bicentennial,* 2 vols. (New York: Josiah Macy, Jr., Foundation, 1976), 1: 269–70.

80. See Edward T. Reichert, "Some Forms of Apparatus Used in the Course of Practical Instruction in Physiology in the University of Pennsylvania," *Penn. Med. Bull.* 14 (1901): 121–32.

from the more acute financial constraints on the laboratory teaching of physiology.

Finally, and most fundamentally, before laboratory teaching of physiology could occupy a secure place in the curriculum, educators had to be convinced of both the medical value of physiological knowledge and the utility of this teaching method. The philosophy of the German university, which substantially influenced American educators after the Civil War, coupled with the emerging zeitgeist of scientific medicine and the concomitant belief in the value of science for improving medical practice, greatly aided the cause of the proselytizers of the physiology laboratory.

The rising status of physiology in the last third of the nineteenth century in part reflected the belief of medical educators in the clinical utility of physiological knowledge. Like Morgan in the 1760s and Drake in the 1820s, late-nineteenth-century physiologists argued that the student must understand the body's normal function before studying its morbid function and ways of restoring normality.[81] Physiology, therefore, was an essential prerequisite to pathology and therapeutics. More pervasive, however, was the belief that since medicine had become scientific, clinicians needed a knowledge of physiology to practice "scientific medicine." Physicians lauded physiology as "the most highly developed rational discipline in medicine"[82] and "the fountain head of American medicine."[83] John A. Benson, professor of physiology at the College of Physicians and Surgeons of Chicago, wrote in 1896:

> To the practicing physician . . . physiology is an absolute *sine qua non*, and he must pay strict attention to this branch before he can hope to become a diagnostician, a pathologist or a therapeutist. . . . When any individual has[,] without such thorough and complete study, attained even considerable success in medical practice, he remains an empiricist and can never be considered a scientific physician.[84]

With the coming of "scientific medicine," no physician could properly practice modern medicine without a thorough education in physiology.

The growth of the laboratory method of teaching physiology further profited from the conviction that in the laboratory a medical student acquired not only concrete physiological knowledge but also a conceptual tool that would enable him to "find his way through the constantly aug-

81. H. P. Bowditch, "The Study of Physiology," *U. Penn. Med. Bull.* 17 (1904): 131–32.
82. Porter, "The Teaching of Physiology in Medical Schools," p. 649.
83. Sewall, "Henry Newell Martin," p. 328.
84. John A. Benson, "The Value to the Medical Student of Physiologic Study," *J. AMA* 27 (1896): 622.

menting horde of facts and draw vicarious profit from those who are face to face with the mysteries of nature."[85] Laboratory experience taught the student how to think like a physiologist—"how to draw and comprehend deductions from personally recognized conditions, how to explain to himself and reason out for himself the relations of abstract and concrete causes and appreciated results, and the bearings thereof."[86] By developing "the scientific habit of thought," laboratory instruction provided a means of dealing with the immense body of physiological knowledge emerging from research laboratories.[87] Porter wrote in 1898 that the rise of the teaching laboratory was grounded in

> the conviction that the mass of knowledge in every department of medicine is grown so huge as to overwhelm both professor and student. The only refuge lies in a thorough mastery of the scientific method. The medical student must acquire power rather than information. Only thus will he be able to hold a steady course through the baffling winds and cross currents of a veritable sea of knowledge.[88]

This, in the perception of many medical educators, was the principal educational value of laboratory teaching in physiology.

The pattern of instruction in physiology at Harvard was, of course, representative of only the best and most progressive American medical schools; yet it ultimately affected the programs of all medical schools in America. There were, however, critics of the Harvard model who objected to it on both philosophical and practical grounds. Charles D. Smith, professor of physiology at the medical school of Bowdoin College, argued in 1895 that the best methods of teaching physiology "in the average school with average students" were recitations from textbooks, laboratory demonstrations, and didactic lectures. Since the average student had no intention of becoming a physiologist, laboratory demonstrations were sufficient:

> At no time should we lose sight of the fact that our business is to assist in the training of men who are to be physicians, hence experimental work in the direction of discovery should not be a part of the student's task. Neither his time nor capacity admit it.[89]

85. Porter, "The Teaching of Physiology in Medical Schools," p. 650.
86. Benson, "The Value to the Medical Student of Physiologic Study," p. 623.
87. William Henry Welch, "The Evolution of Modern Scientific Laboratories," *Bull. Johns Hopkins Hosp.* 7 (1896): 22; Murray Galt Motter, "Medical Education, with Special Reference to the Subject of Physiology," *J. AMA* 44 (1905): 1734.
88. Porter, "The Teaching of Physiology in Medical Schools," p. 652; John C. Cardwell, "The Method of Teaching Physiology," *Phila. Med. J.* 6 (1900): 767–68.
89. Charles D. Smith, "The Best Method of Teaching Physiology," *Bull. Am. Acad. Med.* 2 (1895): 530.

Critics further argued that the cost of equipment and the amount of an instructor's time taken up made laboratory teaching impractical. Questions of desirability and financial feasibility severely restricted the progress of laboratory teaching of physiology in most American medical schools.

By 1896 William Welch was able to write that "every properly e-quipped medical school has a physiological laboratory."[90] Many schools, however, still could not afford to offer this sort of training in physiology. After inspecting American medical schools in 1907, the American Medical Association's Council on Education reported that "the weakest point in the equipment and teaching facilities of medical schools is, naturally, the lack of laboratories and equipment." For most schools the expense of "good, well-equipped laboratories" was prohibitive.[91] A more complete appraisal of the state of physiology instruction in American medical schools appeared three years later, when Abraham Flexner published his report, *Medical Education in the United States and Canada.*

After personally inspecting 155 medical schools, Flexner judged only about 30 of them adequately equipped to offer proper laboratory instruction in the basic medical sciences.[92] In schools like Johns Hopkins and Harvard extensive laboratory facilities and full-time laboratory instructors provided medical students with excellent instruction in physiology. In the more numerous schools of middle rank, however, laboratory facilities for physiology were often inferior to those for anatomy, chemistry, and pathology. And in the "frankly mercenary schools" the teaching of physiology was abysmal.

The medical department of Willamette University in Salem, Oregon, for example, which claimed to teach physiology "experimentally," kept its laboratory apparatus "in a physician's downtown office." When Flexner inquired about the equipment used in teaching experimental physiology at the Eclectic Medical College of New York, "a messenger was despatched to fetch it, and did—a safety-razor case, containing a small sphygmograph." In Chicago and St. Louis, where the law required schools in "good standing" to own certain equipment in experimental physiology, Flexner found it "displayed prominently on tables, brand-new, like samples shown for sale on a counter; the various parts had never been put together or connected." At such schools laboratory instruction was "frankly impossible."[93]

The ideology of medical education Flexner articulated in his report

90. Welch, "The Evolution of Modern Scientific Laboratories," p. 21.
91. "Secretary's Report, Council on Medical Education," *J. AMA* 48 (1907): 1705.
92. Flexner, *Medical Education,* p. 89.
93. Ibid., pp. 85–86.

placed a premium on physiology and the laboratory method of teaching it. He adamantly defended the value of physiological knowledge for the prospective physician:

> It is the business of the physician to restore normal functioning: normal functioning is thus his starting-point in thought, his goal in action. The physiological laboratory enables the beginner to observe the functions of the body in operation and to ascertain how they are affected by varying conditions,—a wholesome discipline for two reasons: it banishes from his mind metaphysical principles, such as vital force, depression, etc.; it tends, in exhibiting the infinite subtlety and complexity of the physiological mechanism, to emphasize normal conditions rather than medication as ultimately responsible for its orderly working.[94]

Laboratory experience in physiology trained the student to think like a scientist, curing him "once and for all of mystical and empiric vagaries." Using the curriculum at Johns Hopkins as his model, Flexner recommended that the student spend the first year of the four-year program studying exclusively physiology (including physiological chemistry) and anatomy (including embryology and histology). About 450 hours would be devoted to physiology, and the principal source of instruction was what the student himself did in the laboratory.[95] As a result of the reforms catalyzed by Flexner's report,[96] after 1920 instruction in physiology aimed at transforming the student into a medical scientist as well as a practitioner.

The general structure of the undergraduate medical curriculum, reorganized along the lines defined by Flexner, remained intact from about 1920 to 1950.[97] In the early 1950s, however, medical educators began questioning both the objectives and methods of training physicians. By the 1960s this reevaluation had given rise to a "counter-revolution against the Abraham Flexner model of medical education,"[98] characterized by a deemphasis on basic medical science in the education of physicians and a redefinition of the aims of the educational program. The most visible

94. Ibid., p. 63; see also p. 54.
95. Ibid., pp. 20–27, 52–89; Cooper, "Undergraduate Medical Education," p. 271.
96. Hudson, "Abraham Flexner in Perspective," pp. 545–61; Bordley and Harvey, *Two Centuries of American Medicine*, p. 165; Cooper, "Undergraduate Medical Education," p. 270.
97. John Field, "Medical Education in the United States: Late Nineteenth and Early Twentieth Centuries," in C. D. O'Malley, ed., *The History of Medical Education* (Los Angeles, Berkeley and London: University of California Press, 1970), p. 511.
98. Maurice B. Visscher, "The Decline in Emphasis on Basic Medical Sciences in Medical School Curricula," *Physiologist* 16 (1972): 43.

cause of this retrenchment in the scientific training of American physicians was the public's demand for a greater supply of practically trained general practitioners. The Carnegie Commission on Higher Education, part of the foundation that sponsored the 1910 Flexner report, formalized popular demands in its 1970 *Recommendations,* calling for a compression of the medical school program from four to three years. Tellingly, this influential report also concluded that extensive laboratory experience in physiology held no great value for medical students.[99] The watchword of this counterrevolution was relevance.

The effects of this counterrevolutionary ideology were to reduce the number of hours devoted to teaching physiology, to curtail or eliminate laboratory instruction in physiology, and to diminish considerations of clinical applications from basic physiology courses.[100] At the beginning of the 1950s the average American medical school allotted approximately 260 hours to course and laboratory work in physiology, but between 1961 and 1971 the mean number of hours assigned to lectures, conferences, demonstrations, and laboratory exercises in physiology declined by an average of 31 percent, with a maximum decrease of 70 percent. Required laboratory instruction suffered most severely, falling from over 100 hours in 1952 to a mean of 45 hours in 1971. By 1971 ten medical schools had entirely abandoned assigned student laboratory work in physiology.[101]

Concurrent with these structural changes in the curriculum were shifts in the orientation and content of preclinical instruction in physiology. While much of the medical student's time shifted from the sciences to clinical work, basic science departments became less preclinical and more purely scientific, approaching physiology as an autonomous biological science rather than as the handmaiden of clinical medicine.[102] Physiologists sought to teach principles and concepts rather than a body of facts and their applications to medical practice. The core of physiology courses remained the functions of the major organ systems—infused with ample quantities of biochemistry and biophysics—but a prime objective of instructors was to teach the medical student to "think physiologically" and

99. Ibid., pp. 47–52; Vernon W. Lippard, "Trends in the Medical Curriculum," in idem, ed., *The Changing Medical Curriculum* (New York: Josiah Macy, Jr., Foundation, 1972), p. 17.

100. A. C. Ivy, "Teaching of Physiology to Medical Students During the First Half of the Twentieth Century," *Physiologist* 7 (1964): 33.

101. Visscher, "The Decline in Emphasis on Basic Medical Sciences," pp. 43–45, 48; Mary E. Cunnane, "Recent Trends in Medical Education: Report of a Survey," in Elizabeth F. Purcell, ed., *Recent Trends in Medical Education* (New York: Josiah Macy, Jr., Foundation, 1976), pp. 1–17; D. Harold Copp, "Physiology in the Curriculum," in Purcell, *Recent Trends in Medical Education,* p. 153; Lippard, "Trends in the Medical Curriculum," p. 13.

102. Ivy, "Teaching of Physiology to Medical Students," p. 33.

instill in him an appreciation for the methods of science. Laboratory instruction focussed on enhancing appreciation of the attitudes of science, developing skills in observation, and teaching the principles of scientific inference.[103]

The trend to teach basic physiology as a biological science with only minimal reference to its clinical applications reflected the changing interests and outlooks of physiology teachers and the great increase in knowledge of physiological phenomena emerging from the so-called biological revolution. As physiologists who taught in medical schools became more specialized and focussed their efforts increasingly on research, their principal activities bore progressively diminishing resemblance to their teaching. As their own interests strayed further from topics of immediate medical application, they often became disinclined to relate basic physiology to the concerns of the clinician. Thus two cultures emerged within the field, and within medicine generally: the scientific and the clinical.[104]

The deemphasis of physiology in the medical school curriculum, however, may have been in part more apparent than real. At the same time that they were reducing the required basic science courses, medical schools were also introducing extensive elective programs that often occupied a year or more of the curriculum.[105] Thus interested students could devote a substantial amount of their time to the study of physiology. Moreover, twenty-five schools had adopted interdisciplinary teaching by 1974, integrating instruction in physiology with other basic sciences.[106] In the "core-elective curriculum," which represented a marked divergence from the educational format of 1920 to 1950, schools required fewer hours in courses labeled physiology but gave considerable physiology instruction in interdisciplinary or elective courses.[107] Furthermore, much of the teaching of applied physiology shifted from the classroom to the clinic,

103. George H. Acheson, "Content and Aims of Physiology, Biochemistry and Pharmacology Courses," in Julius H. Comroe, ed., "Report of the First Teaching Institute, Association of American Medical Colleges," *J. Med. Educ.* 29, no. 7, pt. 2 (1953): 20–34.

104. Ivy, "Teaching of Physiology to Medical Students," pp. 33–34; Douglas M. Knight, "The University in American Society," in Douglas M. Knight and E. Shepley Nourse, eds., *Medical Ventures and the University* (Evanston, Ill.: Association of American Medical Colleges, 1967), p. 14; Lippard, "Trends in the Medical Curriculum," pp. 10–19; Emanuel Suter, "The Two Cultures in Medical Education," in Lippard, *The Changing Medical Curriculum,* pp. 65–78; Robert R. Wagner, "The Basic Medical Sciences, the Revolution in Biology and the Future of Medical Education," *Yale J. Biol. Med.* 35 (1962): 1–11.

105. Cooper, "Undergraduate Medical Education," p. 285.

106. Ibid.; Cunnane, "Recent Trends in Medical Education," p. 4.

107. Field, "Medical Education in the United States," p. 522; Alexander Leaf, "Integrating and Regrouping Courses in the Basic Medical Sciences," in Lippard, *The Changing Medical Curriculum,* pp. 54–64.

freeing instructors of preclinical physiology to focus more narrowly on physiology as a basic science.[108]

Medical educators from the colonial period to the twentieth century generally agreed that the practitioner should have some conception of how the healthy human body functions before attempting to restore the diseased organism to health. The status they accorded physiology in the education of aspiring physicians, however, fluctuated greatly. From an important but clearly not central place in educational programs before the late nineteenth century, the status of physiology peaked in the early twentieth century, when basic physiology became the epitome of medical science, and declined only in recent decades. Yet in the perception of both medical educators and clinicians, physiology—of all the basic medical sciences—has remained the most immediately relevant to the training of the American physician.[109]

108. Visscher, "The Decline in Emphasis on Basic Medical Sciences," p. 52. See also Lee A. Forstrom, "The Scientific Autonomy of Clinical Medicine," *J. Med. & Phil.* 2 (1977): 8–19.
109. Comroe, "Report of the First Teaching Institute, Association of American Medical Colleges," p. 107; Edra L. Spilman and Helen W. Spilman, "A Pair Comparison Study of the Relevance of Nine Basic Science Courses," *J. Med. Educ.* 50 (1975): 667–71.

Chemistry

JAMES WHORTON

FOR much of the period of medical education in America, chemistry has appeared the younger brother of the curriculum, a subject from which significant contributions were expected in the future, but which for the present seemed unaccomplished, awkward, even an embarrassment. As with family affections, opinions about the medical utility of chemistry have run a gamut from enthusiasm to scorn, yet throughout its history as part of the medical curriculum, two fundamental attitudes are easily distinguishable. Chemistry has regularly been cited as the essential preclinical science, the body of knowledge and mode of thinking absolutely prerequisite to an understanding of physiology and pathology, and to the prescription and preparation of remedies. These claims to consequence, however, have just as regularly been contested by a pragmatic segment of the profession doubtful that the relevance of chemistry was being properly demonstrated by its teachers, or even that chemistry had much present relevance for medicine, or, finally, that the subject would ever be of any use to the practitioner. Evolving from a general chemistry with little discernible medical content (from the colonial period to the mid-1800s) into the jumble denominated medical chemistry by the later 1800s and then into the biochemistry of the present century, chemical instruction in American medical schools has had the most checkered of fortunes, and not until its final stage of growth did it command the respect given other subjects in the curriculum.

Nothing less than a turbulent career might have been predicted from the way chemistry gained entrance into medicine. Because of its associations with alchemy and with Paracelsus, iatrochemistry was at first pelted with as much vituperation as any idea in the history of medicine. Once the smoke of the Galenist-Paracelsian wars lifted for good, however, chemistry became an ally of medicine. Its techniques were essential for pharmacy, and its concepts of ferment, acid and alkali suggested theoretical mechanisms for physiology and pathology. Thus as eighteenth-century medical teaching coalesced around distinct subjects, chemistry was recognized as one of the required chairs for a medical faculty. The most brilliant occupant of one of these chairs, Glasgow and Edinburgh's Joseph Black, proclaimed the new respectability and promise of chemistry at the time when medical schools were being founded in America:

> A Century has not yet elapsed since it [chemistry] wore a garb which rendered it disgustful. Cultivated in ages of Barbarity and Superstition it made its appearance void of all ornaments of polite Literature and Taste, but tainted with all the folly and Credulity of the times. . . . But it is now simple and familiar in its language, more extensive in its views, and dedicated to the Improvement of the essential and ornamental arts of Life.[1]

This useful subject was nevertheless largely ignored in the colonies before the appearance of medical colleges. Some instruction in chemistry was offered at Harvard College as early as 1687,[2] and the course in natural philosophy instituted by William Smith at the College of Philadelphia in 1756 included chemistry, fossils and agriculture.[3] But it was chiefly as part of the medical curriculum that chemical education passed through its formative years in America. A chemistry professor, James Smith, was

1. Quoted by John Read, "Joseph Black, M.D., the Teacher and the Man," in Andrew Kent, ed., *An Eighteenth Century Lectureship in Chemistry* (Glasgow: Jackson, 1950), p. 89.
2. I. Bernard Cohen, "The Beginnings of Chemical Instruction in America," *Chymia* 3 (1950): 21.
3. H. S. Van Klooster, "The Beginnings of Laboratory Instruction in Chemistry in the U.S.A.," *Chymia* 2 (1949): 1. For further information on the general development of chemical education in America, see Lyman Newell, "Chemical Education in America from the Earliest Days to 1820," *J. Chem. Educ.* 9 (1932): 687–95; C. A. Browne, "The History of Chemical Education in America between the Years 1820 and 1870," ibid., pp. 696–728; Harrison Hale, "The History of Chemical Education in the United States from 1870 to 1914," ibid., pp. 729–44; and F. B. Dains, "Advances in the Teaching of Chemistry Since 1914," ibid., pp. 745–50.

among the founding faculty of King's College Medical School,[4] and while
the only earlier medical department, that of the College of Philadelphia,
existed four years without a formal chair of chemistry, the subject figured
in the school's program from the start. John Morgan's inaugural discourse
stressed the importance of "Pharmaceutic Chymistry,"[5] and his first general course attempted to present as much of the science of chemistry as
could "conveniently be admitted."[6] Unfortunately, the course schedule of
three lectures a week for three to four months did not permit the convenient admission of much chemistry. Morgan's lectures, in fact, were but a
watered version of the course he had taken with William Cullen at Edinburgh: a description and classification of chemical substances with attention to their uses not only in medicine, but in metallurgy, ceramics and
agriculture as well, all presented without benefit of apparatus for demonstrations. The superficiality of Morgan's course may have provoked Benjamin Rush's comment, during his campaign for the chemistry professorship in Philadelphia, that "I should like to teach chemistry . . . because I
think I could show its application to medicine . . . in a stronger light than
ever has yet been done."[7] Already, it seems, chemistry instructors were
straining to give a clear demonstration of their subject's pertinence, and
even the self-assured Rush's performance fell short of his promise. The
chemical lectures he delivered from 1769 on were, as a matter of fact, well
below the quality of the instruction he had received abroad, though they
remain the best source for an understanding of the content of medical
chemistry in the colonial period. Rush faced the same difficulty that other
American chemistry teachers of the day did, a complete absence of American texts and a shortage of European ones. For those who could obtain
them, he recommended such standards as Robert Boyle, Hermann Boerhaave, and Pierre Macquer, but the need to provide a basic source for all
students led him to publish, in 1770, the first American text, a syllabus of
his own lectures.[8]

    4. Van Klooster, "The Beginnings of Laboratory Instruction in Chemistry," p. 3. Smith's
introductory lecture on the subject, it was reported at the time, was one which "for elegance
and sublimity met with universal approbation."
    5. John Morgan, A Discourse Upon the Institution of Medical Schools in America (1765;
facsimile ed., Philadelphia: University of Pennsylvania Printing Office, 1965), p. 10.
    6. Quoted by Whitfield Bell, Jr., John Morgan: Continental Doctor (Philadel-
phia: University of Pennsylvania Press, 1965), p. 133. Morgan's chemistry lectures, characterized by Bell as "superficial," are described, pp. 134–35. Also see Joseph Hepburn,
"Notes on the Early Teaching of Chemistry in the University of Pennsylvania, the Central
High School of Philadelphia, and the Franklin Institute of Pennsylvania," J. Chem. Educ. 9
(1932): 1577; and Henry Klickstein, "A Short History of the Professorship of Chemistry at
the University of Pennsylvania School of Medicine, 1765–1847," Bull. Hist. Med. 27
(1953): 43.
    7. Quoted by Klickstein, "A Short History of the Professorship of Chemistry," p. 51.
    8. Benjamin Rush, Syllabus of a Course of Lectures on Chemistry (1770; facsimile ed.,

In his introductory remarks, Rush submitted that an acquaintance with chemistry was indispensable to medical practice: "It is impossible to make ourselves acquainted with the nature and laws of the Animal Aeconomy without it."[9] Subsequent classes, however, did little to further such an acquaintance, offering mostly a presentation of inorganic chemistry closely patterned after the lectures of his Edinburgh teacher, Black.[10] A discussion of apparatus preceded an analysis of the phenomena of heat and mixing and descriptions of specific groups of substances and types of reactions: for example, salts, earths (a section which began "Of the Deluge"), metals, waters, and calcination and combustion. The course, to be sure, concluded with sections on the "chemical history" of vegetable and animal substances, but these seem to have comprised little more than a listing of various solids and fluids, organic tissues and secretions. An appendix on vegetable and animal pharmacy made the medical usefulness of chemical knowledge somewhat clearer, but as a whole Rush's lectures display the failing that was to plague medical school chemistry professors through the next century. In all fairness, Rush said about as much as was known about physiological chemistry at the time; that he considered such little information a justification of his assertion that chemistry was indispensable to the physician, reflects that faith in the *future* progress of the science which would frequently have to sustain its embattled advocates through the nineteenth century.

While Rush covered his subject thoroughly, he might have presented it with greater effect. His lectures, "taught in such a manner as to be intelligible to the private Gentleman and enquiring artist, as well as the student of medicine,"[11] were only scantily supplemented by demonstrations. In a day when schools provided no laboratory facilities for students, illustrative experiments by the lecturer were a valuable pedagogical tool, and Rush lagged somewhat behind the European standard by offering at most ten demonstrations per course. These were, moreover, of a very simple nature, the generation of hydrogen from iron filings and sulfuric acid, or of "fixed air" from sulfuric acid and marble, being as

---

Philadelphia: Friends of the University of Pennsylvania Library, 1954). Also see Wyndham Miles, "Benjamin Rush: Chemist," *Chymia* 4 (1953): 37, for an excellent discussion of Rush's course. Rush's recommended texts were Robert Boyle, *The Sceptical Chymist* (Oxford: Davis and Took, 1680); Hermann Boerhaave, *A New Method of Chemistry*, 2 vols. (London: Longman, 1741); and Pierre Macquer, *Elements of the Theory and Practice of Chymistry*, 2 vols. (London: Millar and Nourse, 1764).

9. Quoted by Klickstein, "A Short History of the Professorship of Chemistry," p. 53.

10. For discussion of Black's lectures, see Read, "Joseph Black, M.D.," pp. 78–79; and Douglas McKie, "On Thomas Cochrane's MS Notes of Black's Chemical Lectures, 1767–8," *Ann. Sci.* 1 (1936): 101.

11. Rush, *Syllabus of a Course of Lectures*, p. 5.

sophisticated as any. Nevertheless, as one of his students remarked, "So little was the science pursued at that time in the United States, that this simple exhibition occasioned a numerous assemblage of medical students."[12] The assemblage had their chemical understanding expanded still further by occasional homework assignments which had to be turned in to the professor.

This didactic approach, lectures reinforced by demonstrations and student assignments and recitations, remained the basic format for chemical teaching until the later 1800s. The content of chemical courses, on the other hand, changed drastically before even the 1700s ended, a consequence of the chemical revolution occurring in Europe. Rush's lectures had advocated the phlogiston theory, and there is no evidence that his opinions were altered by Lavoisier,[13] but his successors in the teaching of medical chemistry were most instrumental in getting the new understanding of combustion adopted in the United States.[14] James Woodhouse, professor of chemistry at the University of Pennsylvania from 1794 until 1809 (who had been offered the position, incidentally, only after the diehard phlogistonist Joseph Priestley declined), and Samuel Latham Mitchill, his contemporary at Columbia, took the lead in presenting the "French chemistry" to American students. The new courses continued exhaustively broad, Mitchill's presentation of the "antiphlogistic system" being typical: "The course comprises not only the classification and arrangement of natural bodies, but also treats a great variety of facts, which form the basis of scientific Medicine, rational and experimental Agriculture, and the application of these fundamental truths, as principles to explain useful Arts and Manufactures."[15] The lectures were open to all, though attended primarily by medical students, and were illustrated with specimens and experiments. As with Rush's course, "a Syllabus and a Nomenclature have been published by the Professor, for the information of the students and the public."[16]

Woodhouse's classes in Philadelphia were similar, though buttressed probably with a greater use of experiment. His strong emphasis on labora-

12. Quoted by Miles, "Benjamin Rush," p. 52. Other demonstrations performed by Rush included dissolving camphor in alcohol and NH_4CL in H_2SO_4, mixing oil and water by shaking, and lowering the temperature of water by dissolving KNO_3 in it.
13. Ibid., p. 54.
14. Sidney M. Edelstein, "The Chemical Revolution in America from the Pages of the 'Medical Repository,' " *Chymia* 5 (1954): 155.
15. Quoted by Byron Stookey, *A History of Colonial Medical Education in the Province of New York, with its Subsequent Development (1767–1830)* (Springfield, Ill.: Thomas, 1962), p. 241.
16. Ibid.

tory work attracted many students whose chief interest was chemistry rather than medicine, while for both groups of pupils he supplied a *Young Chemist's Pocket Companion,* apparently the first published laboratory handbook for American chemistry students.[17] Its descriptions of one hundred experiments were accompanied by pictures of apparatus and instructions for assembling a "portable laboratory." Woodhouse's little handbook heralded an instructional device which was to remain popular throughout the nineteenth century, the catechismal "pocket companion" of questions and answers on theoretical as well as experimental chemistry: a supplement to lectures, a handy reference, and a digestible item for cramming.

Woodhouse's students were even occasionally admitted to his private laboratory, a small room on the lower floor of Surgeon's Hall, in which he carried out researches in metallurgy, combustion, respiration, and plant chemistry.[18] The laboratory was also used to prepare demonstrations for his students, demonstrations which must have been instructive if the talented experimenter Priestley actually complimented his dexterity.[19] The most skillful mechanics sometimes blunder, of course, and one of Woodhouse's slips from perfection demonstrates that even eighteenth-century chemical instruction could have its light moments. Benjamin Silliman was witness to an attempt to suffocate a hen under a bell jar filled with hydrogen, an illustration of the irrespirability of the gas. No sooner had the hen been confined, Silliman recalled, than it

> gasped, kicked, and lay still. "There, gentlemen," said the Professor, "you see she is dead"; but no sooner had the words passed his lips, than the hen with a struggle overturned the bell glass, and with a loud scream flew across the room, flapping the heads of the students with her wing, while they were convulsed with laughter.[20]

Undoubtedly entertainment was often an intended effect of demonstrations, it being appreciated that spectacular transformations impressed a lesson more deeply than did bland ones. It may be safely assumed that the approach to demonstrations taken by Harvard Medical School's first chemistry professor, Aaron Dexter, was to an extent shared by all his colleagues struggling to maintain student interest in an abstruse subject. Oliver Wendell Holmes characterized Dexter's "not wholly uninstruc-

17. Edgar Fahs Smith, *Chemistry in America* (New York: D. Appleton, 1914), p. 76. Also see Newell, "Chemical Education in America," p. 685.

18. George Corner, *Two Centuries of Medicine: A History of the School of Medicine, University of Pennsylvania* (Philadelphia: Lippincott, 1965), p. 47.

19. Smith, *Chemistry in America,* p. 106.

20. Quoted, ibid., p. 105.

tive" demonstrations as "marked by startling precipitations, pleasing changes of color, brilliant corruscations, alarming explosions and odors innumerable and indescribable."[21]

As startling as precipitations may be, the chief subject for demonstration, and lecture, at the close of the eighteenth century, was pneumatic chemistry. The study of gases, many believed, had not just sparked the chemical revolution, but had also fulfilled the expectation that chemistry would assume increasing significance for medicine. Thomas Beddoes's studies in England of the curative effects of different gases seemed for a period to open new vistas in therapy (another of Woodhouse's experiments which failed was his attempt to duplicate Humphry Davy's experiences with laughing gas).[22] A great deal more exciting, and long lasting, was Lavoisier's oxygen theory of respiration and body heat, work that augured a new era for animal chemistry. President Wheelock of Dartmouth was perhaps not an exception among the attendants of chemical lectures; he is supposed to have left Nathan Smith's one-man medical course one day and gone directly to chapel where he prayed, "O Lord! We thank Thee for the Oxygen gas, we thank Thee for Hydrogen gas; and for all gases."[23]

The animal chemistry which came to the fore in chemical instruction around 1800 was by no means limited to the physiological and therapeutic functions of gases. Few were so enthusiastic as Woodhouse, who once proclaimed (after a sultry day confined to his laboratory) that "by chemical agency alone, he would produce a human being."[24] Nevertheless, medical students were frequently assured that the analysis of animal solids and fluids was the key to clarifying the last mysteries of physiology and pathology.[25] Thus while chemistry courses continued to donate the bulk of their time to fundamentals (which now included such phenomena as the participation of light and caloric in reactions, galvanism, and chemical affinity), the discussion of animal chemistry was given additional time, and

21. Quoted by William Frederick Norwood, *Medical Education in the United States Before the Civil War* (Philadelphia: University of Pennsylvania Press, 1944), p. 172.

22. Smith, *Chemistry in America*, p. 104.

23. Norwood, *Medical Education in the United States*, p. 189. For good measure, Wheelock is supposed to have given thanks for the cerebrum, cerebellum, and medulla oblongata as well.

24. Smith, *Chemistry in America*, p. 107.

25. See, for example, Felix Pascalis's 1802 oration before the Chemical Society of Philadelphia, an organization founded by Woodhouse and patronized by the city's physicians and medical students. Smith, *Chemistry in America*, pp. 69–70. Also see Joseph Youle, *An Inaugural Dissertation on Respiration: Being an Application of the Principles of the New Chemistry to that Function* (New York: T. and J. Swords, 1793), for an example of speculative animal chemistry among medical students.

sometimes a new dimension—function, as distinct from composition. Students at New York's College of Physicians and Surgeons in the early 1800s, for instance, learned not just about the chemical constituents of blood, chyle, lymph, saliva, and urine, but also the current opinions about the chemical complexities involved in respiration, digestion, assimilation, and decomposition of dead bodies.[26]

The extent to which instruction in animal chemistry was carried, of course, depended on the professor, and if some were inclined to expand the new area to its outer limits, others were determined to restrain what they regarded as scientific presumption. The resurgent vitalism of the early 1800s made many wary of placing much faith in chemical physiology, and such reservations necessarily influenced the teaching of chemistry to medical students. All agreed that chemistry was required by pharmacy, but when the question of physiology arose, the sentiments of the irascible Charles Caldwell could find support. The ambitions of animal chemistry made it seem to him a branch "not of science, but of blunders and balderdast—which identifies man in function with a German stove, or a Belgian beer-barrel."[27] Others agreed that man must be more than "a hydro-phosphorated oxyde of azote,"[28] and this skepticism about the validity of animal chemistry was a vital force depressing the popularity of chemistry in the medical curriculum.

The subject's irrelevancy in many eyes is clearest in the debate at Caldwell's alma mater, the University of Pennsylvania, over a successor to Woodhouse. Ostensibly the controversy swirled around the question of whether the new professor should be a physician or a chemist (in itself a sign of the determination to make the course applicable to medicine), but a strong undercurrent welled from the argument that chemistry was not a necessary chair in a medical faculty.[29] Opposition to chemistry per se was somewhat submerged in 1809, when the physician John Redman Coxe was appointed over the much more qualified chemist Robert Hare. But when Coxe resigned in 1818, the debate was renewed, and the matter of the legitimacy of medical chemistry rose quickly to the surface. Nathaniel Chapman, professor of theory and practice, branded chemistry as "orna-

26. Stookey, *A History of Colonial Medical Education*, pp. 249–50.

27. Quoted by William S. Middleton, "Charles Caldwell: A Biographic Sketch," *J. Med. Educ.* 34 (1959): 984.

28. Quoted by Herbert S. Klickstein, "Charles Caldwell and the Controversy in America over Liebig's 'Animal Chemistry,'" *Chymia* 4 (1953): 135.

29. The controversy is discussed in the two articles by Klickstein previously cited, plus a third by that author, "An Early American 'Discourse on the Connexion Between Chemistry and Medicine,'" *Lib. Chron.* 16 (1950): 64. Also consult Edgar Fahs Smith, *The Life of Robert Hare* (Philadelphia: Lippincott, 1917), pp. 57–58.

mental" rather than medically "useful," and proposed that students should be exonerated from attending chemical lectures.[30]

The best reply to such sentiments came from Thomas Cooper, an unsuccessful candidate for the vacated professorship. His "Discourse on the Connexion Between Chemistry and Medicine" reveals how the more sanguine medical chemists justified their subject.[31] Chemistry, Cooper argued, is not just fundamental to pharmacy and physiology, but is also required for the understanding of diseases such as gout and rickets, for diagnosis through urinalysis, and for the detection of public health dangers, industrial hazards, adulterants in drugs, and poison in crime victims. Certainly not the least reason for studying chemistry was that its application in manufactures, arts and domestic economy had made it a part of general education, and there seemed a danger the public might soon understand the subject better than physicians. Cooper's appeal has been credited with "convincing his hearers of their error,"[32] but if so, it was a fleeting conviction. The applicant who was appointed to the chair of chemistry, Hare, was at first not allowed to participate in the examinations of students for degrees, nor to sign their diplomas, and he felt the need to defend his subject throughout his career.[33]

As a professor at the nation's largest medical school, Hare probably taught chemistry to more students than anyone else in the country in the first half of the century. His classes of three to four hundred pupils met in the best-equipped lecture room–laboratory the period could afford, one outfitted with the latest apparatus, running water, and an enormous hearth in which were located a blast furnace, evaporating ovens, and sandbaths.[34] Unrivalled as a demonstrator, Hare used numerous experiments as frames around which to mold his lectures. He strove to increase the instructiveness of his demonstrations by providing students with a *Compendium* of his course which gave minute explanations of the principles, equipment and procedures involved, explanations which presumably would be studied before attendance at the demonstration.[35] The *Compendium*, which passed through four editions between 1828 and 1840, is educational for later generations as well, presenting the content

30. Klickstein, "A Short History of the Professorship of Chemistry," p. 64.
31. Idem, "An Early American 'Discourse.' "
32. Smith, *Chemistry in America*, p. 137.
33. See Smith, *The Life of Robert Hare*, pp. 485–88; and Klickstein, "A Short History of the Professorship of Chemistry," p. 67.
34. A detailed description, including a drawing, of Hare's lecture room may be found in *Am. J. Sci.* 19 (1831): 26.
35. Robert Hare, *A Compendium of the Course of Chemical Instruction in the Medical Department of the University of Pennsylvania* (Philadelphia, 1828).

of what was for the day a model course in medical chemistry. After comparing modern definitions of the science, Hare proceeded to discuss chemical affinity, crystallization, the effects of heat and light, specific gravity, pneumatic chemistry, combustion, alkalinity, acidity, and metals. With the groundwork thus laid, he advanced into the realm of vegetable chemistry, presenting the methods of organic analysis and information on the elemental and proximate compositions of plants (including heavy emphasis on the therapeutic significance of the recently isolated alkaloids). Discussion of vinous and acetous fermentation served as a bridge to animal chemistry, but the appearance of the subject at page 286, only twenty pages from the *Compendium*'s end, suggests how little weight could still be given physiological chemistry. A listing of the physical-chemical properties of the blood and other common animal substances was followed by his one discussion of a physiological process—respiration and the production of body heat. Reviewing the experiments of theorists along the line from Lavoisier through César Despretz, Hare accepted that most of the heat of the body could be accounted for by a combustion of carbon and hydrogen, but proposed that the balance must come from a vague "fixation of the fluid matter of the blood."[36] Some cursory comments about animal liquids and solids completed his lectures.

That the content of the standard medical school chemistry course of the first half of the nineteenth century was predominantly inorganic chemistry, and rather elementary at that, is verified by a survey of the handbooks used by students to prepare for examinations. Purchasers of David Condie's 1824 *Course of Examinations*, for instance, memorized more than twenty pages of questions and answers on inorganic phenomena, but only six on organic chemistry, and even then the organic section was diluted. As an example, the question "What is the sebacic acid?" was flanked by "What is steel?" and "What are the tests of iron?"[37] Robert Hooper's *Examinations* of 1832, combining chemistry and pharmacy in the same section, leaned toward definitions: of elements, techniques, and processes. A sample "theoretical" question, one of the few relating to organic chemistry, exposes the level of chemical sophistication expected of medical students:

Q. What is the theory of the formation of benzoic acid [by reacting lime with gum benzoin, then adding hydrochloric acid]?

A. The lime during the boiling takes the benzoic acid from the gum

36. Ibid., p. 300.
37. David Condie, *A Course of Examinations . . . Adapted to the University of Pennsylvania and the Other Medical Schools in the U.S.* (Philadelphia: James Webster, 1824), p. 116. The chemistry section of the examinations covers pp. 93–122.

benzoin; the benzoate of lime thus formed is held in solution by the water; upon the addition of muriatic acid, the lime abandons the benzoic acid, to combine with the muriatic acid; the benzoic acid, from its insolubility, is precipitated. . . .[38]

An edition of Hooper issued more than a decade later, in response to the demands of physicians and students, was basically unchanged.[39]

The popularity of such texts as George Fownes's *Manual of Elementary Chemistry* and Robert Kane's *Elements of Chemistry* lends further witness to the dominance of inorganic chemistry, and when it is considered that few professors had the knowledge, facilities, and pedagogical flair of a Robert Hare, it is easy to see why chemistry was generally considered by mid-century to be the course most contemned by medical students and abused by professors. In 1857 Hare, then of emeritus status, protested that "those who are authorized to grant medical degrees, ought not to leave it to the option of the students, whether or not to be ignorant of chemistry."[40] But a few years before, a leading journal had advised that

> with the return of the lecture season, it should be a subject of earnest solicitude in our medical schools to improve the courses on chemistry. They are essential, yet often the most neglected. The faculties of these institutions seem too generally to undervalue that department. Perhaps this may in some measure be due to the second-rate men who not infrequently conduct that branch. What has become of all the enthusiasm that used to be felt for medical chemistry? This is not the first occasion that has been sought for rousing the public sentiment in regard to a branch that has been sinking for years, from an elevated position in schools of medicine, till it is almost forgotten. Energetic men should be put into the drowsy chairs, in the hope that we might soon have many to be proud of as chemists, and that there might [be] a revivification and reorganization of the dying out chemical character of the country.[41]

Yet, as if in reaction to this lethargy, chemistry was already extending itself into areas so tangibly applicable to medicine as to generate new enthusiasm for presenting the subject to medical students. Excitement

38. Robert Hooper, *Examinations in Anatomy, Physiology . . . for the Use of Students* (New York: B. and S. Collins, 1832), p. 154.

39. Robert Hooper, *Examination in Anatomy, Physiology . . . for the Use of Students* (New York: Langley, 1846).

40. Quoted by Klickstein, "An Early American 'Discourse,' " p. 77. Robley Dunglison, *The Medical Student: or, Aide to the Study of Medicine* (Philadelphia: Lea and Blanchard, 1844), was one of the many others who noted that "the department of medical science to which the least importance is apt to be attached by the student, is *Chemistry*" (pp. 215–16).

41. "Medical Chemistry," *Boston Med. & Surg. J.* 45 (1852): 106.

over the recent growth of toxicology, pharmacology, and especially animal chemistry (after the publication of Justus von Liebig's book of that name in 1842) led during the 1840s to the formulation of the chemistry course that would characterize the second half of the century, the subject to be specifically designated medical chemistry. The trend toward this new title represented a significant alteration of curricular nomenclature. In 1849 approximately half of the country's medical schools taught a course entitled simply chemistry; about one-third presented the subject in conjunction with pharmacy, and the remainder offered such combinations as chemistry–botany, chemistry–physiology, chemistry–materia medica–medical jurisprudence–obstetrics, and medical chemistry–toxicology.[42] By 1880 *medical chemistry* was the term in general use.[43]

The protagonists of the new orientation are reminiscent of Rush. They had high ambitions to show chemistry's application to medicine "in a stronger light," but their achievements were disconcertingly modest. The fault lay partly with the science itself, which had not really progressed to a point of extensive usefulness to medicine, and partly with professors who defensively overstated the medical implications of the subject.[44] Their self-conscious groping for relevance created hodgepodges that might include most or all of the ingredients of physiological chemistry, toxicology, urinalysis, quantitative analysis, and "sanitary chemistry."

Finally, blame for the failings of medical chemistry can be placed on the structure of medical education, specifically its lax admission standards. The study of toxicology or urinalysis presupposed a thorough grounding in general chemistry, but few medical students before 1900 could be expected to have obtained this before matriculation. Hence professors of medical chemistry had to continue teaching general chemistry, and usually found themselves with little time left for the more advanced subject. Nor did the late-century extension and grading of the curriculum entirely remove the difficulty. By 1890 most schools offered chemistry as a two-year course, general in the first year, medical in the second, but the former still took too much time. The introductory course, based most frequently on Fownes's *Manual*, had to include a survey of physics as

42. *Trans. AMA* 2 (1849): 284–85.
43. Frank Wigglesworth Clarke, "A Report on the Teaching of Chemistry and Physics in the United States," in U.S. Bureau of Education, *Circular of Information, 1880, no. 6* (Washington, D.C.: Government Printing Office, 1880), pp. 145–56, gives a detailed exposition of chemistry courses at American medical schools.
44. As an example, consider D. P. Gardner, who began his discussion of the "relation of chemistry to the vital force" with the rhapsodic declaration that chemistry "tinges the vapors and the waters with brightness; it gives life to the cold clods of the valley; it endows the impalpable with power" (*Boston Med. & Surg. J.* 37 [1848]: 466; ibid., 38 [1848]: 197–98.

well, and organic chemistry was often not broached before the second year.[45] The tediousness of such a course for students bent on accumulating information needed to practice medicine can be imagined, though chemistry teachers often failed to appreciate the students' viewpoint. A Chicago professor was quite proud of his remedy for the common student belief that chemistry was "of minor importance": he had them spend much of their first year writing and balancing equations at home and at the blackboard. This activity taught students how to think.[46]

Students responded to such courses predictably. Asked to study a subject which seemed unrelated to medicine, in textbooks remarkable only for their "appalling dryness," "the student generally neglects the dryer branches for the two he thinks will be the most immediately useful, so that practice of medicine and surgery crowd chemistry . . . to the wall with a majority of every class."[47] The attitudes of Louisville students in the 1860s seem to have been only too typical:

> In the department of chemistry, the professor was one of those delightful, easy-going teachers, sensible enough to realize the fact that no student at the university was interested in his subject beyond the demonstration of incompatibles and in those mysterious substances which, when united, either produce a brilliant display of colors or an explosion. Those which exploded with the loudest report were most applauded. The two hours a week which were devoted to this confusing branch of science were usually spent by four-fifths of the class in studying the geography of Louisville. If we had a text-book recommended to us, the name of its author has long since disappeared in the granular metamorphosis of my memory cells.[48]

Thus prepared, students entered the second-year course on medical chemistry, most likely taking either John Bowman's *Practical Handbook of Medical Chemistry*, or, later in the century, John Attfield's *Chemistry: General, Medical and Pharmaceutical*. Even this advanced book, however, was largely introductory. Most of its six hundred pages dealt with inorganic chemistry, and only the last third took up such subjects as vegetable and animal chemistry (description of compounds), organic analysis for normal constituents and for poisons, examination and analysis

45. Clarke, *A Report on the Teaching of Chemistry and Physics*, pp. 145–46.
46. J. Wesener, "The Methods of Teaching Chemistry Employed in the College of Physicians and Surgeons of Chicago," *Bull. Am. Acad. Med.* 1 (1894): 521.
47. U.S. Bureau of Education, *Report of the Commissioner of Education* (Washington, D.C.: Government Printing Office, 1870), p. 386.
48. J. Wyeth, "A Medical Student in 1867," *Proc. AAMC* 19 (1909): 24.

of urine and calculi, and pharmaceutical preparations. The lecturers using these texts were inclined to focus on physiological and pathological chemistry, the bulk of attention being directed toward the normal composition of blood, saliva, gastric juice, bile, urine, and so forth, and to the detection of abnormalities in these fluids. Urinalysis received special stress, and textbooks specifically on that subject were often required.[49]

The era of medical chemistry was also marked by the introduction of laboratory instruction. The value of personal chemical experimentation had been recognized since the eighteenth century, and students had all along been encouraged to acquire a "portable laboratory" for study at home. Occasionally, exceptional students might be taken into a professor's private laboratory, but the apparent impracticability of offering laboratory training to hordes of students had kept the chemical apparatus of medical schools generally confined to the hands of professors. There was some agitation early in the 1800s for the adoption of laboratory courses for college chemistry students, culminating in the 1824 opening of Amos Eaton's laboratory at Rensselaer.[50] But medical students interested in experimentation were left to their own devices until past mid-century. Such devices were not necessarily inadequate, as demonstrated by the opportunities offered Philadelphia students after 1849. Alfred Kennedy, formerly chemistry professor at the Philadelphia College of Medicine, opened in that year his Philadelphia College of Chemistry, an institution designed expressly to supplement the didactic lectures of the city's medical schools.[51] Whether or not the instruction offered there exceeded that of Edinburgh, as Kennedy estimated, it was, by American standards, quite advanced. Students met three evenings a week for two months to attend an hour lecture-demonstration, then repeat the experiment in groups of five. By the end of the term, they would identify at least fifty unknowns, "a prominence having been given to the study of poisons and of the falsifications of medicine."[52]

Kennedy's school was the first bright reflection of that sentiment that slowly moved the medical schools themselves to offer laboratory facilities to their students. These were at first scattered and modest (such as the six-desk analytical lab opened at Harvard in 1853),[53] but by the 1870s

49. See Victor Vaughan, *Lecture Notes on Chemical Physiology and Pathology* (Ann Arbor, Mich., 1879), for an outline of a good medical chemistry course. Textbooks are discussed fully by Clarke, *A Report on the Teaching of Chemistry and Physics*, pp. 157–58.
50. Van Klooster, "The Beginnings of Laboratory Instruction in Chemistry," pp. 7–8.
51. Alfred Kennedy, *Practical Chemistry, a Branch of Medical Education* (Philadelphia: Mifflin, 1852).
52. Ibid., p. 9.
53. Harvard University, *The Harvard Medical School, 1782–1906* (Cambridge, Mass.,

laboratory instruction was becoming common nationwide.[54] In 1889 a United States Bureau of Education survey found that 80 percent of the medical colleges responding claimed to make laboratory experiments obligatory for their chemistry students.[55] The amount of laboratory study varied considerably from school to school, ranging from none to elective to required courses providing one to two hours in the lab for every hour in class (up to four hours of laboratory work per week).[56] The level of lab instruction naturally varied much as well, but at its best could be rather demanding. The course on medical chemistry at such schools as Yale, Jefferson, or the University of Michigan attempted laboratory illustrations of the composition of animal tissues, metabolic and digestive processes, activity of ferments, composition of foods, urinalysis, and the detection of poisons.[57]

At the other end of the spectrum, laboratory work could be deplorable, even nonexistent. Twenty years after the survey cited above, Flexner found that in the schools of the lowest order (those he categorized as "frankly mercenary"), "the laboratories are of the most elementary description,—sometimes active and in good order . . . oftener in utter disorder. . . . [At one school] a single set of reagents is provided for the entire class; [at another] there is no running water at the desks; [at still others] laboratory teaching . . . is hardly more than make-believe. . . . Occasionally there is nothing at all." Of the lecture content of such courses, he noted simply that "it never rises above a fair high school level and often falls far below it."[58]

These, like the other disclosures of the Flexner Report, were hardly revelations to progressive medical educators. Dissatisfaction with the chemistry course had, in fact, been mounting almost since the introduction of the distinctive program of medical chemistry. The heterogeneity of the course had been the initial cause for dismay, but as physiological

---

1906), p. 33. See *Trans. AMA* 3 (1850): 47; and ibid. 4 (1851): 443–46, for an indication of the mid-nineteenth-century concern to provide laboratory instruction for medical students.

54. See Clarke, *A Report of the Teaching of Chemistry and Physics*, pp. 145–46.

55. U.S. Bureau of Education, *Report of the Commissioner of Education, 1888–1889* (Washington, D.C.: Government Printing Office, 1889), pp. 1186–87. The institution of laboratory teaching was recognized by the bureau as "the most noteworthy innovation of the decade," and regarded as a significant factor generating pressure to lengthen the course of medical education (U.S. Bureau of Education, *Report of the Commissioner of Education, 1889–1890* [Washington, D.C.: Government Printing Office, 1890], p. 890).

56. Ibid., 1897–1898, pp. xcix–xcx.

57. Ibid., 1889–1890, p. 891; "Medical Schools of Philadelphia," *Boston Med. & Surg. J.* 103 (1880): 373; Wesener, "The Methods of Teaching Chemistry," pp. 521–24.

58. Abraham Flexner, *Medical Education in the United States and Canada* (New York: Carnegie Foundation for the Advancement of Teaching, 1910), pp. 86–87.

chemistry matured and established itself as a core for advanced chemical instruction, medical chemistry ceased to appear such a grab bag. Then complaints came to be levelled chiefly at the first year's tuition. The trouble with the standard medical school course, it was appreciated, was that it was too elementary; by dwelling so long on inorganic chemistry, it gave such little and late attention to the science's medical applications that these were easily overlooked by students. As sentiment for a graded curriculum and stiffer entrance requirements grew, the suggestion that inorganic chemistry be dropped from the curriculum and made a prerequisite became increasingly frequent. The American Medical Association's Committee on Medical Education proposed such action as early as 1867,[59] and two years later submitted that the move would constitute "an entire revolution in the present teaching of medical colleges. . . . Then instead of a chemistry adapted to the scholar of an ordinary high school, the student would learn that of the pathologist and the physician."[60] The editors of the *New York Medical Journal* spoke to the same point, and with more frankness. "General chemistry," they observed, "is one of the useless appendages of a medical education—an extra limb, in short, which may be removed without detriment to the body at large, while its removal will add to the symmetry and usefulness of what remains."[61]

Removal of this vestigial organ of the curriculum was by no means a simple operation, any more than was the general upgrading of medical education during the period. By 1890 a basic knowledge of a number of subjects from botany and physics through French was frequently listed as a requirement for admission to medical school, but chemistry was not among these.[62] In the following two decades, introductory chemistry did find adoption as a prerequisite—about fifty schools claimed to require a high school course in 1907[63]—but enforcement of entrance standards was, as Flexner documented, not always conscientious. Hence there continued appeals for a more sophisticated medical chemistry.

The most cogent analysis of the subject's shortcomings was probably that of William Warren of Washington University Medical School. Finding still by 1909 that the average medical student considered chemistry to be "relatively of slight importance to medicine,"[64] Warren suggested the

59. "Report of the Committee on Medical Education," *Trans. AMA* 18 (1867): 367.
60. Ibid. 20 (1869): 141.
61. "The Study of Chemistry in Medical Schools," *N.Y. Med. J.* 41 (1885): 610.
62. *Report of the Commissioner of Education, 1889–1890*, p. 876.
63. "Council on Medical Education," *J. AMA* 48 (1907): 1703. Also see ibid., 50 (1908): 1638–39.
64. William Warren, "The Study of Chemistry in Medical Schools," *St. Louis Med. Rev.* 58 (1909): 235.

fault was not with the subject or its teachers, but with a curriculum that allotted only two years to chemistry, and then required that the whole field from inorganic through physiological and toxicological chemistry be packed into this period. Under such conditions, "the teachers may be good, but the teaching is in the depths."[65] His solution of making general chemistry a prerequisite and including only biological chemistry and toxicology in the medical curriculum was hardly a new one, but its repetition at so late a date points up the slowness of the profession to respond to chemical education's chronic complaint. "As long as we continue to teach the entire subject of chemistry in our medical schools, the prevailing opinion of chemistry will exist and we shall turn out men who will be incompetent as far as dealing with chemical problems is concerned."[66]

Chemical incompetence among practitioners might well be assumed even without Warren's indictment, or the anecdote of F. W. Clarke about the physician who ordered sodium carbonate and hydrochloric acid on the same prescription because he "wished to produce the effects of both remedies."[67] Too many schools tailored their courses to the demands of the state board examinations, and these, generally lenient at the time, could have insultingly indulgent chemistry sections. The Ohio examination of 1903, for instance, paraded an astonishing nonchalance about the subject:

1. Define chemical incompatibility and give examples.
2. Give chemical formula of three acids.
3. Describe 'K' and its principal salts.
4. How is a salt formed?
5. Describe 'Na' and its principal salts.
6. Differentiate organic and inorganic chemistry and give an example of each.
7. Explain the difference between a carbonate and a bicarbonate.
8. Give formulas and describe calomel and biochlorid.
9. Give tests for acids and alkalies.
10. Give tests for arsenic.

It is surely no commendation of medical chemistry to note that 91 percent of the examinees achieved the passing grade of 75.[68]

In seeming contradiction to such indications of the low state of medical

---

65. Ibid., p. 236.
66. Ibid.
67. Clarke, *A Report on the Teaching of Chemistry and Physics*, p. 146.
68. *J. AMA* 41 (1903): 383, 435. In 1907, the Vermont licensing board considered it essential for physicians to know at what time of the year ozone is most abundant in the atmosphere (*J. AMA* 49 [1907]: 961).

school chemistry is the assertion often made during the early years of this century that physiological chemistry was the best taught of the preclinical courses.[69] The apparent paradox, however, merely indicates the transition from that catchall, medical chemistry, to modern biochemistry. Chemical teaching had suffered all along from a lack of conviction that the subject was medically important—even Thomas Cooper, the staunchest of medical chemistry's defenders, had acknowledged in 1818 that the discipline was in its infancy, and commentators through the rest of the century had, at best, agreed. But Cooper had also predicted it was "the infancy of Hercules,"[70] and by 1900 Hercules was beginning to flex his muscles.

The transition from the speculative animal chemistry deduced from organic formulae (characteristic of the Liebig period) to the physiological chemistry that strove to pry into chemical processes with the tool of physiological experimentation occurred in Europe in the 1870s.[71] In name, physiological chemistry was adopted by American medical professors about the same time, but in fact their early essays at the subject were merely glamorized animal chemistry, catalogues of chemical structure rather than analyses of chemical function.[72] Ironically, instruction in truly physiological chemistry developed not within the medical school, but as part of one of the first premedical programs established in the country. In 1869 Yale's Sheffield Scientific School introduced a course of "Studies Preparatory to Medical Studies," which put considerable emphasis on the biological sciences while also including much general and organic chemistry. Gradually increased attention was paid biological chemistry until in 1874 Russell Chittenden was appointed assistant in physiological chemistry. The following year's opening of the Sheffield's Laboratory of Physiological Chemistry launched his remarkable career in training research scientists in the new field, yet the laboratory also attracted considerable numbers of undergraduates looking for solid premedical training. By Chittenden's telling, it was the "astonishing records" compiled at various medical schools by graduates of his course which hastened the curricular shift from "medical" to "physiological" chemistry.[73]

69. Also noted by Saul Jarcho, "Medical Education in the United States, 1910–1956," *J. Mt. Sinai Hosp.* 26 (1959): 348.

70. Klickstein, "An Early American 'Discourse,' " p. 71.

71. Russell H. Chittenden, *The Development of Physiological Chemistry in the United States* (New York: Chemical Catalog Co., 1930), pp. 21–22, discusses the early years of physiological chemistry in Europe and America.

72. H. Newell Martin, *Am. Chem. J.* 1 (1879): 57; Russell H. Chittenden, "The Importance of Physiological Chemistry as a Part of Medical Education," *N.Y. Med. J.* 58 (1893): 372.

73. Russell H. Chittenden, *History of the Sheffield Scientific School of Yale University,*

However effective a catalyst Chittenden was (and he surely influenced medical school chemistry by training professors as well as students), an extraordinary transformation did occur in the first decade of this century. On the eve of that period the editor of the *Journal of the American Medical Association* complained of the shallowness of courses in physiological chemistry and of the lack of people competent to teach deeper ones;[74] by 1911 the same courses could be positively eulogized.

> Physiologic chemistry and experimental pharmacology, as given in our best schools, are, I believe, the most satisfactory of our laboratory courses. Presented, in most instances, in a vigorously scientific manner, with the student carrying on exact quantitative estimations and using graphic methods of registering results, and himself frequently the object of experiment, these courses fulfill all the rules of the experimental method. . . . [Such courses] give a knowledge of the fundamental principles of metabolism and of practical physiologic chemistry which was not dreamed of by the student of ten years ago.[75]

To be sure, the tribute contained a joker, the phrase "as given in our best schools," and in justice such praise for even the best schools must be modified. Those ten years were the climactic period in the reform of medical education generally, and their coincidence with the emergence of a mature biochemistry makes advances in the teaching of the subject less than startling. Further, physiological chemistry was still offered as a rule only in the second year, and the average first year course included much inorganic chemistry and physics.[76] This elementary course was at last on its way out, but not until the 1920s could it be said that medical school instruction in chemistry was virtually limited to biochemistry, with the

---

1846–1922, 2 vols. (New Haven: Yale University Press, 1928), 2:427. The transition from medical chemistry to biochemistry was also marked by the adoption of research as a standard activity of the faculty. As was appreciated early, an environment "in which knowledge is seethingly advanced" is conducive to more efficient learning by students (Lewellys F. Barker, "Some Tendencies in Medical Education in the United States," in James McKeen Cattell, ed., *Medical Research and Education* [New York: Science Press, 1913], p. 241). Nevertheless, the subject of biochemical research is not so directly pertinent to biochemical teaching as to merit detailed treatment here. See Chittenden, *The Development of Physiological Chemistry;* Thomas Wormley, "Address on Medical Chemistry and Toxicology," *Transactions of the International Medical Congress of Philadelphia, 1876* (Philadelphia, 1877), pp. 49–72; and Graham Lusk, "The Chemistry of Physiology and Nutrition," *J. Am. Chem. Soc.* 48 (1926): 153.

74. "The Chair of Physiologic Chemistry," *J. AMA* 31 (1898): 612–13.

75. Richard Pearce, "The Experimental Method: Its Influence on the Teaching of Medicine," in Cattell, *Medical Research and Education*, p. 103.

76. R. Cole, "Chemistry," *Proc. AAMC* 18 (1908): 88.

course finally being promoted to the first year of study.[77] In the process, the status and scope of biochemistry grew immeasurably. The professorship of medical chemistry became the department of physiological chemistry or of biochemistry (though sometimes it was combined with pharmacology or physiology). By 1940 more than thirty departments had four or more faculty members, and nearly all had at least two.[78] The faculty still complained of having to do remedial teaching, but now it was knowledge of organic chemistry and quantitative analysis that had to be refreshed, and once done, an unprecedented range of subjects could be explored.

In 1908, as biochemistry seemed to be coming into its own, a study of the average medical school chemistry course had found that physiological chemistry was limited to one lecture per week for the second half of the second year, accompanied by six hours a week in the laboratory. The subjects covered in these approximately one hundred hours were sugars and proteins, practical nutrition, ferments and enzymes, and the various body fluids (especially urine).[79] But already the course had to accommodate expanding information, a need to improve laboratory facilities, and declining requirements to teach introductory chemistry. Thus while the basic orientation of medical school chemistry teaching was not to change through the rest of the period under discussion, the content of the course, and consequently the time given it, grew dramatically. By 1945 the average biochemistry course involved 240 hours of lecture and laboratory.[80] With a kind of poetic justice, many of the increased hours had been added at the expense of anatomy,[81] the subject which in the nineteenth century had been so absorbingly practical as to make chemistry appear worthless to many students.

77. H. T. Clarke, "Premedical Requirements in Chemistry," *J. AAMC* 5 (1930): 134.

78. Council on Medical Education and Hospitals of the American Medical Association, *Medical Education in the United States, 1934–1939* (Chicago: American Medical Association, 1940), p. 131.

79. The term *average* is more misleading than usual here, since the extremes of content and course time were very widely separated in the early 1900s. In 1903, two schools allotted only 180 hours or less to chemistry, eleven gave the subject 200 to 300 hours, nineteen provided 300 to 400 hours, five gave 400 to 500 hours, three offered 500 to 600 hours, and one, Miami Medical College, assigned a full 652 hours to chemistry ("Medical Schools of the United States," *J. AMA* 41 [1903]: 461). An "ideal" number of hours for the time was 420 (*Proc. AAMC* 19 [1909]: 93). For a comparison of the content of chemistry courses at various schools, see Flexner, *Medical Education in the United States*, p. 90.

80. Gordon Pritham, "Survey of Courses and Construction of Tests in Biological Chemistry," *J. Chem. Educ.* 22 (1945): 84. For a similar study made several years later, see Pritham, "Survey of Courses in Biochemistry," *J. Chem. Educ.* 31 (1954): 482–83.

81. John Field, "Medical Education in the United States: Late Nineteenth and Twentieth Centuries," in Charles D. O'Malley, ed., *The History of Medical Education* (Berkeley and Los Angeles: University of California Press, 1970), p. 511; Willard Rappleye, "Major

Equally striking as an indicator of change is the fact that by mid-century more than two-thirds of the course time was spent in the laboratory.[82] This had in fact been the case at a few schools since the turn of the century, the better courses of that period having offered animal demonstrations (such as the creation of diabetes by extirpation of the pancreas) and experiments on fellow students (nutrition and calorimetry were particularly exploited), in addition to the standard analyses of tissues and secretions.[83] Many students, of course, had no opportunity for such sophisticated investigations, nor did the improvements in education consequent to Flexner quickly eliminate schools with inadequate laboratories. In his second survey (1925), Flexner was happy to find that new laboratories "have sprung up, and superior equipment, often costly and elaborate has been provided in so many universities . . . that all cannot be enumerated." Nevertheless, he admonished, America's laboratory situation was still "highly uneven"; a number of schools muddled through with obsolete facilities, so that "in range of quality, in distance between best, inferior, and worst, no country in the world resembles the United States."[84] An American Medical Association study published fifteen years later still found room to complain, citing one-third of the country's medical schools for having biochemistry labs which were unsatisfactory by reason of being underequipped or overcrowded.[85]

On the whole, however, biochemical instruction was being radically altered by the availability of laboratories. The 1932 report of a committee appointed by the Association of American Medical Colleges even recommended *decreasing* the quantity of laboratory work to give students more time to read and reflect, but also noted with approval the recent trend away from lectures toward more demonstrations and experiments, such as studies relating to exercise, fatigue, diet, acid-base equilibrium, and respiratory quotients, performed by students on themselves.[86] There re-

---

Changes in Medical Education during the Past Fifty Years," *J. Med. Educ.* 34 (1959): 685.

82. Pritham, "Survey of Courses" (1945), p. 84.

83. Pearce, "The Experimental Method," p. 103.

84. Abraham Flexner, *Medical Education: A Comparative Study* (New York: Macmillan, 1925), pp. 172, 173, 191.

85. *Medical Education in the United States, 1934–1939*, p. 129.

86. Association of American Medical Colleges, *Final Report of the Commission on Medical Education* (New York: Association of American Medical Colleges, 1932), pp. 184–87. There had by then been rising concern for several years about the congestion of the curriculum brought about by increasing laboratory work (for example, see J. Scane, "The Five-Year Course," *Proc. AAMC* 20 [1910]: 47). Ray Wilbur, "Altering the Medical Curriculum," *J. AMA* 88 (1927): 724, ironically noted that "when the laboratories came along they were captured in an educational sense by clinical medicine, but they now have captured their captor."

mained, nevertheless, considerable variation in the amount and kinds of activity assigned to the laboratory. Lab instruction in the country's sixty-six four-year medical schools was thus characterized in 1940:

> Approximately 4/5 of the departments [of biochemistry] stressed instruction in quantitative analysis. Slightly less than 1/2 emphasized the chemical aspects of metabolism, nutrition and diet or vitamins. Twenty-four departments utilized human tissues or fluids, and 27 used animal materials. Unknown specimens were utilized in laboratory teaching by 26 departments. Animal experimentation was not attempted frequently nor were hormones always fully discussed.[87]

Behind these generalizations about content and facilities, of course, stood an assortment of formats for the presentation of material. There appears to have been a general inclination to divide subject matter into discrete units and give written (and occasionally oral) examinations on completion of each portion of the course.[88] What attempts there were at pedagogical innovation were inspired primarily by medical educators' one major reservation about biochemistry: the ability of professors to demonstrate its clinical significance. Robert Hare's appointment to the University of Pennsylvania medical faculty had been delayed nine years, it will be recalled, by the reluctance of the school to have chemistry taught by a man without medical training. Faculties of a century later were no less worried about the presentation of biochemistry by Ph.D.'s instead of M.D.'s. The subject had originated in America in a university setting, Yale, and was first taught to graduate students, but as the utility of physiological chemistry for medicine became increasingly apparent, the discipline had been appropriated by medical schools. This at first excited fears that biochemistry would be subverted to purely medical ends, that urinalysis would be given more weight than metabolism and the full value of the science be lost.[89] As there was a shortage of M.D.'s qualified to teach the more specialized chemistry, though, just the opposite embarrassment occurred. Biochemistry came to be taught by nonclinical personnel who stressed theory at the expense of clinical applications.[90] Most departments attempted to compensate for their lack of clinical expertise

87. *Medical Education in the United States, 1934–1939*, p. 133.
88. Ibid.
89. See Albert Matthews, "The Scope and Present Position of Biochemistry," *American Naturalist* 31 (1897): 276; Chittenden, *History of the Sheffield Scientific School*, 2:438; Joseph Fruton, "The Place of Biochemistry in the University," *Yale J. Biol. Med.* 23 (1951): 307.
90. *Medical Education in the United States, 1934–1939*, pp. 130–31; Joseph Gast, "The Teaching of Medical Biochemistry," *J. AAMC* 23 (1948): 235–38.

by having a member of the department of medicine deliver some of the lectures; and a new style of textbook, the "clinical or applied biochemistry," was being issued by the 1930s. Several schools developed imaginative teaching programs to close the distance between pure and clinical biochemistry,[91] but some gap still remained at the end of the 1950s. As was observed by W. W. Westerfield in 1953, "The greatest weakness in biochemical training for medical students today lies in the . . . area of tying together the clinical problems with the applicable fundamental biochemistry."[92] Without making light of this continuing difficulty, however, it might be suggested that the frustration is still a victory of sorts. It stems only from a lack of teachers qualified to clarify in detail the links between chemistry and medicine, whereas for much of chemistry's history as a medical subject, many had doubted that any such links existed.

91. For examples, see M. R. Everett, "A Method of Presenting Biochemistry in Harmony with Modern Medicine," *J. AAMC* 10 (1935): 344–46; Sidney Bliss, "Teaching of Biochemistry to Medical Students," ibid. 14 (1939): 50–52; W. Knowlton Hall, "The Teaching of Applied Biochemistry to Medical Students," ibid. 23 (1948): 385–90.

92. W. W. Westerfield, "Biochemistry in Medical Education," *J. Med. Educ.* 28 (1953): 29.

Materia Medica and Pharmacology

DAVID L. COWEN

MATERIA MEDICA, one of the "two most important branches" of medicine which the new College of Philadelphia proposed to offer, made its formal debut in American medical education with a series of lectures by Dr. John Morgan, scheduled to begin November 18, 1765. Morgan's aims and aspirations served as a model for the teaching of the materia medica for the next 125 years, until the new science of pharmacology began to take over. "The authors to be read in the Materia Medica will be pointed out," Morgan said in describing his course. "The various Substances made use of in Medicine will be reduced under Classes suited to the principal Indications in the cure of Diseases."[1] This straightforward approach sometimes gave way in the nineteenth century to facile taxonomic arrangements of plants or alphabetical arrangements of drugs.

"Similar virtues in different Plants, and their comparative powers," Morgan continued, "will be treated of, and an Enquiry made into the different Methods which have been used in discovering the Qualities of Medicines; the virtues of the most efficacious will be particularly insisted

1. William Frederick Norwood, *Medical Education in the United States Before the Civil War* (Philadelphia: University of Pennsylvania Press, 1944), pp. 63–64.

upon."[2] It would be interesting to know the nature of these enquiries, for William Cullen, under whom Morgan had studied, had been critical of three approaches sometimes used: noting the effects of a drug when given to "brute animals," mixing the drugs with freshly drawn blood, and injecting the drugs into the veins of "living brutes."[3] Though there had indeed been some experimentation by 1765, Anton Störck had not yet completed his investigations, and the work of William Withering, François Magendie, and Claude Bernard lay in the future. Morgan's flicker of pharmacological interest was probably satisfied by the empirical approach, characteristic of the whole of the materia medica and exemplified in Cullen's comment that "since the use of ipecacuanha [as an emetic] has become known, the squills have been more rarely used."[4]

"The Manner of preparing and combining [medicines] will be shown by some instructive Lessons upon Pharmaceutic Chemistry . . . and Pharmacy,"[5] Morgan said. Here the Philadelphia doctor was recognizing the intimate connection between medicine and chemistry on the one hand and pharmacy on the other. These relationships were also to characterize the teaching of materia medica for many years.

Morgan's statement also promised "some critical Lectures upon the chief Preparations contained in the Dispensatories of The Royal College of Physicians at London and Edinburgh."[6] In these he would point out limitations on the teaching of materia medica resulting from the fact that although the official pharmacopoeias had already undergone some cleansing, the traditional and the empirical still dominated their content. The Edinburgh *Pharmacopoeia* then official—the fifth edition of 1756—contained a list of some 375 vegetable simples and another list of animal simples that, though reduced to 29, still included bees, stag's horn, bezoar stone, snails, earthworms, millipedes, cuttlefish bone, and the viper. Polypharmaceuticals continued to characterize the compositions, and although ancient theriacs had been eliminated, a Theriaca Edinensis of 10 ingredients remained.

Finally, Morgan promised that his whole series of lectures would "be illustrated with many useful Practical Observations of Diseases, Diet and Medicines."[7] Morgan thus voiced a desideratum constantly sought thereafter, the teaching of the materia medica as a vital and integral part of medicine rather than a mnemonic exercise.

2. Ibid.
3. William Cullen, *A Treatise of the Materia Medica*, 2 vols. (Dublin: White, 1789), 1:122–23.
4. Ibid., 2:400.
5. Norwood, *Medical Education*, p. 64.
6. Ibid.
7. Ibid.

We have only an inkling of Morgan's success in attaining these goals. Benjamin Rush, who attended Morgan's lectures, was so unimpressed by the course that in 1796, when Morgan was no longer teaching materia medica, he advised a student that he would lose nothing by not attending lectures on the subject.[8]

Materia medica was an integral part of the curriculum of every American medical school established in the next one hundred years. Only a few schools, however, were able to afford the luxury of a chair devoted solely to materia medica;[9] more commonly it was taught along with another, often unrelated, course. Despite the obvious importance of botany to materia medica in that age and the fact that Adam Kuhn's original chair at Pennsylvania in 1768 was in materia medica and botany, few schools put the two fields of study together.[10] When the two were joined, it undoubtedly reflected the special interests of the faculty.[11] Botany did appear in the medical curriculum in conjunction with other courses, however,[12] and probably in some cases it was included in the materia medica course without appearing in the title of that course.[13] Sometimes there were

8. William D. Hoyt, Jr., "A Young Virginian Prepares to Practice Medicine, 1796–1800," *Bull. Hist. Med.* 11 (1942): 584.

9. A survey of medical school histories and related literature revealed at least nineteen schools with separate chairs of materia medica at some time during the nineteenth century. Some noted figures held such posts: Adam Kuhn, Benjamin Smith Barton, David Hosack, Robley Dunglison, Jacob Bigelow, W. P. C. Barton, Nathaniel Chapman, John Syng Dorsey, John R. Coxe, and Charles Lee.

10. Among them Yale in 1810 (Harold S. Burr, "The Founding of the Yale Medical School," *Bull. Med. Libr. Assoc.* 34 [1946]: 177); Brown in 1811 (Seebert J. Goldowsky, "Beginnings of Medical Education in Rhode Island," *R. I. Med. J.* 38 [1955]: 498); Harvard in 1816 (Thomas Francis Harrington, *The Harvard Medical School*, 3 vols. [New York: Lewis, 1905], 1:416); Transylvania from 1817 to 1857 (Norwood, *Medical Education,* p. 292; Henry D. Shapiro and Zane L. Miller, eds., *Physician to the West: Selected Writings of Daniel Drake* [Lexington: University Press of Kentucky, 1970], pp. xxxvi–xxxvii); Dartmouth in 1821–1824 (William A. R. Chapin, *History: University of Vermont College of Medicine* [Hanover: Dartmouth, 1951], p. 126); Jefferson in 1828–1830 (Norwood, *Medical Education,* p. 103); Miami (Ohio) University Medical Department in 1831 (ibid., p. 310); and Wisconsin in 1854 (William S. Middleton, "First Medical Faculty of the University of Wisconsin," *Wis. Med. J.* 54 [1955]: 380).

11. Kuhn, Benjamin Smith Barton, W. P. C. Barton, and Jacob Bigelow especially.

12. Botany was apparently taught with materia medica and pharmacy at Western Reserve in 1844 (Frederick C. Waite, "The Beginning of Institutional Medical Education in Cleveland," *Bull. Acad. Med. Cleveland* 31 [1946]: 11), with these two and chemistry at the Worthington Medical College in 1830 (Jonathan Forman, "The Worthington Medical College," *Ohio St. Arch. & Hist.* 50 [1941]: 377), with medical chemistry at Boston in 1874 (Boston University School of Medicine, *Announcement, 1873–74* [Boston: Boston University School of Medicine, 1873]), and, as medical botany, with materia medica and therapeutics at the Eclectic College of Cincinnati from 1859–1871 (Ralph Taylor, "Formation of the Eclectic School in Cincinnati," *Ohio St. Arch. & Hist.* 51 [1942]: 284–85).

13. The first announcement of the Female Medical College of Philadelphia in 1850 noted that Professor Dickeson, professor of materia medica and therapeutics, would include in his lectures "such instructions in Botany as the time will permit" (Gulielma Fell Alsop,

independent lectures or courses in it.[14] The same was true of chemistry[15] and pharmacy.[16] Each appeared in a joint professorship with materia medica at times, but chemistry eventually went its own way and pharmacy was absorbed by materia medica.

As the nineteenth century progressed, however, materia medica most frequently joined with therapeutics.[17] When John J. Abel went to the University of Michigan in 1891 and began transforming materia medica into pharmacology, he occupied the chair of materia medica and therapeutics.[18] At a few medical schools a third and even a fourth subject were added to the responsibilities of the professor of materia medica and therapeutics.[19]

Frequently, especially when schools were opened on a shoestring, economics or the unavailability of competent faculty dictated that materia medica be taught by faculty members whose interests obviously lay elsewhere. Sometimes the responsibility for it fell to a veritable polymath who could discourse on virtually any medical topic.[20] In 1820 at

History of the Women's Medical College, Philadelphia, Pennsylvania, 1850–1950 [Philadelphia: Lippincott, 1950], p. 21).

14. At Brown in 1811 (Henry R. Viets, "Medical Education—Old Purposes and New Methods," *R. I. Med. J.* 27 [1944]: 153); and Worthington in 1838 (Jonathan Forman, "The Worthington School and Thompsonianism," *Bull. Hist. Med.* 21 [1947]: 777).

15. The combination of materia medica and chemistry was found at King's College in 1767 (Byron Stookey, "Colonial Medical Schools," *Bull. N.Y. Acad. Med.* 40 [1964]: 273); Harvard in 1782, where the combination prevailed at least until 1811 (Harrington, *The Harvard Medical School*, 1:287, 295, 302; and Thomas Edward Moore, Jr., "Early Years of the Harvard Medical School: Its Founding and Curriculum, 1782–1810," *Bull. Hist. Med.* 27 [1953]: 537); and Pennsylvania in 1819 (Norwood, *Medical Education*, p. 78). At Dartmouth in 1797 "Chemistry and Materia Medica" was one of the three original general fields offered (ibid., p. 187). At the University of Virginia a "School of Chemistry and Materia Medica" was established in 1827 and the two subjects were taught by the same professor until 1853 when a "School of Chemistry and Pharmacy" was established (Chalmers L. Gemmill and Mary Jeanne Jones, *Pharmacology at the University of Virginia School of Medicine* [Charlottesville: Department of Pharmacology, University of Virginia, 1966], pp. 30, 57). In the 1840s the combination of chemistry and materia medica was also to be found at Rush Medical College (Norwood, *Medical Education*, p. 341).

16. At Pennsylvania Samuel Griffitts was appointed to the chair of materia medica and pharmacy in 1789. The same chair was listed in 1835 and 1850 (Norwood, *Medical Education*, pp. 78, 83; Joseph Carson, *A History of the Medical Department of the University of Pennsylvania* [Philadelphia: Lindsay and Blakiston, 1869], pp. 160, 179). There was a professor of materia medica and pharmacy at the Pennsylvania College of Medicine in 1839 (Norwood, *Medical Education*, p. 94).

17. A survey of medical school histories and related literature revealed at least twenty-six schools where the materia medica–therapeutics combination was utilized.

18. "A Century of Medical Education at the University of Michigan," *J. Mich. St. Med. Soc.* 49 (1950): 584.

19. These subjects included physiology, diseases of women and children, midwifery and jurisprudence together, chemistry, anatomy, obstetrics, laryngology, jurisprudence, and pharmacy.

20. See n. 19.

Dartmouth there was a professorship in the theory and practice of physic, materia medica, and botany.[21] Four years later Thomas Jefferson envisaged a chair at the University of Virginia covering "anatomy, surgery, physiology, pathology, materia medica, pharmacy, and the history of the progress and theories of medicine."[22] Robley Dunglison, the twenty-six-year-old Englishman who took the post, no doubt felt relieved when he moved to the University of Maryland in 1833 and found that his new chair embraced only materia medica, therapeutics, hygiene, and medical jurisprudence.[23]

That materia medica was often thrown together with such unrelated fields[24] suggests these relationships were either matters of convenience or the result of a rather disparaging attitude toward the course. When J. P. Emmet succeeded Dunglison at Virginia, materia medica was a "new" subject to him.[25] In at least four instances[26] the task of teaching materia medica fell to the dean or registrar. The situation at the University of Michigan at mid-century reveals much about attitudes toward materia medica and the facility with which it was mixed and matched with other courses. In 1850 Dr. Silas H. Douglass was listed as "Professor of Chemistry, Pharmacology, and Materia Medica" and Dr. Jonathan A. Allen appeared as "Professor of Therapeutics, Materia Medica, and Physiology." In 1854 Dr. Alonzo B. Palmer was added to the staff as "Professor of Materia Medica, Therapeutics, and Diseases of Women and Children." Later Palmer transferred to the chair of pathology and the practice of medicine, and by 1861 Douglass had become "Professor of Chemistry, Mineralogy, and Pharmacy."[27]

21. Carleton B. Chapman, *Dartmouth Medical School: The First 175 Years* (Hanover: University Press of New England, 1973), p. 26.

22. Norwood, *Medical Education*, p. 263.

23. Gemmill and Jones, *Pharmacology at Virginia*, pp. 11–12; Norwood, *Medical Education*, p. 90. At Vermont, in 1826, Joseph A. Gallup was teaching the institutes of medicine, materia medica, clinical practice, and obstetrics (Frederick C. Waite, *The Story of a Country Medical School* [Montpelier: Vermont Historical Society, 1945], p. 48). At William and Mary, in 1841, John Millington was expected to teach anatomy, physiology, materia medica, and pharmacy in the first session, and the anatomy of the nerves and organs of sense, pathology, therapeutics, operations of surgery, and a continuation of materia medica and pharmacy in the second session (Norwood, *Medical Education*, p. 260).

24. These included mineralogy, the theory and practice of medicine, jurisprudence, pathology, histology, embryology, and, with some frequency, obstetrics.

25. Gemmill and Jones, *Pharmacology at Virginia*, p. 29.

26. The College of Physicians and Surgeons in New York (1811) (Norwood, *Medical Education*, p. 117); the Medical Academy of Georgia (1829) (ibid., p. 276); the Pennsylvania College of Medicine (1845) (ibid., p. 95); and the Atlanta Medical College (1855) (ibid., p. 280).

27. "Century of Medical Education at the University of Michigan," p. 579; Norwood, *Medical Education*, p. 351.

The patterns John Morgan set for the teaching of materia medica prevailed throughout most of the nineteenth century, as descriptions of courses in that century bear out. In 1820 Daniel Drake, to whom materia medica was of great importance in conducting medicine "on scientific principles," thought that the subject should teach the "selection, preparation and administration of medicines."[28] The Harvard statutes in 1831 provided that "the lectures on Materia Medica consist of the history of various articles used in Medicine,—their preparation, form and properties, as well as their doses and application to the treatment of disease."[29] The University of Virginia described its course in 1846/47 as "a detailed account of the medical agents, in their commercial history, physical properties, chemical habitudes, pharmaceutical preparations, doses and medical applications."[30]

Such examples, which could be multiplied, show that the course in materia medica was a kind of cataloguing process. (One is tempted to describe the lectures as an oral dispensatory.) The presentations, moreover, sometimes followed the arrangement of the pharmacopoeia. At the New York Medical College in 1860 the "drugs were presented with particular reference to their botanic arrangement and action,"[31] and as late as 1902 discussants at a meeting of the Section on Materia Medica, Pharmacy, and Therapeutics of the American Medical Association pleaded that drugs "be arranged according to their therapeutic value, rather than in alphabetical order."[32]

Commonly included in courses on materia medica was the preparation of drugs, that is, pharmacy. Occasionally, as we have noted, materia medica and pharmacy were combined in one chair; but even when they were not, the course in materia medica usually included instruction in pharmacy. Indeed, medical students were so eager for instruction in that field that some at the University of Maryland in the 1840s asked Professor David Stewart of the Maryland College of Pharmacy for permission to attend his lectures. Permission was "cheerfully granted."[33] Pharmacy, materia medica, and therapeutics were among the courses mandated in the AMA's 1847 standards for medical curricula.[34]

28. Daniel Drake, *An Inaugural Discourse on Medical Education* (Cincinnati: Looker, 1820), pp. 6, 13.
29. Harrington, *Harvard Medical School*, 2:484.
30. Gemmill and Jones, *Pharmacology at Virginia*, p. 42.
31. Linn J. Boyd, "New York Medical College," *N.Y. St. J. Med.* 57 (1957): 576.
32. Warren B. Hill, "The Place and Importance in the College Curriculum of Materia Medica," *J. AMA* 39 (1902): 547; and discussion by Horatio C. Wood, Jr., ibid., p. 550.
33. George E. Osborne, "David Stewart, M.D.: First American Professor of Pharmacy," *A. J. Pharm. Educ.* 23 (1959): 221.
34. William G. Rothstein, *American Physicians in the Nineteenth Century* (Baltimore: Johns Hopkins Press, 1972), p. 115.

While there is some validity to C. B. Chapman's claim that materia medica was s "more Pharmacy than Pharmacology" in the mid-nineteenth century,[35] the close relationship between materia medica and therapeutics continued. Though Dunglison, for example, contended in 1837 that therapeutics was of equal importance to materia medica, he defined the latter as teaching "the properties of the tools or agents with which the physician has to fulfill his remedial indications, and [pointing] to the mode in which such agents can be applied with greatest advantage."[36] The National Medical College of Washington promised in 1850 to give "especial attention . . . to Physiological action, and Therapeutic adaptation of remedies. Their *Modus Operandi* will be fully discussed."[37] Such a promise was either bravado or naiveté. More realistic was the description of the course in materia medica at Virginia in 1846/47. It included not only "the detailed account of medicinal agents," but also "General Therapeutics or an account of the effects of the various classes of remedies on the organism, and their modus operandi *so far as understood*," and "Special Therapeutics or the application of these agents to individual diseases, as *supported by experience* or the *theory* of a particular disease."[38] The italics, which have been added, reveal the limitations of the science at that time.

Regardless of how much pharmacy, therapeutics, chemistry, or botany it contained, the course in materia medica was always taught didactically, as Carl A. Dragstedt reveals in describing his experience at Northwestern.[39] The lecture notes of eighteenth or nineteenth-century students in materia medica are remarkably similar to textbooks. Professors often read their lectures. J. P. Emmet of Virginia wrote in 1827 that he took "a great deal of pains" with his lectures and wrote "them out at length."[40] When Asa Fitch complained that William J. Macneven's lectures at the Rutgers Medical College were "too learned for me,"[41] he was probably commenting on the detail and dryness of the course. The most telling comment, however, came from Benjamin Rush in 1796, when he explained to a student that he would lose nothing by not attending lectures on materia medica because "they are entirely such as Dr. Cullen has delivered in his

35. Chapman, *Dartmouth Medical School*, p. 70.
36. Gemmill and Jones, *Pharmacology at Virginia*, p. 14.
37. Circular of the National Medical College, Washington, D.C., 1850 (National Library of Medicine [NLM], Bethesda, Md.).
38. Gemmill and Jones, *Pharmacology at Virginia*, p. 42.
39. Carl A. Dragstedt, "The Department of Pharmacology: Northwestern University Medical School," *Quart. Bull. Northw. Univ. Med. Sch.* 26 (1952): 61.
40. Gemmill and Jones, *Pharmacology at Virginia*, p. 29.
41. Samuel Resneck, "A Course of Medical Education in New York City in 1828–29," *Bull. Hist. Med.* 42 (1968): 559.

writings."[42] Not all instruction in materia medica was poor—James Graham at the Cincinnati College of Medicine and Surgery was called an "excellent" teacher[43]—but learning the subject was almost universally a feat of memorization. On his arrival at Northwestern in 1926 Carl Dragstedt was challenged by a colleague, "in an apparent effort to assess [his] qualifications," to better his record of listing 654 cathartics![44] But the course in materia medica was not always a test of endurance against tedium and poor lectures. Collections of specimens or materia medica cabinets were quite commonplace, and the use of drawings, paintings, live specimens, and models was not unusual.[45]

There is little evidence that materia medica required or encouraged laboratory work. As early as 1832 the Virginia catalogue announced that "there is attached to this school, a very extensive apparatus and laboratory in which the students are occasionally permitted to see the operations and perform experiments,"[46] but the program included chemistry and pharmacy as well as materia medica. (This announcement preceded a boast that "a free use is made of the blackboard in these as well as in almost all other classes in the University.")[47] Where the program included toxicol-

42. Hoyt, "A Young Virginian Prepares," p. 584.

43. Norwood, *Medical Education*, p. 321.

44. Dragstedt, "Department of Pharmacology: Northwestern," p. 61.

45. In 1818 at Harvard, the "collection of specimens of the materia medica" was considered an "auxiliary to the several courses of medical instruction" (Harrington, *Harvard Medical School*, 1:423). The National Medical College of Washington advertised in 1850 that it had a cabinet "enriched with Specimens of all the Drugs and Preparations of the Pharmacopoeia" (Circular, 1850 [NLM]). At Virginia the cabinet, furnished at the professor's expense, had been used so much by 1851 that it was reported to be worn out and in need of replacement. The college provided an annual appropriation of twenty-five dollars to "purchase additional specimens," and its collection "of all the crude drugs and all the preparations which have been dealt with in the lectures" was still in use from 1885 to 1893 (Gemmill and Jones, *Pharmacology at Virginia*, pp. 45, 64–65, 77). At Michigan a materia medica "museum" was established in the late 1850s for the exhibition of "pure, rare, and expensive chemicals used in therapeutics" (Thomas V. Abowd, et al., "Our Heritage: A History of the Medical School," *U. Mich. Med. Center J.* 33 [1967]: 185).

George B. Wood at the Philadelphia College of Pharmacy and the University of Pennsylvania exhibited, in the 1830s, "living specimens of medicinal plants from all parts of the world, grown in his own private garden . . . for that special purpose" (George W. Corner, *Two Centuries of Medicine: A History of the School of Medicine, University of Pennsylvania* [Philadelphia: Lippincott, 1965], pp. 125–26; J. Hampton Hoch, "A Survey of the Development of Materia Medica in American Schools and Colleges of Pharmacy," *A. J. Pharm. Educ.* 12 [1948]: 150). Others resorted to the use of drawings, as at the Female College of Philadelphia in 1850 (Alsop, *Women's Medical College*, p. 21). Virginia used "accurate coloured drawings and paintings" in 1846 and 1851 (Gemmill and Jones, *Pharmacology at Virginia*, pp. 42, 45). In 1875 the Philadelphia College of Pharmacy boasted of sixty-five structural models and the use of a stereoptican to illustrate lectures in botany and materia medica (Hoch, "Development of Materia Medica," p. 152).

46. Gemmill and Jones, *Pharmacology at Virginia*, p. 31.

47. Ibid.

ogy, laboratory demonstrations occasionally took place. The Iowa Medical College promised in the 1850s to "present to the class unlabelled poisons for analysis, and supply them with the necessary equipment so that they may succeed in detecting the various poisons."[48] In 1869 the University of Michigan also provided some laboratory work in toxicology.[49] And beginning with Harvard's curricular reforms in 1870, "clinical and laboratory instruction" purportedly assumed an importance equal to "attendance at lectures."[50] How far this pertained to materia medica is not known.

It has been claimed that the homeopathic "proving" by "exact reiterated experiments on healthy humans," done at Boston University in the 1870s to determine the "pharmacological and pathogenic action of a drug," was "probably the earliest laboratory exercise in pharmacology."[51] Perhaps so, but such provings obviously had their limitations.

By the late 1800s interest in pharmacologic experimentation as part of medical education was growing. The 1887 catalogue of the Western Reserve School of Medicine, for example, mentioned experiments that actually demonstrated the effects of drugs on animals.[52] But most medical schools clung to the old ways. At the Ohio Medical College there was no laboratory requirement beyond dissection until 1888,[53] and none until 1889 at the Medical College of Louisiana.[54]

Traditional courses in materia medica persisted in the nineteenth century despite the impact of therapeutic nihilism coming out of Europe. However, some Americans succumbed to its influence. Jacob Bigelow, for example, lamented at mid-century the fact that the "science of therapeutics, or the branch of knowledge by the application of which physicians are expected to remove diseases, has not, seemingly, attained to a much more elevated standing than it formerly possessed."[55] And Oliver Wendell Holmes's famous dictum that little would be lost if, with few exceptions, the entire materia medica were thrown into the sea, illustrates the point.[56]

48. Ferdinand J. Smith, "Early Medical Education of Keokuk," *J. Iowa St. Med. Soc.* 30 (1940): 177.

49. Hoch, "Development of Materia Medica," p. 153.

50. Hebbel E. Hoff, "Medical Progress a Century Ago: A New Medical Curriculum in America," *Conn. Med.* 36 (1972): 59; Harrington, *Harvard Medical School*, 3:1022.

51. Earl H. Dearborn, "The Development of Pharmacology at Boston University School of Medicine," *Boston Med. Q.* 6 (1955): 34.

52. Frederick C. Waite, *Western Reserve University Centennial History of the School of Medicine* (Cleveland: Western Reserve University Press, 1946), p. 191.

53. Frederick C. Waite, "Medical Education in Ohio," *Ohio St. Med. J.* 49 (1953): 625.

54. Harold Cummins, "Formal Medical Education in New Orleans, 1834," *Bull. Med. Libr. Assoc.* 30 (1942): 306.

55. Walter Artelt, "Louis' amerikanische Schüler und die Krise der Therapie," *Sudoffs Arch. Gesch. Med.* 42 (1958): 300.

56. See Rothstein, *American Physicians*, p. 178.

It seems likely that Bigelow may have had a hand in preparing the "Practical Views on Medical Education" issued by the Harvard medical faculty in 1850. This document contended that

> in Materia Medica there are some thousands of substances and their compounds, which possess what is called medicinal power. Yet it is not probable that any physician effectively reads the one-half or remembers one-quarter, or employs in his yearly practice one-tenth, of the contents of the common dispensatories.[57]

The medical faculty was therefore admonished (in all fields, not merely in materia medica) to condense and abridge, to teach the student "what he can and should master," and to "point out to him the sources, fortunately abundant, from which he may obtain" whatever else he might require.[58]

Although the course at Harvard may have reflected these views, there is little evidence of any radical change in the place of materia medica in the medical curriculum. In fact, the introduction of new and revolutionary drugs like the vegetable alkaloids, the glucosides, the halogens, and, later in the century, the organic and synthetic chemicals, did not alter the basic patterns of instruction in materia medica. New advances in science had little impact. The foundations being laid for modern pharmacology and physiology by François Magendie, Claude Bernard, and Oswald Schmiedeberg and the new rationale for drug therapy emanating from the cellular pathology of Rudolph Virchow did not influence American medical education until the last decade of the century.

Moreover, interest in pharmacological experimentation was scant. In the 1780s John Leigh of Virginia experimented with opium on animals and humans,[59] and in the early 1800s a few dissertations appeared with titles like *An Inquiry into the Modus Operandi of Medicines upon the Human Body*[60] and *Experiments and Observations on the Absorption of Active Medicines into the Circulation.*[61] Although these reflected the scientific limitations of the day, they did indicate the beginnings of a critical and objective approach to the evaluation of drugs—by checking pulse rates, examining saliva, and performing postmortems on dogs, for example.

But neither therapeutic nihilism, nor new drugs, nor interest in pharmacological experimentation seemed to affect the teaching of materia medica. The subject matter was changing, its scientific foundations were

57. Harrington, *Harvard Medical School*, 3:1014.
58. Ibid.
59. V. Robinson, "Drugs," *Dictionary of American History*, 2nd ed., 7 vols. (New York: Scribner's, 1940), 2:171.
60. By William W. Bibb (Philadelphia: Carr and Smith, 1801).
61. By Benjamin C. Hodge (Philadelphia: Maxwell, 1801).

becoming clearer, but, judging from criticisms that persisted into the next century, materia medica remained an empirical and traditional study, didactic in presentation, relying largely on botanical or alphabetical arrangements that depended upon memorization as the chief educational method. One critic in 1901 called the materia medica "a conglomerate heap . . . of dry technical knowledge . . . neither retained nor applied."[62] The lecture system remained inviolate.

The time devoted to materia medica varied from school to school. At mid-century, Boston University required four meetings weekly;[63] Harvard, three.[64] In 1852 the American Medical Association recommended that each school have a chair in materia medica, with not less than sixteen weeks of instruction. Schools that did not comply were to be denied representation in the association.[65]

It would, of course, be a mistake to assume that no changes or improvements were taking place in the teaching of materia medica. Textbooks and reference works necessarily embraced new findings, although the compendious and tedious approach still prevailed. There was a world of difference, however, between David Hosack's 1813 reading list, which required William Lewis's *New Dispensatory*,[66] still basically in its original 1753 form, and the reading list of the University of Virginia in the 1880s, which required the latest *United States Pharmacopoeia*.[67]

The transformation of materia medica into pharmacology, that is, from a didactic and descriptive study of drugs to an experimental and critical course in the operation of drugs, began in the last decade of the nineteenth century. The arrival of John J. Abel as professor of materia medica and therapeutics at the University of Michigan in 1891 marked the turning point. Abel had spent the years from 1884 to 1890 abroad, where his interests had turned to biochemistry and experimental pharmacology.[68] At Michigan he gave the "students the best possible instruction by means of lectures, demonstrations, and quizzes, in the manner [of] my European teachers."[69] In his third year at Michigan he introduced courses on

62. J. R. Jones, "Medical Education," *J. AMA* 37 (1901): 743.
63. Dearborn, "Pharmacology at Boston University," p. 33.
64. Harrington, *Harvard Medical School*, 2:541.
65. David S. Cannom, "Development of Medical Education in the United States," *Conn. Med.* 33 (1969): 127.
66. Circular for Hosack's "Private Medical School," 1813 (New York Academy of Medicine, Rare Book Room, Bd. Pam., vol. 6).
67. Gemmill and Jones, *Pharmacology at Virginia*, p. 77.
68. Charles E. Rosenberg, "Abel, John J.," *D. S. B.* (1970–1976), 1:9.
69. Quoted by William T. Salter, "Medicine as a Science: Pharmacology," *N. Eng. J. Med.* 244 (1951): 138.

"the influence of certain drugs on the metabolism of tissue" and on "the methods of modern pharmacology."[70]

Abel, who was to effect the change from the applied science of materia medica to the biological science of pharmacology (to use his own language),[71] moved on to Johns Hopkins in 1893. There certain chairs, including that in pharmacology, were made full time to increase opportunity for research, and organized laboratory courses were introduced.[72] Abel assumed the responsibility for teaching physiological chemistry to medical students, as well as pharmacology, but at the end of the century he was teaching a lecture and demonstration course in "Practical Therapeutics," offered to third-year students two afternoons a week. It was linked with toxicology and pharmacology and was apparently an early effort at bridging the gap between the preclinical science of pharmacology and clinical medicine.[73] In 1900 toxicology and pharmacology were required courses in the Johns Hopkins curriculum, with second-year students taking six hours of lectures and one hour of recitation. It was at Johns Hopkins that Abel stressed the importance of chemistry and physiology in pharmacology, and it was there that he sought to introduce microanalytic techniques.[74] "The day has long since passed," Abel was later to say, "when he who knows the drugs of the pharmacopoeia and their clinical uses and who is able to set up a kymograph and attach a few registering instruments can claim to be a pharmacologist."[75]

At the University of Michigan the study of pharmacology received a further boost with the arrival of Abel's successor, Arthur R. Cushny, the father of the idea of the biologic assay of drugs. Cushny, who left Michigan in 1905 for University College, London, found that the course in pharmacology was given in the junior year and consisted of daily lectures and demonstrations and weekly quizzes. He expanded the course and developed laboratory pharmacology, which later was to become a required course of eight weeks. For this laboratory course each student was given a work sheet, which collectively formed Cushny's famous *Labora-*

70. Rosenberg, "Abel," p. 10.

71. John J. Abel, "On the Teaching of Pharmacology, Materia Medica, and Therapeutics in Our Medical Schools," in *John Jacob Abel, M.D., Investigator, Teacher, Prophet, 1857–1938: A Collection of Papers by and about the Father of American Pharmacology* (Baltimore: Williams and Wilkins, 1957), p. 57.

72. Richard H. Shryock, *The Unique Influence of the Johns Hopkins University on American Medicine* (Copenhagen: Munksgaard, 1953), pp. 19–20.

73. Alan M. Chesney, *The Johns Hopkins Hospital and the Johns Hopkins University School of Medicine: A Chronicle*, 3 vols. (Baltimore: Johns Hopkins Press, 1943–1963), 1:227; 2:169.

74. Ibid., 2:287; Rosenberg, "Abel," p. 10.

75. Quoted by Thomas D. Darby, "On Teaching Pharmacology and Therapeutics in Our Medical Schools," *Am. Heart. J.* 67 (1964): 147.

tory Guide in Experimental Pharmacology, published in 1905. Cushny's general patterns for the pharmacology program remained essentially unchanged under his successors until 1941.[76]

Abel's description of his basic course in pharmacology as it was given in the last decade of the nineteenth century is revealing. Although he preferred to teach it when students were beginning their clinical studies, they began their work at the conclusion of the first third of their second year. The initial part of the course was devoted to toxicology, which Abel considered "inseparable from pharmacology." The course ran for eight weeks and required two afternoon sessions and a Saturday morning recitation or conference. The afternoon session began with a brief lecture— there was little in the way of didactic lecture—with physiological demonstrations, followed by laboratory work largely chemical in nature. In addition, students received reading recommendations and participated in informal discussions with the instructor.

The remainder of the year was devoted to pharmacology, also partially a laboratory course. The class worked in sections of four, with five or six topics in "artificially contrived" experiments required. Because it was impossible for the class to perform more than six experiments, numerous class demonstrations were necessary "for the rest of the experimental work." Abel believed that the subject of materia medica did not require any special instruction. He did not want to "overburden the student's mind with a multitude of dry details of interest or value solely to the pharmacist or to the student of pharmacognosy." The unnecessarily detailed description of drugs he believed to be out of place in a medical school, and he taught materia medica in direct connection with pharmacology. The instructor allowed himself only "the briefest introduction to the physical and chemical properties of a drug" before beginning "the more important discussion of its pharmacologic action." Those drugs and preparations discussed were placed on a table where the students could examine them; the more important ones were passed from hand to hand.

He could of course not disregard therapeutics in the pharmacology course, but the major responsibility and capability there, he believed, lay with the clinical staff. He recommended a special course in "Practical Therapeutics."[77]

76. "Century of Medical Education at the University of Michigan," p. 584; Abowd, "Our Heritage," p. 186; Richard J. McMurray, "History of the University of Michigan Medical School," *U. Mich. Med. Bull.* 16 (1950): 247.

77. Abel, "On Teaching Pharmacology," pp. 62–70. For a detailed and comprehensive survey of the pharmacology program at Western Reserve in 1902, see Torald Sollman, "The Teaching of Therapeutics and Pharmacology from the Experimental Standpoint," *J. AMA* 39 (1902): 539–46.

The term *pharmacology* was not new when courses in the field began to appear in the late nineteenth century; it had long been used to designate the scientific aspects of pharmacy. Dunglison had used the term more or less synonymously with materia medica. "Therapeutics," he had written in 1837, "is commonly associated with materia medica or pharmacology."[78] In 1828 Jonathan A. Allen had published a book called *A System of Pharmacology,* but it was essentially a work in materia medica.

Moreover, the basic intent of pharmacology was not new. The University of Virginia, even before Abel's influence was felt, described its course in materia medica as laying "particular stress . . . upon the *physiological* action and rational *therapeutical* applications of drugs."[79] In view of the state of pharmacological knowledge at that time, this may have been window dressing, but at least the significance of materia medica was recognized, as indeed it had been even earlier in the century. The term *pharmacology* actually appeared in the titles of courses at Michigan in 1850[80] and at Boston in the 1870s.[81] Nevertheless, it was only after Abel's success at Michigan and Johns Hopkins that emphasis was placed on the effect of drugs on the living organism and that laboratory teaching became common. In the 1890s courses called pharmacology began to appear among the offerings of medical schools throughout the United States.[82]

Since pharmacology, to use Dragstedt's definition, in the "general sense included materia medica, therapeutics, and toxicology"—and involved the "study of the action and fate of drugs in the animal organism" only in the "limited sense"[83]—it was only natural that chairs of pharmacology were often coupled with these and other disciplines: with materia medica;[84] with materia medica and toxicology;[85] with physiology;[86] and with materia medica, therapeutics, and physiology.[87]

78. Gemmill and Jones, *Pharmacology at Virginia,* p. 14.
79. Ibid., p. 77.
80. "Century of Medical Education at the University of Michigan," p. 579.
81. Dearborn, "The Development of Pharmacology at Boston University," p. 34.
82. Dragstedt, "Department of Pharmacology: Northwestern," p. 61.
83. Carl A. Dragstedt, "An Historical Consideration of Pharmacology," *Quart. Bull. Northw. Univ. Med. Sch.* 32 (1958): 179.
84. At Western Reserve in 1904 (Waite, *Western Reserve University,* p. 376) and at West Virginia in 1913 (Edward J. Van Liere and Gideon S. Dodds, *History of Medical Education in West Virginia* [Morgantown: West Virginia University Library, 1965], p. 27).
85. At Virginia in 1908 (Gemmill and Jones, *Pharmacology at Virginia,* p. 108) and Texas at Galveston as late as 1922 (*The University of Texas Medical Branch at Galveston: A Seventy-Five Year History* [Austin: University of Texas Press, 1967], p. 118).
86. At Wake Forest in 1910 (Coy C. Carpenter, *Story of Medicine at Wake Forest* [Chapel Hill: University of North Carolina Press, 1970], p. 9).
87. At Oklahoma in 1909 (Mark R. Everett, *Medical Education in Oklahoma: The University of Oklahoma School of Medicine and Medical Center, 1900–1931* [Norman: University of Oklahoma Press, 1972], p. 34).

Not all medical schools promptly followed the new trend. Twenty-five Ohio medical schools inaugurated required laboratory courses between 1888 and 1913, but pharmacology, although it may have been subsumed under physiology, was not separately designated.[88] The Detroit College of Medicine's four-year program included materia medica but not pharmacology in 1895, and a chair of pharmacology and therapeutics was not established until 1913.[89]

Progress, however, was substantial. By the time of Flexner's report in 1910 the twenty-five schools in his "first division"—those requiring or about to require two years of college work for entrance—had four separate laboratories, one of which was the pharmacology laboratory.[90] In the better "second division" schools—those requiring only high school for entrance but taking "extraordinary pains in teaching"—there also were generally four well-equipped scientific departments; one of these was physiology, which included pharmacology.[91] However, the inferior schools in the second division—those "more or less outspokenly commercial" and devoid of a "free scientific spirit"—usually had no pharmacology laboratories. "Their teaching of materia medica and therapeutics is wholly on didactic lines," Flexner reported.[92] Even less satisfactory were the "basely mercenary" schools, where laboratory instruction was "hardly more than make-believe."[93]

Flexner's report, which placed pharmacology in the first two years of "laboratory sciences," recognized that "few even of the best schools are able to cultivate pharmacology to any considerable extent" because of financial considerations. The University of Pennsylvania was complimented for the "excellent fashion" in which its laboratories, including pharmacology, had been provided for since 1904, but Flexner noted that this was exceptional.[94] He went on to champion a full-time faculty in pharmacology. "The needs of pharmacology," he pointed out, "are . . . not different from those of physics; and the pharmacologist can as little make the teaching of pharmacology a side issue to the practice of

88. Frederick C. Waite, "Changes in the Medical Educational Program in Ohio from 1890 to 1910," *Ohio St. Med. J.* 45 (1949): 1085.

89. Fanny Anderson, "History of Wayne University College of Medicine," *Bull. Wayne Univ. Col. Med.* 2 (1955): 66, 70.

90. Abraham Flexner, *Medical Education in the United States and Canada* (New York: Carnegie Foundation for the Advancement of Teaching, 1910), p. 71.

91. Ibid., p. 78.

92. Ibid., pp. 80, 82.

93. Ibid., p. 86.

94. Ibid., pp. 57, 134; Abraham Flexner, *Medical Education: A Comparative Study* (New York: Macmillan, 1925), p. 164.

medicine or the conduct of a drug store as the physicist can subordinate his academic duties to the operation of a trolley line."[95] Flexner's strong brief for pharmacology had its effect, and the surviving schools of medicine all sooner or later fell into line.[96]

The rise of pharmacology meant the decline, although not the disappearance, of materia medica as a subject of study in American medical schools. Despite Abel's dictum that "all unnecessarily detailed description of crude drugs, of their active principles . . . is out of place in a medical school,"[97] despite the opprobrium heaped upon it as "the least progressive of all medical disciplines,"[98] and despite the assertion that it occupied "a minor place" in medical education,[99] materia medica remained a part of the medical curriculum.

Flexner reported in 1910 that in most American schools "the old materia medica held sway; and the tedious description of the appearance, sources, and supposed virtues of an infinite number of drugs, roots and herbs, occupied a chair tenanted by a practitioner of long experience." Fifteen years later he was still able to find some American and many British and French schools "in which the old-fashioned teaching of materia medica has not yet been replaced by modern pharmacology."[100]

But inexorably materia medica courses were being absorbed into pharmacology courses, although initially the change from materia medica to pharmacology may have been nominal.[101] By 1953 a study of thirty-one departments of pharmacology reported that they were devoting only 4.7 percent of their time to materia medica, pharmacy, and prescription writing.[102] Yet as late as 1961 some contended that too much time had been and was still being devoted to materia medica. On the other hand, some teachers continued to find a great deal for their students to learn in the field. A prominent pharmacologist in 1961 thought students "should

95. Flexner, *Medical Education in the United States and Canada*, p. 60.

96. E.g., Hahnemann in Philadelphia attributed the establishment of a laboratory in physiology and pharmacology in 1910 to Flexner's activity (William A. Pearson, "History of the Hahnemann Medical College, 1898 to 1948," *Hahnemann Monthly*, 83 [1948]: 53).

97. Abel, "On the Teaching of Pharmacology," p. 68.

98. Carl F. Schmidt, "Pharmacology in a Changing World," *Ann. Rev. Physiol.* 23 (1961): 3.

99. Hill, "Place and Importance in the College Curriculum of Materia Medica," p. 546.

100. Flexner, *Medical Education: A Comparative Study*, pp. 158, 168.

101. At Northwestern, for example, the pharmacology students were taught in 1908 "to recognize various herbs and plants . . . [their] action . . . toxicities, and indications" (John A. Wolfer, "Reminiscences of My Medical Student Days at Northwestern Fifty Years Ago," *Quart. Bull. Northw. Univ. Med. Sch.* 28 [1954]: 86).

102. Julius H. Comroe, Jr., et al., eds., *The Teaching of Physiology, Biochemistry, Pharmacology: Report of the First Teaching Institute, Association of American Medical Colleges . . . 1953* (Chicago: Journal of Medical Education, 1954), p. 116.

know . . . the parts of plants, their pharmacopoeial preparations [and] their therapeutic activities."[103]

Although pharmacology seemed to have a "boundless opportunity" to "rationalize materia medica and therapeutics" and to provide an escape from the "concerted adherence to dogmas based on a superficial understanding of complex physiological principles,"[104] the teaching of pharmacology did not prosper. It remained inadequate in many schools and absent in others.[105] "The chairs of pharmacology during the first two decades of this century were poorly supported, and the newly appointed professors in many if not most cases were viewed with condescension by their colleagues [and] with indifference, hostility or contempt by the clinicians," wrote Carl Schmidt, who joined the department of pharmacology at Pennsylvania in 1919.[106] The fact that pharmacology had become a satellite of physiology and biochemistry contributed to this situation.[107] Students "began to yawn and even groan during their courses in pharmacology,"[108] and economy-minded administrators, responsive to such reactions, tucked pharmacology into the physiology or biochemistry department.[109] This satellite relationship,[110] described by some as "symbiosis" and by others as "parasitism,"[111] continued in various schools for a considerable time.[112] Schmidt believed that what Oswald Schmiedeberg had called the "Negative Phase of Pharmacology" did not end until 1919, but others placed pharmacology's "darkest days" in the 1930s.[113]

103. Ko Kuei Chen, "The Role of Pharmacology in the Medical Curriculum," in Ko Kuei Chen, ed., *The American Society for Pharmacology and Experimental Therapeutics, Incorporated: The First Sixty Years, 1908–1969* (Washington, D.C.: Judd and Detweiler, 1969), p. 113.

104. Flexner, *Medical Education in the United States and Canada,* p. 64; Darby, "On Teaching Pharmacology," p. 145.

105. Saul Jarcho, "Medical Education in the United States, 1910–1956," *J. Mt. Sinai Hosp.* 26 (1959): 348.

106. Schmidt, "Pharmacology in a Changing World," pp. 3–4.

107. William T. Salter of Yale found that there had been "an apathetic attitude among pharmacologists, which amounted to frank decadence." He thought that the subservience of pharmacology to physiology had placed limitations on new fields of research (Salter, "Medicine as a Science: Pharmacology," p. 136).

108. Ibid., p. 137.

109. Ibid.

110. In Flexner's second-division "better" schools there were usually four departments, one of which was physiology in which pharmacology was included.

111. Dragstedt, "Department of Pharmacology: Northwestern," p. 62.

112. In the 1930s, for example, pharmacology and physiology were taught as one course at Duke (James F. Gifford, Jr., *Evolution of a Medical Center: A History of Medicine at Duke University to 1941* [Durham: Duke University Press, 1972], p. 111).

113. Schmidt, "Pharmacology in a Changing World," p. 4; Maurice H. Seevers, "Projection to the Future," in Chen, *The American Society for Pharmacology and Experimental Therapeutics,* p. 209.

Several factors influenced the development of pharmacology and consequently the status and the teaching of that discipline in the three decades between 1920 and 1950. First was the brilliant work of a handful of scientists who followed Abel and Cushny: Robert A. Hatcher, Arthur S. Loewenhart, S. J. Meltzer, Henry G. Barbour, Torald Sollmann, C. F. Schmidt, and A. N. Richards, for example.[114] Second was the impact of biochemistry and, later, the tremendous achievements in organic and physical chemistry and in biophysics.[115] Third was the series of drug explosions, the arsphenamines, insulin, synthetic ephedrine, and vitamins at first; then the sulfas, the antibiotics, steroids, antihistamines, antihypertensives, and diuretic, psychotropic, and cardiac drugs.[116]

Pharmacology underwent a radical change from an essentially critical science seeking to test old remedies into a field interested in pharmacodynamics and the mechanisms of action at the cellular level, as well as in drug characteristics like potency, speed of action, rate of absorption, and rate of elimination. A new "rational pharmacology" emerged, potentially capable of developing made-to-measure medicinal agents, and new specialties like biochemical pharmacology and molecular pharmacology took their place in medical education.[117]

Courses in pharmacology thus received a new orientation. The objectives of the course at Boston University in the 1940s and 50s were "to stimulate the student to acquire a basic knowledge of drugs and their use; to aid him in integrating pharmacology with biochemistry, physiology, anatomy, pathology, and microbiology, and to develop in him a rational approach to therapeutics."[118] At Virginia the course description laid greater emphasis on analysis and interpretation of data obtained in the laboratory, on changes in structure and function, and on the action of drugs.[119]

Also in this period the introduction of graduate education in pharmacology reflected both the increasing importance of pharmacology in medical practice, industry, and medical education, and the constant flow

114. See Salter, "Medicine as a Science: Pharmacology," p. 139.
115. Ibid., pp. 137, 140; Allan D. Bass, "Expansion and Change of Direction of the Discipline," in Chen, *The American Society for Pharmacology and Experimental Therapeutics*, p. 155; Seevers, "Projection to the Future," ibid., p. 210; and C. Heymans, "Pharmacology in Old and Modern Medicine," *Ann. Rev. Pharmacol.* 7 (1967): 6.
116. Walter Modell, "The Basis for the Choice and Use of New Drugs," *Gen. Prac.* 20 (1959): 129; and D. W. Woolley, "The Revolution in Pharmacology," *Perspect. Biol. & Med.* 1 (1958): 174–97.
117. Ibid.
118. Quoted in Dearborn, "The Development of Pharmacology at Boston University," p. 36.
119. Gemmill and Jones, *Pharmacology at Virginia*, p. 117.

of new knowledge into the science of pharmacology. In the 1920s and 1930s a few schools pioneered in awarding Ph.D. degrees in pharmacology.[120] This met with some opposition from medical pharmacologists who insisted that the subject was a medical discipline requiring medical training.[121] However, few physicians entered pharmacology, and the increasing need for pharmacologists, combined with government support, spurred the development of graduate programs.[122] By 1951 there were twelve university departments with "organized programs for graduate training."[123] The new medical schools of the 1960s occasionally provided for such graduate programs in new facilities separate from the medical school.[124]

The impact of graduate programs on pharmacology is evident in a 1953 survey, which indicated that 51 percent of the teachers of pharmacology held Ph.D. or Sc.D. degrees, another 17 percent held both Ph.D. and M.D. degrees, 30 percent held only M.D. degrees, and 2 percent had no doctorates.[125] In 1968 members of the Society for Pharmacology and Experimental Therapeutics holding Ph.D. degrees outnumbered those with M.D. degrees two to one. It is significant, however, that of the eighty-four chairmen of pharmacology departments, thirty-six had M.D. degrees, eighteen had both M.D. and Ph.D. degrees, but only thirty had the Ph.D. alone.[126]

In 1953 the report of the First Teaching Institute of American Medical Colleges dealt with the teaching of physiology, biochemistry, and pharmacology. According to this report, the aim of courses in pharmacology was now the creation of "disciplined rather than stuffed minds" and the development of the capacity to use rather than simply to acquire facts. The student was to learn to question rather than to accept, and to "evaluate claims of therapeutic success and to make intelligent use of new ideas and new drugs."[127] As cliché-ridden as these statements may appear, they

120. Neil C. Moran, "Clinical Pharmacology—Old Wine in New Bottles?," *Clin. Pharmacol. Ther.* 12 (1971): 421.

121. Chen, "The Role of Pharmacology in the Medical Curriculum," p. 116.

122. Seevers, "Projection to the Future," p. 210.

123. Salter, "Medicine as a Science: Pharmacology," p. 137.

124. Penn State, for example (Vernon W. Lippard and Elizabeth F. Purcell, eds., *Case Histories of Ten New Medical Schools* [New York: Josiah Macy, Jr., Foundation, 1972], p. 354).

125. Comroe, *Report of the First Teaching Institute*, p. 130.

126. A. R. McIntyre, "Flexner, Pharmacology, and the Future," *J. Clin. Pharmacol.* 8 (1968): 279.

127. George E. Acheson, "Content and Aims of Physiology, Biochemistry and Pharmacology," in Comroe, *Report of the First Teaching Institute*, p. 24.

do indicate a basic change taking place in American medical education.

Pharmacology courses were almost universally taught in the second year of the medical curriculum in order to make use of preliminary studies in chemistry and physiology. [128] Faculty preference was heavily in favor of making pharmacology the last preclinical course, [129] and many favored giving the course in the third or fourth year, after the student had been exposed to clinical problems. [130]

The number of scheduled course hours in pharmacology was generally high. [131] Three-fifths of the schools still included prescription writing, materia medica, and pharmacy among the topics covered, with 4.7 percent of the lecture time being devoted to them. [132] Toxicology was included in almost 70 percent of the schools, which devoted 5.7 percent of the lecture time to it. The remaining lecture topics, all on specified drug classes, indicated that the largest proportion of time, 16.6 percent, was devoted to chemotherapeutic agents and antibiotics; 10.7 percent to autonomic drugs; 9.1 percent to endocrines; 7.9 percent to cardiovascular drugs; 6.7 percent to analgesics and antipyretics; and 6.4 percent to general anesthesias. [133] Almost 25 percent of laboratory time was devoted to autonomic drugs, over 20 percent to central-nervous-system depressants, 9.4 percent to "general pharmacology," and 8 percent to cardiovascular drugs. [134] In 43 percent of the schools students were required to do from one to twenty experiments, and in 45 percent of the schools from twenty-one to forty experiments. [135] In only 21 percent of the schools were the students required to report a complete description of purposes, methods, results, and conclusions; 31 percent required only a brief statement of results, 21 percent a single data sheet, 12 percent a data sheet and a statement of results, and 15 percent required no report. [136]

Another index of the growth of pharmacology—and of its continued association with physiology—was the number of full-time faculty: a total

128. Out of seventy-six schools, one taught pharmacology in the first year, two taught it in both the first and second years, and the remaining seventy-three taught it in the second year (Comroe, *Report of the First Teaching Institute*, p. 121).
129. Out of 617 responses, 155 selected pharmacology and 291 selected pharmacology with another course or other courses (ibid., p. 120).
130. Acheson, "Content and Aims," ibid., p. 32.
131. Ten schools scheduled between 101 and 140 hours, 15 between 141 and 180 hours, 19 between 181 and 220 hours, and 18 over 220 hours (Comroe, *Report of the First Teaching Institute*, p. 113).
132. In thirty-one out of fifty-two schools (ibid., p. 116).
133. Ibid.
134. In fifty-one pharmacology departments (ibid., p. 117).
135. In sixty pharmacology departments (ibid., p. 154).
136. Ibid., p. 156.

of 269 in pharmacology and 75 in pharmacology and physiology in 76 medical schools in the United States.[137] Accompanying this growth were new techniques and methods. Biostatistics appeared more frequently in pharmacology than in physiology laboratories, and "Quantitiative Pharmacology" developed "apace."[138] Even more significant was the popularity of "project teaching" and "conference teaching." The former, in use at one institution since 1947,[139] consisted of special laboratory assignments in which students worked on a long-term "chronic experiment" rather than on a short "classical study," or in which a student selected, designed, performed, and reported on a research project.[140] Although project teaching was not without its critics, the evidence seems to indicate that it met with considerable enthusiasm.[141]

The student conference, hardly a radical innovation,[142] was in use at Boston University in the 1940s or 1950s,[143] and took its place alongside the lecture and laboratory in the teaching of pharmacology. The conferences were intended to be discussion sessions, covering lecture and laboratory materials and, rarely, text assignments; they were not recitation or quiz sections.[144] However, the large size of many conference groups[145] suggests that the term *conference* was sometimes only a euphemism. General reaction was, nevertheless, favorable.[146]

Two recurring problems of educational procedure concerned pharmacologists in 1953. One was the correlation and integration of pharmacology with other basic sciences; the other related to the extent to which pharmacology courses should be clinically or therapeutically oriented.

Despite the preference of two-thirds of the delegates at the 1953 First

137. Ibid., p. 128.

138. Ibid., pp. 27, 28; Salter, "Medicine as a Science: Pharmacology," p. 141.

139. The school was unnamed (Comroe, *Report of the First Teaching Institute*, p. 178).

140. Victor E. Hall, "Teaching and Learning Techniques," in Comroe, *Report of the First Teaching Institute*, pp. 79–80; Comroe, ibid., p. 178.

141. It was estimated that 20 percent of the laboratory courses devoted time, ranging from 5 percent to 55 percent, to project teaching (Comroe, ibid., p. 119).

142. Torald Sollmann used conferences as a teaching device in 1902 ("The Teaching of Therapeutics and Pharmacology," p. 541); and at Buffalo, in the same year, Eli H. Long contended that he "did not teach by lecturing but by conferences with the students" (symposium discussion, *J. AMA* 39 [1902]: 550).

143. Nine conferences per semester of groups of six students were provided for. One faculty member was involved and the conference was ungraded (Dearborn, "The Development of Pharmacology at Boston University," p. 36).

144. Hall, "Teaching and Learning Techniques," in Comroe, *Report of the First Teaching Institute*, p. 87.

145. Only 28 percent of the pharmacology departments had fifteen or fewer students in a conference and 22 percent had over thirty (Comroe, ibid., p. 158).

146. Hall, "Teaching and Learning Techniques," in ibid., p. 86.

Teaching Institute of American Medical Colleges for separate courses in biochemistry, physiology, and pharmacology,[147] and despite the fact that 40 percent of department chairmen reported little or no consultation with other preclinical departments,[148] a considerable effort toward integration was noticeable by the early 1950s.[149] "Coordinated," "conjoint," and "parallel" courses were available, departmental lines disappeared, and new courses on "cellular function" embraced the totality of the basic sciences.[150] It is not easy to separate goals from reality, but there was a realization that science, and medical science in particular, should not be compartmentalized. As the pendulum reversed itself, pharmacology once again merged with the other basic sciences.

The second problem, the relationship of pharmacology to clinical studies, was not restricted to pharmacology; other preclinical sciences also had to contend with it. In 1876 Theodor Billroth wrote that the art of using and choosing drugs should not be included in pharmacology lectures but should be discussed in the clinic.[151] Later, Abel contended that the teaching of pharmacology should not ignore the clinical uses of a drug.[152] But even in his day the correlation of pharmacology with clinical medicine was "apt to be feeble," and it remained so at least until the 1940s.[153] It is rare to find a professor, like J. A. Waddell of Virginia (1911–1945), being praised by a student for the "good deal of emphasis on the clinical application" of drugs.[154]

How much clinical orientation should be given and who should give it were much-debated questions. Pharmacologists were wary. A precondition of their interest in clinical medicine was its noninterference with the usual subject matter; they wanted everything pertinent, even if not clinically applicable, to be covered.[155] Nevertheless, almost every department chairman in 1953 recognized the desirability of emphasizing pharmacology's contribution "to the understanding of clinical disorders," and there was a "strong tendency" to select clinically useful and promising drugs as examples in pharmacology courses.[156] "Practical Pharmacology," "Clinical

147. Comroe, ibid., p. 124.
148. Ibid., p. 123.
149. H. G. Weiskotten, "Continuing Evolution of the Medical Curriculum," *J. AMA* 145 (1951): 1127.
150. Comroe, *Report of the First Teaching Institute*, pp. 167–71.
151. T. Z. Csáky, "Clinical Pharmacy and Pharmacology: Friends or Foes," *J. Med. Educ.* 48 (1973): 906.
152. Abel, "On Teaching Pharmacology," p. 62.
153. Jarcho, "Medical Education in the United States," pp. 348–60.
154. Gemmill and Jones, *Pharmacology at Virginia*, p. 119.
155. Acheson, "Content and Aims," in Comroe, *Report of the First Teaching Institute*, p. 21.
156. Ibid., p. 33; Comroe, ibid., pp. 110, 119.

Correlations," and other attempts at "vertical correlation" gradually entered the curriculum, albeit not without friction and not without failures.[157]

In 1959 Chauncey Leake defined the intellectual problems of pharmacology as being essentially chemical and biological, embracing (1) the dose-effect and time-concentration relations of drugs; (2) localization and biological site of action of chemicals; (3) mechanisms of absorption, distribution, fate, and metabolism, and excretion of chemicals in living material; (4) the mechanisms of actions of chemicals on living material; and (5) the relations between chemical constitution and structure and biologic action.[158] A highly technical and scientific structure is evident, but it is also clear that to "pure" pharmacologists, clinical applications were somewhat beyond their realm.

In the late 1960s and early 1970s the movement toward integrated courses gained renewed emphasis. It was a time of self-analysis and reform for medical education, and a spate of new medical schools struggled to outdo one another in the search for relevance and economy of effort. Curriculum experimentation abounded.[159]

The basic sciences of the preclinical years, including pharmacology, were combined in a variety of interdisciplinary forms. In 1962 one commentator on the revolution in biology and its impact on medical education contended that the philosophy and techniques of biochemistry, physiology, microbiology, and pharmacology were "all but indistinguishable" and recommended that, while separate lectures should be devoted to each, the laboratory work for all should be consolidated. This was not only logical; it would shorten the formal preclinical curriculum.[160] Such proposals went beyond mere theorizing,[161] and by 1973 twenty-one schools had interdisciplinary programs in the basic sciences.[162]

157. Eugene W. Landis, "Interrelationships," in Comroe, ibid., pp. 45–48; Comroe, ibid., pp. 172–75.

158. Chauncey D. Leake, "The Status of Pharmacology as a Science," *Am. J. Pharm. Educ.* 23 (1959): 174.

159. See Lippard and Purcell, *Case Histories,* and, by the same editors, *The Changing Medical Curriculum* (New York: Josiah Macy, Jr., Foundation, 1972).

160. Robert R. Wagner, "The Basic Medical Sciences: The Revolution in Biology and the Future of Medical Education," *Yale J. Biol. Med.* 35 (1962): 8.

161. See, e.g., Stuart C. Cullen, "University of California School of Medicine, San Francisco Medical Center," *Calif. Med.* 111 (1969): 494; Clifford Grobstein, "University of California, San Diego School of Medicine," in Lippard and Purcell, *Case Histories,* p. 109; Alexander Leaf, "Integrating and Regrouping Courses in the Basic Medical Sciences," in Lippard and Purcell, *The Changing Medical Curriculum,* pp. 54, 60.

162. Maurice B. Visscher, "The Decline in Emphasis on Basic Medical Sciences in Medical School Curricula," *The Physiologist* 16 (1973): 47.

118   David L. Cowen

The effects of this were a decline in the time allotted to preclinical studies and a gradual disappearance of the traditional division of the curriculum into two preclinical and two clinical years.[163] In the process classical pharmacology declined, along with other preclinical sciences. A survey of course and laboratory hours for pharmacology in American medical schools indicated that lecture time varied from 180 to 220 hours in the academic year 1952/53, was at 162 in 1966/67, and lay between 101 and 140 in 1972. Similarly, pharmacology laboratory hours, between 41 and 60 in 1952/53, dropped to fewer than 20 in 1971/72. Moreover, in the latter years 25 percent of the schools provided "no assigned time for laboratory instruction in pharmacology" whatsoever.[164] (Some studies had shown that laboratory work in pharmacology, though of "some value," could be "dispensed with without adverse influence upon student knowledge" or grade performance.)[165] In the academic year 1974/75 about one out of every six American medical schools did not include a required course in pharmacology in its curriculum.[166]

Pharmacologists understandably lamented the tendency to neglect their field.[167] Some blamed the attrition on a fallacious reductionism that held that major scientific problems could be solved "by focusing on smaller and smaller sub-units,"[168] that is, on the whole concept of the interdisciplinary approach. Others blamed it on the clinicians, whom the pharmacologists had long accused of being loathe to confer with them,[169] and with whom relations had often been "far from satisfactory."[170]

The process of integration and retrenchment in pharmacology was intimately related to the development of clinical pharmacology. The delineation of *clinical pharmacology* as a distinct body of knowledge dates from 1952, when Dr. Harold Gold in the United States and Dr. John H.

163. Ibid.; Lippard and Purcell, *The Changing Medical Curriculum*, p. 13.
164. Visscher, "The Decline in Emphasis," pp. 48, 45.
165. Avram Goldstein, "A Controlled Comparison of the Project Method with Standard Laboratory Teaching in Pharmacology," *J. Med. Educ.* 31 (1956): 374. See also J. B. Kahn, Jr., "The Pharmacology Laboratory: Tool or Sacrament?," *J. Med. Educ.* 40 (1965): 870–77; and H. G. Mandel, et al., "The Value of Laboratory Teaching in Pharmacology," ibid. 46 (1971): 69–77.
166. Based on a survey of the data in *1974–75 AAMC Curriculum Directory* (Washington, D.C.: American Association of Medical Colleges, 1974).
167. E.g., Chauncey D. Leake, "The Teaching of Pharmacology: Report of the Meeting of the Western Pharmacology Society," *J. Med. Educ.* 43 (1968): 850; and Louis Lasagna, "The Clinical Pharmacologist as a Servant of Society," *Canad. Med. Assoc. J.* 97 (1967): 112.
168. Ibid.
169. Visscher, "The Decline in Emphasis," p. 52; Salter, "Medicine as a Science: Pharmacology," p. 137.
170. Chen, "The Role of Pharmacology in the Medical Curriculum," p. 117.

Gaddum in England introduced the term as it came to be used.[171] Earlier the phrase had referred to qualitative, often subjective, observations on the effects of drugs on man. Gold saw it as an independent academic discipline, a field based on objective, scientific methods: the use of controls, the double-blind design, and statistical analysis.[172] By 1967 the American Society for Pharmacology and Experimental Therapeutics had established a Division of Clinical Pharmacology.[173]

The demarcation between classical and clinical pharmacology was difficult and tortuous. There were those who contended that the general pharmacologist had "no business" with practical procedures and that clinical relationships should be left for the clinical situation; the general pharmacologist was to deal with principles and concepts.[174] Some clinical pharmacologists went even further and expressed a willingness to teach the basic science to their clinical students. In any event, the clinical pharmacologists wanted departments separate from the basic pharmacology departments.[175]

Reasonable heads prevailed and the processes of "vertical integration" begun in the 1950s gained momentum. Referring to general and clinical pharmacology, Maurice H. Severs declared in 1969 that "both come first."[176] And indeed working relations between the two did develop. Clinical demonstrations, for example, supplemented the basic pharmacology course, but the most frequently used program of vertical integration placed the teaching of some basic pharmacology in the clinical program.[177]

By 1969 thirty-five colleges were offering programs in clinical pharmacology.[178] Class exercises included controlled clinical trials and utilized computers, television, tapes, and the "POMR"—the problem-oriented medical record.[179] (Similar teaching devices appeared in basic pharmacol-

171. Harry Gold, "Clinical Pharmacology—Historical Note," *J. Clin. Pharmacol.* 7 (1967): 310.
172. Ibid.; George B. Koelle, "Major Research Events in Pharmacology, 1940–1970," *Federation Proc.* 30 (1971): 1408.
173. Bass, "Expansion and Change of Direction," p. 156.
174. Acheson, "Content and Aims," in Comroe, *Report of the First Teaching Institute*, p. 22.
175. Moran, "Clinical Pharmacology," p. 423.
176. Seevers, "Projection to the Future," p. 215.
177. Duncan E. Hutcheon, "The Society-to-Cell Concept as Applied to the Teaching of Pharmacology," *J. Clin. Pharmacol.* 11 (1971): 162; Richard Penrose Schmidt, "Comparative Role Development," *J. Med. Educ.* 48 (1973): 958; Lippard and Purcell, *The Changing Medical Curriculum*, pp. 58, 69–70.
178. Frederick Wolff, "The Myth of Clinical Pharmacology," *New Eng. J. Med.* 280 (1969): 391.
179. See George E. Nelson, "The Problem-Oriented Medical Record and Teaching of

ogy courses as well.)[180] Critics, however, abounded. One called clinical
pharmacology a "myth";[181] another dubbed it an "academic laugh-in."
The latter asked, "How far has academe really risen to meet the challenge . . . in pharmaceutical therapeutics?" and replied, "About one
Ångström unit."[182] In the opinion of the critics, so little time was devoted
to clinical pharmacology that instruction was superficial.

The continuing flood of new drugs and the constant progress of science
multiplied the problems of pharmacology in the 1960s and 1970s. During
these decades pharmacology became even more closely correlated with
biochemistry and biophysics. Biochemical pharmacology gained in importance and challenged the classical biochemistry courses.[183] One
course, planned for the new medical school at Brown in 1963, demanded
expertise in physical science, enzymology, and biophysics.[184] There were
even suggestions that classical pharmacology be abandoned in favor of
biochemical pharmacology.[185] Molecular pharmacology required ties with
chemistry, physical chemistry, and mathematics. Its development reflected the rapid application of such advances as radioisotope labeling, gas
chromotography, fluorescence and infrared spectroscopy, nuclear magnetic resonance, mass spectrometry, X-ray diffractometry, and electron
microscopy. Its notable successes in certain areas—for example, the
characterization of genetic material—gained it prestige.[186]

The process of specialization and differentiation is reflected in the
number and variety of pharmacology courses offered in medical schools.
At George Washington in 1974, for example, medical students could take

Clinical Pharmacology," *J. Clin. Pharmacol.* 12 (1972): 375–81; G. B. Leslie and D. H.
McClelland, "The Exchange of Video-Tape Recordings for Teaching Physiology and Pharmacology," *Med. & Biol. Ill.* 22 (1972): 27–29; S. Fred Brunk, et al., "A Teaching Format in
Clinical Pharmacology: Comparison of Two Exanthines and a Placebo," *J. Clin. Pharmacol.*
13 (1973): 121–26; and Norman Kahn and J. Thomas Bigger, Jr., "Instruction in Phar-
macokinetics: A Computer-Assisted Demonstration System," *J. Med. Educ.* 49
(1974): 292–95.
    180. See Thomas H. Holmes, "Some Observations on Medical Education," *Psychosom.
Med.* 31 (1969): 269; and Hugh J. Burford and Frank T. Stritter, "Evaluation of a Teaching
Program in Medical Pharmacology," *J. Med. Educ.* 49 (1974): 236–43.
    181. Wolff, "The Myth of Clinical Pharmacology," pp. 390–91.
    182. Edward A. Carr, Jr., "A Short Course in Clinical Pharmacology," *Clin. Pharmacol.
Ther.* 11 (1970): 459.
    183. Heymans, "Pharmacology in Old and Modern Medicine," p. 6; Seevers, "Projection
to the Future," p. 211.
    184. Ibid., p. 211; Lippard and Purcell, *Case Histories*, p. 45.
    185. Seevers, "Projection to the Future," p. 212.
    186. Koelle, "Major Research Events," p. 1408; Bass, "Expansion and Change," p. 156;
Heymans, "Pharmacology in Old and Modern Medicine," p. 6.

not only the required lecture-laboratory-conference course in pharmacology, but any one of seventeen additional electives in the field.[187]

Despite these developments, however, classical pharmacology, though hardly as important in time or emphasis as it had been, did not disappear. Ninety-nine of one hundred nineteen American medical schools in 1974 required a pharmacology course, and one other school included the subject in an integrated course. Sixty-nine schools put it in the second year, nineteen in the first year, ten in both years, and one in the third year. In only three instances did *clinical pharmacology* appear in the title of a required course.[188] Moreover, in spite of its new scientific foundations, pharmacology had freed itself from affiliation or amalgamation with physiology departments. By 1969 only one major school still had a combined department, and it was planning to separate the two fields.[189]

But pharmacology instruction was not always successful. One critic in 1968 flatly denied that "today's pharmacology courses really worked." The young medical graduate was ill informed about drugs, he asserted, and pharmacology instruction needed to "be made more effective."[190] Another forceful critic accused medical schools of taking "the surrealist position that the appropriate response to a need for more teaching about drugs is to gut their own pharmacology departments." He predicted a "new Ice Age in drug therapy" if the trend continued.[191]

This state of affairs reflected both the tremendous expansion in medical knowledge and its concomitant crowding of the medical curriculum, and the increasing emphasis, regretted by many, on a practical pharmacology that taught "to cure." Pharmacology, it was feared as the 1970s approached, was in danger of being reduced "to a sort of empiric indoctrination in the spirit of the materia medica of seventy-five years ago."[192]

---

187. George Washington University, *Bulletin: School of Medicine, 1973–74* (Washington, D.C.: George Washington University, 1973).

188. Based on a survey of *1974–75 AAMC Curriculum Directory.*

189. Bass, "Expansion and Change," p. 157.

190. Harold Hodge, "The Pros and Cons of Innovations in Teaching Pharmacology," *Proc. West. Pharmacol. Soc.* 11 (1968): 13.

191. Carr, "A Short Course," p. 459. With regard to the inadequacy of the training of physicians in pharmacology, see also Wolff, "The Myth of Clinical Pharmacology," p. 390; and Thomas H. Maren, "Role of Pharmacology in Physician Education," *J. Med. Educ.* 48 (1973): 465.

192. Hodge, "The Pros and Cons of Innovation," p. 13.

Pathology

RUSSELL C. MAULITZ

PATHOLOGY as the study of the "seats and causes of disease" has a history stretching back long before the beginnings of American medical education. But pathology as an organized human activity, a socially defined set of roles and approaches to the physician's work is—unlike, let us say, surgery—of recent vintage in America and abroad.[1] Writing the history of the teaching of this subject in America thus raises some interesting definitional questions.[2] Does one begin with what has become recognizable in the twentieth century as pathology, a cluster of theoretical and instrumental agendas subsuming everything from forensic toxicology at the practical level, to "B" and "T" lymphocyte differentiation at the research level? That is, does one adopt a presentist posture in order to trace in retrospect all those strands that have been woven together into what appears a seamless mesh? Or does one rather seek out the meaning of pathology as it was taught under radically different pedagogical rubrics during the eighteenth, nineteenth, and twentieth centuries?

1. Esmond Long, *A History of American Pathology* (Springfield, Ill.: Charles C. Thomas, 1962), is the standard work on the subject.
2. The standard works in the history of pathology do not, and probably need not, concern themselves with such definitional questions. For a guide to those writings, see

Adopting either of these historical approaches discloses only a part of the overall picture of an evolving discipline. But both point to development of the study of pathology as a critical—some would say *the* critical—step by which the student of the medical sciences becomes a student physician. "In pathology," to quote one recent historian of medical education, "the student at last began to feel like a doctor, as he examined diseased organs, grossly and microscopically, and attended autopsies on patients who had died in the hospital."[3] In this essay I shall use both historical approaches to describe the integration and the ultimate—if only partial—disintegration of pathology.

The mechanism that brought pathology into focus as a subject of prime importance for the medical student, legitimizing the claims of certain proponents of the new scientific medicine—who called themselves pathologists—to special and exclusive expertise in their field, was quite literally a converging lens: the objective of the improved microscope. In the middle of the nineteenth century, microscopes were brought into the United States in ever increasing numbers, particularly in the post–Civil War period. Hordes of young medical students who finished their training with a European *Wanderjahr* learned microscopy as a symbol of the new ideology of scientific medicine. As American manufacturers stretched to catch up with the new optical technology, achromatic microscopes were pressed into service in the education of American physicians.[4] The microscope was introduced into the medical school curriculum not so much for the histological analysis of normal tissues, as for the cellular pathology of diseased organs. Elevated to the level of a theoretical paradigm by Rudolf Virchow, cellular pathology was both intellectually predictive and socially legitimating for its practitioners—who in turn became its teachers.[5]

The microscope thus created both the field of vision and the institutional niches for men who presented themselves as academic pathologists. They became the stewards of that discipline which combined and correlated the macroscopic findings of the postmortem dissection with the microscopic findings of cellular injury or aberrancy, the histo-pathology of disease. They posited the various mechanisms, operating at the esoteric level of the living cell, by which such correlative changes might occur in

Long, *A History of American Pathology*.

    3. Vernon W. Lippard, *A Half-Century of American Medical Education* (New York: Josiah Macy, Jr., Foundation, 1974), pp. 9–10.

    4. See James H. Cassedy, "The Microscope in American Medical Science," *Isis* 67 (1976): 76–97, for an extremely useful treatment of this subject.

    5. I have dealt with the German program in my article "Rudolf Virchow, Julius Cohnheim, and the Program of Pathology," *Bull. Hist. Med.* 52 (1978): 162–82.

different disease processes. In doing this the pathologists interposed themselves firmly and almost permanently between the other traditional basic sciences and the clinical setting that they subserved more directly than anyone else based in the laboratory. Long before Abraham Flexner wrote his report, and well into the second half of the twentieth century, pathologists thus assumed a unique position in the education of the student physician. The pathologist might not have been able to promote his field as the cornerstone of the graduate physician's clinical education or indeed of clinical health care. But he argued quite successfully that in the education of the nascent clinician, the undergraduate medical student at mid-career, his subject was the entrance to the wards. The pathologist undertook the role of interlocutor between clinic and laboratory. Thus pathology both as a part of the medical curriculum and as a science remained in focus for nearly a century until, in the decades after World War II, it began once again to blur. Despite the incursions of bacteriology, which it had developed and then merged with in an uneasy relationship that ended in separation, pathology had remained a self-conscious and self-contained discipline for nearly a century.[6] With the appearance of molecular biology, biophysics and immunology, the service, teaching, and research strands of pathology began to unravel. What had remained a stable discipline for decades ruptured and began to disintegrate.[7]

BEFORE CONVERGENCE: 1765–1847

The historical process by which pathology became a unitary subject in the medical curriculum began in the mid-nineteenth century, when it assumed the stable contours by which the modern physician recognizes it. Not surprisingly, then, pathology had seldom previously been taught under the aegis of one professor. The integrity of pathology as a subject in the curriculum necessarily awaited the development of the science and its technology. The problem becomes clearer when one considers a basic definitional issue: as the science or study of disease, pathology displays a central and consistently useful ambiguity or tension between the *causes* and the *results* of disease. The microscope made it possible for the medical student to understand certain processes, such as neoplasia or acute suppuration, in terms of certain other concrete principles that served as both cause *and* effect. The malignant transformation of cells and cell-

---

6. See "Consolidation and Aggrandizement, 1884–1939," below.
7. See "Epilogue: The Late Twentieth Century," below.

mediated inflammation are but two examples. However, for the better part of the first century of the Republic, pathology, taken as the study of the *causes* of disease, was taught as part of the domain of the professor of the theory and practice—or of the "institutes"—of medicine. The *results* of disease, in turn, were often in the domain of the professor of surgery, or, adjunctively, of pathological anatomy. It was the surgeon whose livelihood depended on (and made possible) the most fine-grained appreciation of the structure of the body parts in the diseased as well as the healthy state.[8]

In the early decades of the Republic it was thus not unusual to find the teaching of anatomy, surgery, and pathological anatomy closely allied. Even before the development in the 1760s of the first formal medical curriculum in the colonies at the College of Philadelphia, these subjects were naturally linked.[9] Those who, like Thomas Cadwalader, had undergone a medical apprenticeship in America and finished their education in Europe were skillful as prosectors and hence qualified to teach normal and pathological anatomy to the extent that their surgical education allowed. But the medical student's exposure to the expertise of such anatomically knowledgeable preceptors was often limited by the availability of bodies for autopsy demonstration, a problem that persisted well into the nineteenth century, when a series of anatomy acts made the requisite cadavers more widely available. In the eighteenth century the use of autopsy in teaching depended on the sudden availability of the remains of a politically undesirable figure or the body of an executed criminal.[10]

Such matters were only marginally improved at first by the institution of formal medical curricula. In the College of Philadelphia, for example, Benjamin Rush held forth on causal (later known as "general") pathology as part of the course in the institutes of medicine.[11] For Rush and most of

8. This relationship continued to obtain, of course, well into the era of scientific medicine beginning in the 1870s.
9. A survey of the essential works on the history of the nation's oldest medical school will necessarily begin with the model institutional history by George Corner, *Two Centuries of Medicine: A History of the School of Medicine, University of Pennsylvania* (Philadelphia: Lippincott, 1965); his "Notes and References" (pp. 324–46) comprise a useful bibliographic essay. For a brief early view, see E. H. Clarke, "Practical Medicine," in the 1876 centenary collection *A Century of American Medicine* (reprint ed., Brinklow, Md.: Old Hickory Bookshop, 1962), pp. 3–72.
10. See the useful short overview by the distinguished historian to whom this volume is dedicated: W. F. Norwood, "Medical Education in the United States before 1900," in C. D. O'Malley, ed., *The History of Medical Education* (Berkeley and Los Angeles: University of California Press, 1970), pp. 463–99.
11. The history of the institutes of medicine as a case study in the life cycle of a discipline

his successors, the institutes consisted of aspects of physiology and therapeutics in addition to the more theoretical part of pathology. In Rush's
case this amounted to the promulgation of a unitary approach to disease
causation, owing much to the Edinburgh physicians William Cullen and
John Brown, as well as to general eighteenth-century views on the stimulation and irritability of nerves and vessels.[12]

Missing from Rush's lexicon was the anatomical viewpoint, the localistic
approach of surgeons. This critical element was to make morbid anatomy
and pathological anatomy a central subject in the medical education of the
first half of the nineteenth century. The reception first of pathological
anatomy in this period and then of cellular pathology a half-century later,
both deriving from technical and intellectual impulses from abroad (France
and Germany respectively), was possible because of the relatively free
crossover between the formal education of physicians and surgeons.
America provided, therefore, an ideal laboratory for an infusion of the
teaching of subjects which, like pathological anatomy, demanded a recep-
tivity in the student toward both the localistic surgical viewpoint and the
"theory and practice of physick."

The most important early impulse from abroad was the pathological
anatomy practiced by Xavier Bichat and his many followers in the Paris
Hospital during the first three decades of the nineteenth century.[13] American medical schools and teaching hospital libraries, lacking indigenous
texts in pathological anatomy, looked to France for insight and instruction. In the first quarter of the century a number of works found their way
into English translation from the continental European (largely but not
exclusively French) literature.[14] Such works tended to polarize along the
theoretical-practical lines, ranging from the treatises of William Cullen
and Johann Blumenbach on the one hand to the works of Xavier Bichat,
Pierre Desault, and Jean Corvisart on the other.[15] Scanning a checklist of
such books reveals the Americans' gaze turning progressively toward the
more localistic French tradition of postmortem dissection as a teaching

---

is yet to be written; it was, however, the subject of an incisive, but apparently as yet
unpublished, Fielding H. Garrison Lecture by Lloyd G. Stevenson.

12. Long, *American Pathology*, p. 17; see also Richard H. Shryock, "The Medical Reputation of Benjamin Rush: Contrasts over Two Centuries," *Bull. Hist. Med.* 45 (1971): 507–52.

13. See Erwin H. Ackerknecht, *Medicine at the Paris Hospital* (Baltimore, Md.: Johns
Hopkins University Press, 1967); and R. C. Maulitz, "A Treatise on Membranes: Concepts
of Tissue Structure, Function, and Dysfunction, from Xavier Bichat to Julius Cohnheim"
(Ph.D. diss., Duke University, 1973), chs. 1–2.

14. Eric Gaskell, "Early American English Translations of European Medical Works,"
Med. Hist. 14 (1970): 300–307.

15. Ibid.

device to link the clinic with theoretical advances. Aware of the relatively freer access of French physicians to dissection and vivisection materials, American medical educators added French texts, both in the original language and in English translation, to their personal and institutional libraries.

Medical students in established eastern medical schools and hospitals enjoyed easier access to such studies than students on the frontier; removed from the port cities of the eastern coast, the latter were largely deprived of such written support for their practical studies in pathology. A few such students attended early schools founded in Lexington, Kentucky, or Cincinnati, Ohio. Because most were trained by apprenticeship, it is difficult to assess the extent of their education in pathology, since it was no doubt largely a sidelight of their training in the institutes or, more particularly, in surgery. Of the elite eastern institutions that acquired textbooks and other works for their students' studies in pathology, almost none have preserved their early working libraries. Hence the range of texts actually used by the early American medical student is also obscure. Further, medical schools have dismantled their early collections as they revitalized new ones. Of the early Philadelphia teaching institutions' libraries, only that of the Pennsylvania Hospital remains as a valuable clue to the reading habits of the physician-in-training during the late eighteenth and early nineteenth centuries.[16]

The Pennsylvania Hospital provides the historian with another important clue to the teaching of pathological anatomy in these early years. From the colonial period to their ritual formalization in the Flexner era,[17] the clinico-pathological correlations made possible by the mandate of the early hospitals and almshouses—the care of sick, invalided, and poor patients—were an invaluable and otherwise nearly unobtainable lesson for the student physician. Some of these early institutions, such as the Pennsylvania Hospital, developed in time into largely private hospitals; others began as almshouses and evolved into general hospitals serving indigent patients during the ethnic and social transformations of the second half of the century. During the nineteenth and early twentieth centuries these institutions became of prime importance for the practical study of pathological anatomy, first at the macroscopic and later at the microscopic level.[18] Because patients in these hospitals died in great

16. Efforts at preserving and cataloguing other libraries, such as that at Transylvania, are also underway or completed; that of the Pennsylvania Hospital is currently being prepared for publication in a manner which promises to be particularly useful to scholars.

17. "Consolidation and Aggrandizement: 1884–1939," below.

18. On the Chicago setting, and the particular importance of Christian Fenger, see James

numbers of a variety of illnesses, physicians were afforded the opportunity to conduct postmortem examinations of the lesions associated with those illnesses.[19] Many such hospitals developed anatomical museums replete with pathological specimens. The relationship of pathologist and clinician both affected and was affected by the one evolving between teaching and patient-care institutions. Academic pathology was a beneficiary of its practitioners' role in the general hospital long before separate departments of pathology came into being; for many decades this relationship survived the invention in the 1870s of the university hospital.[20]

If the early nineteenth-century hospital was one element in the teaching of pathology, the peripatetic lecturer was another. Men like John Godman and John Delamater, teaching multiple subjects including pathological anatomy in multiple institutions, underscore again the symbiosis of pathologist and clinician already mentioned in connection with hospitals: prior to the existence of separate niches for professional pathologists, both roles could be filled by the same individual. Beyond the developed urban east—and in medical academe this meant for the most part beyond Philadelphia and New York—where early medical curricula could effectively be subdivided, the one-man-band motif seen in the peripatetic professors was prevalent in the first quarter of the century and persisted well into the second before fading out.[21]

John Delamater, for example, taught eleven subjects in nine different schools ranging from the Berkshire Medical Institution of Pittsfield, Massachusetts, to the medical department of Western Reserve University in Ohio. Of the eleven different subjects he taught, only two, general pathology and pathological anatomy, represented areas later to be subsumed by pathology as an integral discipline. Yet in the very nature of his

C. Russell, ed., *History of Medicine and Surgery and Physicians and Surgeons of Chicago* (Chicago: Biographical Publishing Corp., 1922).

19. There is no adequate survey of the development of the American hospital; but see Charles E. Rosenberg, "And Heal the Sick: The Hospital and the Patient in Nineteenth-Century America," *J. Soc. Hist.* 10 (1977): 428–47, and the various individual hospital histories cited by him (see especially n. 2, above). Rosenberg is preparing a longer work on the history of patient care in America which will deal in considerable detail with the social and institutional development of hospitals.

20. On the formulation of the idea of the University Hospital, see Corner, *Two Centuries of Medicine*, pp. 133–53; on the critical period after the Civil War in which this took place, see "Convergence: 1847–1884," below.

21. The peripatetic theme in American medical education is well covered in a number of places, including the works of W. F. Norwood; of especial use also is the beginning section on "Medical Education" in Gert H. Brieger, *Medical America in the Nineteenth Century* (Baltimore, Md.: Johns Hopkins University Press, 1972), pp. 3–42.

intellectual range Delamater typified two important features of the teaching of pathology during this period: first, it was taught by those physicians conversant with the manipulative parts of medical practice, such as surgery or obstetrics; and yet, second, it remained susceptible to division between general pathology, which stressed the proximate and remote causes of disease, and special pathology, which, as pathological anatomy, stressed the local lesions resulting from the various specific disease processes.[22]

Another early professor of pathological anatomy in the Berkshire Medical Institution was the peripatetic and influential Elisha Bartlett. He taught pathological anatomy and other subjects at Pittsfield, Woodstock, Dartmouth, Transylvania, Maryland, Louisville, the University of New York, and the College of Physicians and Surgeons of New York.[23] Similarly, Alonzo Clark taught pathological anatomy in a number of New York and New England medical schools before settling in New York to establish a tradition of education in pathology. Samuel David Gross and Austin Flint, who earned major reputations as educators in surgery and medicine, respectively, were also peripatetics who from the inception of their pedagogical travels laid stress on the importance of pathological anatomy; in the second edition of his *Elements of Pathological Anatomy* Gross lamented, with his usual flair for overstatement, "That America with its great hospital facilities should have no school of pathological anatomy is an anomaly that cannot fail to excite the wonder of the age and amazement of posterity . . . a strange, culpable oversight which should be speedily corrected. . . . I only wish that every medical college in the country were compelled to introduce it in its curriculum of studies."[24]

The peripatetic career by which a knowledge of pathology was disseminated was exemplified as well by John Godman. Godman held forth on pathological anatomy in the dissecting rooms of the Philadelphia Almshouse after his 1818 graduation from the medical school of the University of Maryland, an institution that from its inception had laid particular emphasis on normal and pathological anatomy. From Philadelphia he ventured west, spending a period of time in Cincinnati teaching surgery and surgical pathology under the aegis of Daniel Drake (himself a

22. On Delamater much has been written; see esp. F. C. Waite, *Western Reserve University: Centennial History of the School of Medicine* (Cleveland, Ohio: Western Reserve University Press, 1946), p. 513 and passim.

23. On Bartlett and on medical education in general in this period, see Brieger, *Medical America*, pp. 3–42.

24. Quoted in David Rowlands and Esmond Long, *History of the Pathology Department of the University of Pennsylvania* (Philadelphia: University of Pennsylvania Publications Office, 1978), ch. 1.

peripatetic and a proponent of pathology) at the Medical College of Ohio. Returning to Philadelphia, Godman took over Jason Lawrence's teaching in the Philadelphia Anatomical Rooms. The latter context reflected another, closely related, institutional development in the second and third decades of the century, a development that impinged directly on the dissemination of knowledge in pathological anatomy: the establishment of private anatomy schools like the Tremont Street School in Boston.[25]

Here, at mid-century, Oliver Wendell Holmes was exploring, as William E. Horner had been doing at the University of Pennsylvania in the preceding decade and a half, the utility of the microscope in the study of normal and diseased organs.[26] As early as September 1838 Holmes had given special instruction in the Tremont School with lecture-demonstrations in microanatomy. In 1847 he became Parkman Professor of Anatomy and Pathology at Harvard, exemplifying further a typical linkage with a neighboring discipline; later in the same year he became dean of the medical school, and J. B. S. Jackson became professor of pathological anatomy and curator of the museum, exemplifying in turn the "natural historical" bent of the older macroscopic tradition of morbid anatomy.[27]

In the decades preceding the half-century mark, while Horner, Holmes and others were beginning to discern through a glass darkly the research and teaching value of their new optical instruments, two other developments began to affect the teaching of pathology: the emergence of American textbook publishing in pathological anatomy, providing larger numbers of students with exposure to the subject; and a continued strengthening of the magnetic attraction exerted by Paris.

Slowly and fitfully, in the second quarter of the nineteenth century, American medical education was assuming its own infrastructure and becoming less wholly reliant on European medical culture, even while the latter remained a powerful influence. Typical of the early didactic publishing productions of this period were the treatises on pathological anatomy produced by two of Benjamin Rush's colleagues and successors at the University of Pennsylvania, William Horner and Samuel Jackson. The former, as professor of anatomy, published in 1829 what probably qualifies as the first American textbook of pathology, a *Treatise on Pathological Anatomy*. Three years later his colleague, Jackson, who as professor of the institutes was responsible for physiology and for diagnosis

25. Thomas F. Harrington, *The Harvard Medical School: 1782–1905*, 3 vols. (New York: Lewis, 1905), 2:535–36 and passim.
26. Cassedy, "The Microscope," p. 81.
27. Harrington, *Harvard Medical School*, p. 499.

and treatment as well as general pathology, published his text on *The Principle of Medicine Founded on the Structure and Functions of the Animal Organism*. In it he noted the debt owed to Horner by American medical men, and lamented the underdeveloped role of pathological anatomy in American medical education and practice.[28] While French works in pathological anatomy, notably the *Elements of General Pathology* of Auguste F. Chomel and the monographs on phthisis and similar subjects by Pierre Louis, continued to be translated in the second quarter of the century, American works became more numerous in the 1830s and 1840s. From the publishing capital of Philadelphia, the textbooks of pathology that appeared from the pens of Samuel D. Gross in 1839 and Alfred Stillé in 1848 extended the growing journal literature of Godman, Drake, and others, and the medical lexicography of Robley Dunglison.

From the 1820s on, despite the fact that the Paris School had already passed its moment of greatest intellectual innovation, and despite (or perhaps in part because of) the growing self-reliance of American medical education, English-speaking students from Great Britain and the United States finished their education in Paris under the likes of Chomel and Louis. In search of the clinical patina provided by the French emphasis on physical diagnosis and pathological anatomy, Americans such as George Shattuck, Jr., William W. Gerhard, Alfred Stillé, Henry I. Bowditch, Caspar Pennock, James Jackson, Jr., and Oliver W. Holmes studied under Louis in Paris.[29] The importance of this early intellectual migration did not reside (as would be the case with a later generation's exodus to Germany and Austria) in the sheer numbers of students proceeding to the European continent to acquire the latest clinico-pathological approaches. Rather, American students' exposure in the 1820s and 1830s to Louis and to the Paris School was that of a small elite whose impact after their return was disproportionate to their numbers—precisely because they all returned to teach pathological anatomy in American medical schools and to publish in the field.

CONVERGENCE: 1847–1884

The microscope, in opening a window for medical men on the very small, provided expansive new intellectual and professional vistas. Its use in medical teaching and practice extended during the fourth and fifth dec-

28. Rowlands and Long, *History of the Pathology Department*, p. 2.
29. The still classic exposition is that of William Osler, "The Influence of Louis on American Medicine," in *An Alabama Student and Other Biographical Essays* (New York: Oxford University Press, 1909), pp. 189–210.

ades of the nineteenth century into the various branches of medicine, including pathological anatomy, and became a necessary if not sufficient condition for the infusion of the scientific ethos into medicine.

One should of course be careful not to link this ethos or ideology of science too intimately with any given technology, even if that combination of technology and ideology was to have a decisive influence on the teaching of pathology in late-nineteenth-century American medical schools. Oliver Wendell Holmes returned to Boston from Paris and the tutelage of Pierre Louis, unable to "remember ever hearing one word about the microscope or the results obtained from its employment."[30] Yet by 1847, which may be said to mark the beginning of the maturation of pathology in America, Holmes possessed and used two imported instruments, a Chevalier and an Oberhäuser.

Neither the medical use of the microscope per se nor even the cell theory of Matthias Schleiden and Theodor Schwann was in the 1840s the deciding factor in the recasting of the teaching of pathology. Rather, that pivotal role in the remodelling of pathology was to be played in the 1840s and 1850s by the adoption by American medical educators of cellular pathology. A theoretical system for explaining pathological change based squarely on the use of the microscope, cellular pathology had been elaborated by Rudolf Virchow in the Pathological Institute of Berlin in the mid-1850s. But pathology as an organized discipline in the United States actually had begun in the preceding decade: in 1847 J. B. S. Jackson of Boston and Alonzo Clark of New York both assumed full-time pathology positions in their respective medical schools, Harvard and the College of Physicians and Surgeons.

Jackson, the reticent and patient-shy nephew of the acclaimed clinician James Jackson, was at once the first professional pathologist and one of the last academic pathological anatomists of the old natural historical tradition. That tradition stressed his talents as curator of a museum of morbid anatomy, rather than the talents, as a microscopist, of another likely colleague, Oliver W. Holmes. In New York, however, the same year saw Alonzo Clark appointed to the post of lecturer in physiology and pathology with the recommendation from the board of trustees that

> the subject of physiology is now confined to the professor of anatomy. It has been found, however, that anatomy is required to be taught so minutely, to meet the wants of the students, that it is impossible for the same professor to do justice to the other branch.

30. From Holmes's "Address to the Boston Microscopical Society," quoted in Cassedy, "The Microscope," p. 81.

On the other hand, the recent application of improved microscopes to healthy and diseased structures, together with the great advances in the Department of animal chemistry, and the light it has shed on the constitution of our bodies in health and disease, and upon healthy and disordered functions, leave an hiatus in these Departments so great that, in the unanimous opinion of the Board, a new professorship is required.[31]

Although the professorship was not formally endowed until 1873—during the decade in which pathology truly flowered as an institutionalized subject—Clark's lectures were well received from the outset. The 1852 catalogue of the College of Physicians and Surgeons noted that his course

has been a very important addition to the regular course of instruction, and is the only course of the kind in this country. The lectures on physiology embrace the minute anatomy of the tissues, and are amply illustrated by magnified drawings, and by frequent demonstrations under the microscope. The course on pathology is equally full, and is constantly enriched by the exhibition and demonstration of recent specimens illustrating the various changes produced in tissues and organs by disease.[32]

If one examines the careers in the 1850s of these two proto-pathologists, Jackson and Clark, along with that of Nathan Smith Davis, active in the teaching of pathology at Rush Medical College, several points become apparent concerning a field in transition. Whereas Jackson was responsible almost exclusively for pathology at Harvard, Clark at Columbia was bringing the new microscopy into his teaching even while he continued in the earlier, traditional mode spanning two or more subjects. Davis in Chicago covered the same intellectual spread as did Clark, but returned in the late 1850s to clinical medicine. Well into the twentieth century this was to remain a common alternative career pattern for medical men who combined expertise at the bedside, autopsy table, and microscope bench.[33]

Although German academic pathology grew and prospered in the 1850s and 1860s, it was not until after a lag phase of a decade and a half that

31. In the "Memorial of the Board of Trustees of the College of Physicians and Surgeons to the Regents of Columbia University," quoted in John C. Dalton, *History of the College of Physicians and Surgeons in the City of New York* (New York: College of Physicians and Surgeons, 1888), p. 91; see also John Shrady, *The College of Physicians and Surgeons of New York: A History* (New York: Lewis, n.d.).

32. Dalton, *History of the College of Physicians and Surgeons*, p. 92.

33. On Chicago see Russell, *History of Medicine and Surgery*, and Thomas N. Bonner, *Medicine in Chicago, 1850–1950: A Chapter in the Social and Scientific Development of a City* (Madison, Wis.: American History Research Center, 1957).

American medical educators began concertedly to embrace the new methods in teaching and in research developed by their European counterparts. Then, in the 1870s and 1880s, two trends, both relating to newly emerging patterns of American medical education, began to impinge on the teaching of pathology. The first was a new intellectual wave of eastward migration, this time to Germany and in much larger numbers than the earlier migration to France, of young medical men eager to assimilate the new scientific medicine. The other was the concomitant establishment on American shores, in the space of two decades, of new positions or new departments in pathology at nearly every major medical school. In 1869, more than a decade before the influential Dane Christian Fenger arrived in Chicago to put his stamp on both surgery and pathology at the Rush and Northwestern medical schools, at least one and perhaps both schools were able to appoint professors with primary responsibility for the teaching of pathology, H. F. Chesbrough and J. H. Hollister, respectively. At the Medical College of the Pacific, Edwin Bentley assumed the professorship of descriptive and microscopic anatomy and pathology in 1870. Reginald H. Fitz, an exponent of the new pathology, gained influence (and a department) at Harvard in the late 1870s. At Dartmouth a chair of general pathology was created in 1871. In New Orleans, the Tulane curriculum rested on the obvious if traditional merits of Stanford Chaillé, demonstrator of anatomy since the 1850s, and ushered pathology into a significant place only when it came to include bacteriology after 1889.[34]

In Philadelphia, on the other hand, James Tyson quietly began studying the microscopic appearances of urine and morbid tissues without benefit of study abroad; he consulted with fellow physicians on such matters, as microscopist to the Philadelphia (later Philadelphia General) Hospital, and lectured on microscopy and urinary chemistry (in the process roughing out the contours of chemical pathology) in 1870/71. By 1873/74 Tyson was clinical lecturer on pathological anatomy and histology, but only in 1877/78 did he become professor of general pathology and morbid anatomy.[35] The changes in title reflect more than sterile symbolism: this was a critical decade for pathology. Its evolution was impelled both by new theoretical advances from Germany and by changes closer to home in the American system of higher education, changes allowing greater division of expertise and labor in the academic marketplace.

34. Russell, *History of Medicine and Surgery*, pp. 192–208; also H. E. Ernst, *Harvard Medical School, 1782–1906* ([Boston: n.p., 1906]); Carleton B. Chapman, *Dartmouth Medical School: The First 175 Years* (Hanover, N.H.: University Press of New England, 1973); and L. R. Chandler, *Pioneering in Health* (San Francisco: Stanford Associates, n.d.).
35. Rowlands and Long, *History of the Pathology Department*, ch. 1.

No doubt some of the changes in the purview and title of those charged with teaching pathology were cosmetic and did not reflect what the medical student learned. Certainly not all of those enjoying new posts and departments had formative training in the German mode of high scientific medicine. But for those who did go to Germany, pathology was the central discipline, the scientific basis of clinical medicine. Training in Germany, however, did not guarantee instant academic success and a host of attentive ears on a young medical scholar's return. Although T. Mitchell Prudden went to Heidelberg and William H. Welch to Strasbourg and Breslau in 1876, the former returned to deaf ears in New York City, while the latter accepted an obscure post at the Bellevue Hospital Medical College. But Welch was persistent; he had proved himself in the German laboratories of two of Rudolf Virchow's most esteemed protégés, Friedrich von Recklinghausen and Julius Cohnheim, men who represented polar approaches to the pathology that Virchow had carefully and programmatically limned. Said Welch:

> I am sure that I could not find a better place [than Breslau] to learn pathology; it seems to flow in at every pore. Cohnheim himself is not a learned man, in the sense in which Virchow commands the whole history of pathology, but . . . he has actually revolutionized every department of pathology to which he had devoted himself.[36]

Armed with both the experimental pathology of Cohnheim and Virchow's grand vision of what pathology could and should be, Welch had returned to the United States determined to enact a similar institutional program. In a step heralded in virtually every historical account of American medical education, he accepted an invitation in 1884 to assume a professorship at a new university in Baltimore, the Johns Hopkins.

CONSOLIDATION AND AGGRANDIZEMENT: 1884–1939

During Welch's first stay in Cohnheim's Breslau, the clinician Robert Koch had made a number of visits to Ferdinand Cohn, while Carl Weigert

---

36. One cannot begin to list all the treatments of Welch, the founding of Hopkins, and the role therein of pathology. But see Thomas N. Bonner, *American Doctors and German Universities: A Chapter in International Intellectual Relations, 1870–1914* (Lincoln, Neb.: University of Nebraska Press, 1963), from which I quote here, p. 113; Owsei Temkin, "The European Background of the Young Dr. Welch," reprinted in *The Double Face of Janus and Other Essays in the History of Medicine* (Baltimore, Md.: Johns Hopkins University Press, 1977), pp. 252–60; Richard H. Shryock, *The Unique Influence of the Johns Hopkins University on American Medicine* (Copenhagen: Munksgaard, 1953); Donald Fleming, *William H. Welch and the Rise of Modern Medicine* (Boston: Little, Brown, 1954); and Simon and James T. Flexner, *William Henry Welch and the Heroic Age of American Medicine* (New York: Viking, 1941; reprint ed., Dover, 1966).

and Paul Ehrlich were already well under way with their bacteriological investigations. Their early work had little impact before 1882, but within a decade Welch was back in Germany from Johns Hopkins to learn more about the newly recognized pathogenicity of bacterial organisms. Thus began the uneasy union in the medical curriculum of two nascent disciplines, one but slightly older than the other. For about a quarter of a century—that is, until World War I—pathology dominated bacteriology in medical school teaching, with the latter enjoying rather looser links with hygiene and clinical teaching.

By the end of the 1880s, the decade in which the promise of Koch and his bacteriological postulates was beginning to become apparent, then, medical school courses in pathology were doubly invigorated by German bacteriology and cellular pathology. Although many, if not most, of the German textbooks of pathology being read in translation by American medical students—Frank Chance's translation of Rudolf Virchow's *Cellular Pathology* (1860), Theodor Billroth's *Surgical Pathology* (1884), Julius Cohnheim's *General Pathology* (1889), and the popular Wood's Library edition of Ernst Ziegler's *General Pathological Anatomy and Pathogenesis*—did not yet emphasize bacteriology, American pathology courses began to incorporate bacteriological insights and findings.

There are student notebooks extant from a variety of institutions that bear out this assertion. One may look beyond William H. Welch's European-modelled Johns Hopkins, at least to those schools that continued to compete with Johns Hopkins in purveying an elite, scientific medical education during the two decades before Flexner. A particularly interesting example of such firsthand accounts of courses of pathology may be found in the durable and varied tradition of medical education in Philadelphia. Surviving notebooks from a variety of courses in the University of Pennsylvania permit, because of that institution's early roots, a vista stretching over a century on the changing place of pathology in the medical curriculum. They also underscore the point that pathology grew out of the various clinical subjects.[37]

Thus in a much earlier era, aspects of pathology had been presented in courses on the institutes and practice of medicine as well as on surgery. Benjamin Smith Barton's lectures on the institutes had been broken down along classical nosological lines, in which "the art of discerning and listing of diseases may be best obtained by an accurate and complete observation of their phenomena, by means of which we may arrange diseases accord-

37. My examination of these MS notebooks was facilitated by the gracious cooperation of the Historical Collections of the College of Physicians of Philadelphia, Mrs. Ellen Gartrell, Curator.

ing to their genera and species."[38] Emphasizing the various fevers that had scourged Philadelphia and other port cities, Barton had where possible included his ideas, based on his scheme of general pathology, of the state of the art of discerning proximate causes and mechanisms of disease. Hence he taught that dysentery "consists according to Cullen of a preternatural constriction of the colon. . . . Hoffman again thinks it depends upon an oscillation or convulsion of the large intestines . . . with which the system sympathisis [*sic*]."[39]

More accessible to the twentieth-century reader are notes of a series of surgical lectures, perhaps delivered by J. R. Coxe at Pennsylvania in 1822/23. The surgeon, too, is concerned with classes of disease— "eresipelas, oedema, burns, mortification, wounds" are contiguous entries and topics to be taken up—but he begins with a long disquisition on inflammation and its treatment from the standpoint of the pathological anatomist: "Nothing is more necessary to the surgeon than the principles of inflammation. . . . Inflammation does not immediately follow the application of the cause: the space of 24 hours sometimes intervening. . . . If Inflammation be not stopped by some of the means above mentioned, it proceeds to a suppuration." Of psoas abscess: "This disease is seated in the cellular membrane under the Psoas muscle where matter is deposited in a cist of the cellular substance."[40]

Three-quarters of a century later pathology was being taught as a unitary subject in the lectures of James Tyson. His 1888/89 course in pathology was completely oriented toward cellular pathology: "The vast majority of diseases reside in the cell."[41] The Virchowian influence is readily apparent. On October 15 he discusses cloudy swelling of the cells and fatty metamorphosis; on October 20 he turns to atrophy and necrosis (seen as a form of nutritional arrest), as well as inflammation. Before moving on to tumors—also a Virchowian rubric—he dwells on the problem of inflammation: acute, granulomatous, tuberculous. He notes in that last category that the tubercle is devoid of blood vessels, and that on "Mar 24, 1882 Koch made comment that the Bacillus tuberculosis was the cause. This is now the accepted belief. It is an infectious disease—one

38. MS notebook (H. Van der Veer) on the institutes and practice of medicine in the University of Pennsylvania, 1814–1815, given by Benjamin Smith Barton (College of Physicians of Philadelphia, Historical Collections), p. 1. Students' names are given in parentheses in subsequent references to notebooks from the same collection.

39. Ibid., p. 139.

40. MS notebook (F. J. LeMoyne) on the course in surgery in the University of Pennsylvania by J. R. Coxe [?], 1822–1823, pp. 1, 5, 17, 41.

41. MS notebook (Joseph McFarland) on pathology in the University of Pennsylvania by James Tyson, 1888–1889, unpaginated. The frontispiece of this notebook bears the student's pictorial sketch of the bust of a suitably avuncular appearing Tyson, beneath which is the inscription: "My dear children . . . you make me feel like a first rate nursery maid."

due to a specific cause."[42] After sixteen lectures on general pathology—
the general causes and mechanisms of disease according to the canons of
cellular pathology—Tyson moves ahead to special pathology, "the
pathological anatomy of the organs," beginning with the blood—its purposes and its dyscrasias (including the anemias with "Osler's classification
of anaemia").

In the next year another student provided a set of "Notes on General
Pathology from the Lectures to the Medical Class of 93 at the University
of Pennsylvania by John Guiteras, M.D." Here a marked increase in
emphasis on bacteriology may be noted, along with a continued stress on
inflammation, "a reaction of the parablastic tissues to the action of irri-
tants," citing Augustus Waller, René "Deutroscher" [*sic*], William Ad-
dison and Julius Cohnheim.[43]

The emphasis on bacteriology is most pronounced, however, in the
period just after the turn of the century, the period when the various
biomedical disciplines were jockeying for position in the American medical curriculum. In the "Outline of Regular and Special Pathology" given
as a set of lectures (and published) at the Medico-Chirurgical College of
Philadelphia by Joseph MacFarland—the pathologist whose attendance
at Tyson's lectures a decade earlier is attested above—"Infection and
Immunity" occupy the first of three parts of the outline. While he did not
make them as voluminous as Part III covering morbid anatomy, MacFarland had advisedly put his Part I on bacteriology, along with his Part II on
"The Pathology of Metabolism" (a nod to another new science, physiological chemistry, on which pathologists had designs), up front where they
would catch the reader or listener freshly and quickly. For a while, then,
pathology and bacteriology were particularly intimate companions in the
medical curriculum.[44]

It is not surprising that when the Committee of One Hundred of the
Council on Medical Education of the American Medical Association reported in 1909 on its model medical curriculum, the subcommittee preparing its section on pathology and bacteriology was chaired by William
H. Welch's former student, the Harvard-based William T. Councilman,
with Welch himself an active member.[45] This report must be viewed in

42. Ibid.
43. MS notebook (J. M. Swan) on general pathology from the lectures to the medical class
of 93 at the University of Pennsylvania by John Guiteras, M.D., unpaginated.
44. MS notebook (M. F. Percival) on the outline of regular and special pathology as
taught by [Joseph MacFarland in] the Medico-Chirurgical College of Philadelphia, 1901–
1905.
45. Councilman's own syllabus was heavily oriented toward bacteriology (W. T. Councilman and F. B. Mallory, *Pathology: Syllabus* [Boston: Fairbanks, 1904]). On the back-

the context of the elaborate feinting and posturing that formed the pre-
lude to the Flexner Report, which was to appear in the following year.
Seen in this light, the 1909 model curriculum report is especially in-
triguing: one may, for example, compare the brief two-page report of
Councilman's subcommittee with page after page of detailed recommendations of others, such as the subcommittee on organic and physiological
chemistry and physiology. The latter specified prerequisites, minimum
hours, optional courses, teaching methods, instructors' qualifications,
equipment and many other features of the proposed program. The
pathologists simply stressed the importance of laboratory teaching and
proper equipment, and let it go at that. Either they felt quite secure in
the curriculum or could agree on little more than the minimum
statement—or both.[46]

What is certain is that in the years around the First World War, pathology and bacteriology began to subdivide and go their separate ways.
Departments of bacteriology and hygiene began to emerge from the
pathology-dominated institutional and curricular forms that had spawned
them.[47] Within thirty years the process of fission was largely complete. At
the end of the 1930s a task force headed by Herman G. Weiskotten
surveyed the sixty-six four-year regular medical schools then accredited
by the AMA Council on Medical Education and Hospitals. Noting that
forty-eight of the schools now had separately budgeted departments of
pathology, they stated flatly that

> although twenty-two schools had combined bacteriology and
> pathology in a single department, in practically every instance in
> which the two subjects appeared to be managed successfully there
> was separate personnel for teaching and research in each subject
> and the support of the combined department was such that neither
> group was seriously handicapped. In other words, the combination
> was largely artificial and bacteriology virtually functioned as a sepa-
> rate and independent department. In other cases the combined

---

ground to the Flexner Report, see Robert H. Hudson, "Abraham Flexner in Perspective: American Medical Education, 1865–1910," *Bull. Hist. Med.* 46 (1972): 545–61.

46. Committee on Medical Education of the AMA, *A Model Medical Curriculum: Report of the Committee of One Hundred*, AMA Bulletin No. 5, 1909, pp. 48–64;
for a school-by-school breakdown on the place of these subjects, with respect to timing
and balance between course offerings, see U.S. Bureau of Education, *Courses
of Study in Medical Schools* (Washington: Government Printing Office, 1899).

47. See, for example, the description of the events leading up to the split between
pathology and bacteriology at Western Reserve by Waite, *Western Reserve University*, p.
390.

department served as a definite hindrance to the development of both subjects from the standpoint of teaching as well as research.[48]

Welch, his students, and his colleagues were able both to establish pathology as a useful and "saleable" discipline in the medical school curriculum and to win for it pride of place over virtually all the other basic sciences as the final scientific proving ground for medical students embarking on their clinical careers. It is a story well rehearsed in the annals of medical education. What historians have understood less clearly about the decades bracketing the turn of the twentieth century is the manner in which pathology and clinical medicine continued to interpenetrate in the medical curriculum.

The various ways in which this relationship was preserved may be seen in a number of cases. Pathology's delicate poise between the laboratory and the clinic was reflected in the career patterns of those who taught it and in the teaching forms they devised to support it. In New York, for example, while Mitchell Prudden elected the laboratory as his primary venue, Francis Delafield straddled the laboratory and the clinic. Like Prudden and Welch, Delafield had furthered his medical training with study trips to England and the Continent, and like them he had returned convinced of the Virchowian wisdom: pathology was the backbone of medical research and medical education. But unlike his contemporaries, Delafield retained his interest in bedside medicine; as an internist he therefore emphasized and lectured to his students at the College of Physicians and Surgeons on the importance of the connection between pathology and clinical medicine.[49]

William Osler was of a similar persuasion. In Montreal and later in Philadelphia Osler performed autopsies and formulated his cases in terms of clinico-pathological correlations, which he drilled into his students in rounds and in his writing. The title page of his earliest monograph (1878) bears the dictum of the English pathologist Samuel Wilks: "Pathology is the basis of all true instruction in practical medicine."[50] At the turn of the century Osler was to reminisce about this early vantage point: "From the chair of the Institutes of Medicine at McGill, both physiology and pathology were taught . . . I soon found that my chief interest was in the pathological part of the work." Four years later he noted that "no more instructive work is possible than carefully demonstrated specimens illus-

48. Herman G. Weiskotten, et al., *Medical Education in the United States, 1934–39* (Chicago: American Medical Association, 1940), pp. 155, 161.

49. Long, *History of American Pathology*, pp. 136–37.

50. Quoted in the useful article by Howard B. Burchell, "Osler: In Quest of the Gnostic Grail in Morbid Anatomy," *J. Hist. Med.* 30 (1975): 235–49; p. 237.

trating disturbance of function and explanatory of the clinical symptoms." And six years later (1909), again: "As is our pathology so is our practice; what the pathologist thinks today, the physician does tomorrow."[51]

As Eugene Opie was later to reemphasize, Osler turned easily, at Old Blockley and in subsequent sites where he attended on the wards, from the postmortem room and microscope to the bedside. His seminal text on *The Principles and Practice of Medicine*, a milestone in the pedagogical history of internal medicine, was an outgrowth of his conviction about the intimate relationship between the two disciplines.[52]

Perhaps the most influential teaching tool devised to shore up the relationship between the clinicians' and pathologists' viewpoints emerged from neither Baltimore nor Philadelphia, but rather from Boston. In 1900 Walter Bradford Cannon of the Harvard Medical School, a man who would come to symbolize the link between clinical medicine and another of the basic sciences, physiology, published an article suggesting a correlative approach to "case methods of teaching systematic medicine."[53] Ten years later Dr. Richard Cabot modified Cannon's suggestions and established the Case Records of the Massachusetts General Hospital, more widely and generically known as the Clinico-Pathologic Conference. The CPC became a fixture in most of the medical schools of the United States between 1910 and the Second World War, persisting in many locales down to the present time—if only, as was often the case, in attenuated form. For decades the CPC was, however, a major event— often *the* major event—in the intellectual life of the American medical school, satisfying a variety of social needs: it focussed the attentions of attending and student physician alike, encouraging them to match wits in reaching the pathologic diagnosis. And it cemented the special relationship between pathologist and clinician, who were, despite their overt attempts to stump one another in the conference exercise, joined in the symbiosis of scientific medicine.[54]

EPILOGUE: THE LATE TWENTIETH CENTURY

The notion that pathology was the scientific basis of medicine had served, even after bacteriology was shorn away and given separate-but-equal status in the curriculum, as the field's claim to preeminence among the

51. Ibid., pp. 237–38.
52. Eugene L. Opie, "Osler as a Pathologist," *Bull. Hist. Med.* 23 (1949): 321–26.
53. Walter B. Cannon, "Case Medicine of Teaching Systematic Medicine," *Boston Med. & Surg. J.* 142 (1900): 31–36.
54. "CPCs on Matters Gray and White" [editorial], *N. Eng. J. Med.* 280 (1969): 384.

medical schools' basic science subjects. After Flexner the other basic sciences began making and documenting the appropriateness of similar claims; this process continued to gain momentum, particularly in the era of big science which began after World War II. The status of pathology as most favored discipline in the training of young physicians was eroded in the research sector as the National Institutes of Health and other sources distributed funds to many competing biomedical disciplines. Here one should recall that there is a complex and reflexive relationship between the research, teaching, and service functions of those who "profess" the various disciplines. Pathology after World War II began to suffer from an unravelling of those functions. Preclinical teaching in pathology began to recede from the leading edge of pathological research, which was progressively more concerned with immunopathology and subcellular injury.

While those responsible for the pathology segment of the "new curricula" in postwar medical education valiantly attempted to incorporate the new findings into their teaching, they often found themselves besieged on several flanks at once. Teaching hospitals often arrogated to themselves the service functions of pathology departments, leaving the teaching and research flanks financially and administratively exposed. Immunology and molecular biology on the research side were hardly the preserve of pathologists alone, and curriculum committees found them to be inappropriately reduplicated in the curriculum. This led, in turn, to revamped curricula in which the basic sciences lost, by and large, required teaching hours. Responding to this challenge, academic pathologists in many cases eliminated or cut back on special pathology in the required curriculum. Surveys of pathology organ by organ and system by system became elective courses for subsequent medical school years, although they often remained quite popular. The required course in pathology, emphasizing theory, was ironically close once again to the general pathology course of a much earlier era. And pathology, in teaching as in research, found itself in an identity crisis from which it continued to strive to recover.[55]

55. A muted view of these changes is given in Rowlands and Long, *History of the Pathology Department*, pp. 83–105; a more pointed assessment is that of H. Popper, "The Identity Crisis of Pathology," *Mt. Sinai J. Med.* 41 (1974): 311–17. See also H. Popper and D. W. King, "The Situation of American Pathology, 1975: Education Problems Yesterday, Today and Tomorrow," *Beitr. Pathol.* 156 (1974): 85–94.

Internal Medicine

EDWARD C. ATWATER

BY an application of the science of acoustics to diseases of the chest, we are now enabled to pronounce with unerring precision upon the nature, location and extent of diseases of the circulatory and respiratory organs, which less than half a century ago were veiled in impenetrable darkness and obscurity." So said the president of the Medical Society of the State of New York to those assembled for the annual meeting of the organization in 1854.[1] Exaggerated as the claim may be, it is hard for us who take for granted the methods of physical examination to appreciate the changes that occurred in medicine in the four decades before the American Civil War.

At the beginning of the nineteenth century there was no stethoscope, no clinical thermometer, no percussion hammer, no ophthalmoscope, no sphygmomanometer, and no useful microscope. Though Hippocrates had

Acknowledgment: Mr. Philip Weimerskirch, history of medicine librarian at the Edward G. Miner Library of the University of Rochester School of Medicine and Dentistry, found many useful source materials; and Miss Sandra Markus, interlibrary loan librarian, was able to obtain for me many materials not available locally. Useful suggestions came from Drs. Lawrence A. Kohn, Donald G. Anderson, and William L. Morgan, Jr.

1. Jenks S. Sprague, "Annual Address," *Trans. Med. Soc. St. N.Y.* (1854): 17.

described the succussion splash of pleural or cavitary effusion more than two thousand years earlier and Leopold Auenbrugger's work on percussion had appeared in 1761, they were generally ignored. In fact, the known methods of physical examination, including direct auscultation by placing the ear on the chest wall, were seldom used or mastered technically; and the significance of the information that could be obtained by such means was obscure. Beyond superficially inspecting a patient and perhaps feeling the pulse, the American physician devoted little time to physical examination.[2] Nor did he attempt to reconstruct the natural history of the patient's illness in any systematic way.

He knew little about what went on within the body, in health or disease. The nature of some functions could be inferred from anatomical knowledge, obtained by dissecting cadavers. However, physiology was in its infancy, and vivisection, later its fundamental technique, was not yet employed. Though Giovanni Morgagni had demonstrated toward the end of the eighteenth century that disease usually produced distinctive changes in specific organs, it was not possible to identify or evaluate these changes in the living patient. Physicians continued to deal with disease and treatment largely in a priori philosophical terms, referring to fever as a disease and unbalanced humors as a cause.

By the end of the nineteenth century physical examination was a highly sophisticated method with an array of bedside instruments. The perfection of the microscope made it possible to go from the organ pathology of Morgagni and the tissue pathology of Xavier Bichat to the cellular concepts of Rudolf Virchow, and the later introduction of the oil immersion lens greatly aided the development of microbiology. The discovery of anesthesia made vivisection practical, thereby providing the physiologist with his most important tool. The microscope and developments in chemistry made it possible to study the morphological and molecular elements of body fluids. All of these advances contributed to the practice of medicine generally. But it was application of the stethoscope, more than anything else, that made internal medicine a separate discipline.

Internal medicine, like most specialties, acquired a separate identity as a result of new technology that required specialized training. The need to learn the methods of physical diagnosis, particularly use of the stethoscope, made individualized bedside teaching necessary and the previously popular grand walking round and the clinical lecture inadequate. Once proficiency in the use of certain tools became essential, the method

2. Dr. Edward A. Holyoke, well-known teacher and physician of Salem, Massachusetts, was an exception. He used direct auscultation in 1793 on a fifty-three-year-old man to diagnose empyema with bronchopleural fistula. An autopsy proved him correct ("Auscultation in Boston in 1793," *Boston Med. & Surg. J.* 58 [1858]: 83–84).

of giving clinical instruction had to change from a passive to an active one.[3]

It was not until the twentieth century, however, that undergraduate instruction at American medical schools regularly included practical clinical training and medical students routinely examined patients carefully and recorded the details of their illnesses. The reasons for this delay were economic and social as well as technological. In order to provide such training there had to be hospitals where large groups of patients could be examined under supervision, a situation that did not exist generally until the end of the nineteenth century. Financial subsidies for medical education were also necessary so that class size could be limited and sufficient faculty provided for individual bedside instruction. Course length had to be increased in order to provide time for clinical instruction. Once these prerequisites were available, the individualized teaching method, called the clinical clerkship, became virtually universal. It has remained the fundamental way of teaching internal medicine.

The "internal" concept itself reflected the fact that the techniques of physical examination, especially auscultation and percussion, made it possible to examine the "inside" of a patient from the outside. In contrast to this, surgery still dealt almost exclusively with the then "external" problems of orthopedics, urology, and superficial tumors. With the coming of anesthesia, asepsis, and the surgical invasion of the body at the end of the century, the surgeon became, in fact, the internist, but the contrary usage was by then established.

The term *internal medicine* came into general use late in the nineteenth century. Before then the great body of medicine, from which surgery and obstetrics had already been separated, was known as physic and its teachers as professors of the theory and practice of physic. The founding of a Society for Internal Medicine in Berlin in 1881, the holding of the first Congress of Internal Medicine in Germany in 1882, and the organizing of the Association of American Physicians in 1885 officially introduced the new term.

In the evolution of the teaching of internal medicine several themes are important: the introduction of a special technology, the development of hospitals for teaching, the delay in providing individual clinical experience for the undergraduate until financial subsidies made it possible to limit class size and increase the number of faculty, and the more recent

---

3. John Ware, who later succeeded James Jackson as Hersey Professor of Theory and Practice of Physic at Harvard, drew attention to this fact in one of his clinical lectures as early as 1835. In clinical attendance, he said, the student must not be passive. Learning physical signs is a slow process except in a hospital with instruction (Ware Papers, Box 2, Francis A. Countway Library, Harvard Medical School, Boston, Mass.).

effect of specialization and graduate training programs on undergraduate clinical instruction.

THE TECHNOLOGY OF INTERNAL MEDICINE

Following the publication of the *Traité de l'auscultation médiate* by René-Théophile-Hyacinthe Laennec in 1819, in which the author described the use of his stethoscope for studying the acoustics of the respiratory and cardiovascular systems, diagnosis became a science. Laennec's contribution was not merely the device that made his observations more precise but also the care with which he made his examination and the way he interpreted his data in terms of anatomical change. By associating particular sounds with structural abnormalities later found at autopsy, it was possible to predict or describe what was occurring internally in organs hidden from view in the living patient.

Unlike Auenbrugger's long-obscure work, Laennec's was soon well known.[4] In 1820 a translation of a French review appeared in an American journal,[5] and the following year an American physician wrote that "the continued use of this instrument has satisfied us more and more of the benefits which may be attained by it." He added, however, that it would take a lot of hard work and practice.[6] Laennec's book itself was published in Philadelphia in 1823, two years after the appearance of an English translation in London. By 1839 there had been nineteen printings in French, German, Italian, and English, four of them in the United States.[7]

In 1824 John Bell, a Philadelphian who had studied with Laennec, published the first American work on the subject of stethoscopy, entitled "Some General Remarks on the Use of the Stethoscope, as an Aid in Forming a Correct Diagnosis of Diseases of the Lungs, Together with Some Observations on the Symptom Called by M. Laennec, Pectoriloquy."[8] That same year, a twenty-two-year-old medical student, Edmund Strudwick of North Carolina, published some reports that included stethoscopic examination of patients he had cared for on the wards of the

---

4. Hippocratic authority and the fact that Auenbrugger had no students to spread the word delayed acceptance of the "New Invention" (Bernhard J. Stern, *Social Factors in Medical Progress* [New York: Columbia University Press, 1927], p. 52). On the other hand, Laennec and those who followed him were active teachers.

5. *Am. Med. Record* 3 (1820): 53–46.

6. *N. Eng. J. Med. & Surg.* 10 (1821): 132–56, 265–93; quotation on p. 293.

7. Henry R. Viets, " 'De l'auscultation médiate' of Laennec," *Arch. Surg.* 18 (1929): 1280–97.

8. *N. Y. Med. & Phys. J.* 3 (1824): 268–81. Only four Americans are known to have studied with Laennec. Another one of them, Samuel George Morton (M.D., University of Pennsylvania, 1820) wrote what William Osler later called "the earliest and one of the best books on phthisis written in America."

Philadelphia Almshouse.[9] Soon American publishers were providing a succession of French and English works on stethoscopy, the former usually translated by Americans who had studied in Paris.[10] Two men, Samuel Jackson, attending physician at the almshouse in Philadelphia, and James Jackson, Hersey Professor of the Theory and Practice of Physic at Harvard, were major sponsors in introducing stethoscopy to America,[11] probably because each of them had students who studied in Paris and returned as "apostles of the school of observation."[12]

The older men found the new technique difficult. James Jackson acknowledged his ears were "old and were not trained early. . . . [Oliver Wendell] Holmes has attended to auscultation more than any other of my (recent) pupils and I often call on him to help me with my ears." To his son he wrote that he did not expect to master the stethoscope, "yet I expect you to do it. It is incomparably easier for you than for me."[13] The senior generation did recognize the instrument's importance. Jackson's colleague, the versatile Jacob Bigelow, wrote in 1839 that "the discoveries of Laennec . . . have constituted the most important acquisition which medical science has received during the present century."[14]

Between 1820 and 1860 almost six hundred young American physicians

9. Edmund Strudwick, "Remarks on the Stethoscope in Relation to Phthisis Pulmonis," *Phila. J. Med. & Phys. Sci.* 8 (1824): 33–52. The Almshouse was predecessor of the famous Philadelphia General Hospital at Blockley, Pennsylvania.

10. Martinet, 1827; Collin, 1829; Williams, 1830; Meriadec Laennec, 1832; Rouanet, 1833; Louis, 1834; Raciborski, 1839; Hope, 1842; Walshe, 1843.

11. Austin Flint, recalling his medical student days at Harvard in 1832, said that James Jackson "was earnestly engaged in the subject of physical exploration. He never failed to carry the stethoscope during his hospital visits, and the signs of cardiac and pulmonary diseases entered largely into his clinical instructions" (Austin Flint, "The Life and Labors of Laennec: An Introductory Address Delivered at the New Orleans School of Medicine, Nov. 14, 1859," *New Orleans Med. and Hosp. Gazette* 6 [1859]: 736–56; see also W. W. Gerhard, *On the Diagnosis of Diseases of the Chest* [Philadelphia: Key and Biddle, 1836], p. xi). Claims of priority for introducing stethoscopy were made by others. A Philadelphia physician wrote that "the stethoscope was introduced into Philadelphia within somewhere about the year of its first publication and that it has been used ever since that time without interruption." A New Englander responded that he had obtained a stethoscope and an 1819 edition of Laennec from France as soon as it had been possible, adding, "I have ever since been as constant to my stethoscope as a Dutchman to his pipe or an Englishman to his umbrella" (see the introduction to Victor Collin, *Manual for the Use of the Stethoscope: A Short Treatise on the Different Methods of Investigating the Diseases of the Chest*, trans. W. N. Ryland [Boston: B. Perkins, 1829]).

12. William Osler, "Memoir of Alfred Stillé," *Trans. Coll. Phys. Phila.*, 3rd ser., 24 (1902): lviii–lxxi; quotation on p. lxi.

13. Letter to H. I. Bowditch, then studying in Paris, quoted in George R. Minot, "James Jackson as a Professor of Medicine," *N. Eng. J. Med.* 208 (1933): 254–58; quotation on pp. 256–57. James Jackson Putnam, *A Memoir of Dr. James Jackson* (Boston and New York: Houghton, Mifflin, 1905), p. 331.

14. Jacob Bigelow, "Brief Rules for Exploration of the Chest, in Diseases of the Lungs and Heart," *Boston Med. & Surg. J.* 20 (1839): 357–69, 373–78, 389–94; quotation on p. 357.

studied in Paris hospitals, especially with P. C. A. Louis, who, after the death of Laennec in 1826, became one of the most popular teachers of the new medicine.[15] From these students came a generation of leaders of the medical profession in America. William W. Gerhard of Philadelphia and Henry I. Bowditch of Boston both wrote books on physical diagnosis that became classics, and Oliver Wendell Holmes won a Boylston Prize for his essay on physical examination of the chest. Caspar Pennock and Edward Mott Moore did early experimental work attempting to correlate physiological function with physical signs in living animals.[16] William Pepper, Alfred Stillé, and George C. Shattuck became leading figures at the University of Pennsylvania and at Harvard.

The students of Louis learned more than auscultation. Some of them also organized a Society for Medical Observation in 1832 and asked Louis to preside. Their purpose was to improve their own abilities as clinical observers by taking a detailed history from the patient, performing a meticulous physical examination, and discussing the findings in pathophysiologic terms. Their group met weekly, with each student in turn presenting a case he had prepared.

> The members were arranged around a table that occupied three sides of the room, and each person had paper and pen or pencil before him. He was prepared . . . to note the most trivial omission or a too inconsiderate deduction made by the reader. Each subsequently criticized the paper from these notes. This was done in the keenest manner. Louis, as President, summed up the result of the meeting by not only criticizing the reader, but also his critics' remarks.

There were no petty quarrels or personal attacks, but also no sentimental

15. The literature on this subject is extensive: William Osler, "Influence of Louis on American Medicine," *Bull. Johns Hopkins Hosp.* 8 (1897): 161–67; Walter R. Steiner, "Some Distinguished American Medical Students of Pierre-Charles-Alexandre Louis of Paris," *Bull. Hist. Med.* 7 (1939): 783–93; Guy Hinsdale, "The American Medical Argonauts: Pupils of Pierre Charles Alexandre Louis," *Trans. & Stud. Coll. Phys. Phila.* 13 (1945–1946): 37–43; Russell M. Jones, "American Doctors in Paris, 1820–1861: A Statistical Profile," *J. Hist. Med.* 25 (1970): 143–57; Russell M. Jones, "American Doctors and the Parisian Medical World, 1830–1840," *Bull. Hist. Med.* 47 (1973): 40–65.

16. W. W. Gerhard, *On the Diagnosis of Diseases of the Chest;* Henry I. Bowditch, *The Young Stethoscopist; or, the Student's Aid to Auscultation* (New York: J. and H. G. Langley, 1846); Oliver W. Holmes, "On the Utility and Importance of Direct Exploration in Medical Practice," in *Boylston Prize Dissertations for the Years 1836 and 1837* (Boston: Little and Brown, 1838), pp. 245–371; Caspar Pennock and Edward Mott Moore, *Report of Experiments on the Action of the Heart, Read Before the Pathological Society of Philadelphia, Oct. 28 to Nov. 4, 1839* (Philadelphia: Merrihew and Thompson, 1839). A typical experiment consisted of rendering a ram unconscious with blows on the head, inserting a bellows through a tracheotomy, opening the chest and placing a stethoscope directly on the heart in an attempt to relate the heart sounds with the observed muscular contractions.

delicacy. All of this was described by Louis in "An Essay on Clinical Instruction," in which he noted modestly that the methods of observation used were "more exact than those of former periods, but less rigorous than those which will succeed."[17] His prediction proved correct.

In the decades that followed, the convenience and precision of physical diagnosis increased. The most notable improvement in the stethoscope was the semiflexible binaural model made popular by George P. Cammann of New York City in 1851, which remained the standard instrument in this country until the development of the combination bell and diaphragm by the Boston engineer R. C. M. Bowles at the end of the century. In 1851 Hermann von Helmholtz elaborated the principle of the ophthalmoscope. The thermometer was adapted to clinical use in the 1870s, when Carl Wunderlich and others began recording temperatures on graphs and using the patterns in a practical way. The explanation of the reflex arc by Wilhelm Erb and Carl Westphal brought the percussion hammer into neurology after 1875. In 1896 the application of an inflatable bladder made the sphygmomanometer—the last of the major tools of bedside examination—practical for the first time. Significant improvements in the achromatic microscope made it possible to examine blood smears and urine sediments.[18]

In addition to these innovations, physicians began applying the stethoscope to acoustical phenomena of the body other than those of respiration. The French surgeon Jacques Lisfranc found that the crepitus produced by movement of fractured bones and the grating sound made by a catheter rubbing against a bladder stone were diagnostically useful.[19] Cardiac murmurs and extrathoracic vascular bruits were also identified. Since many of these conditions were amenable to treatment, the stethoscope was of more varied usefulness in the days before the development of radiography.

As early as 1855 an English manual appeared in the United States outlining the method of collecting and recording historical data still in use today. It described not only percussion and auscultation, but also abdominal, neurological, and psychiatric examinations, and the use of the opthalmoscope, the speculum, and the spirometer. Also included were instructions for performing microscopic and chemical tests on blood and

17. [Henry I. Bowditch], "Louis and His Contemporaries," *Boston Med. & Surg. J.* 87 (1873): 292–95; quotation on p. 293. P. C. A. Louis, *An Essay on Clinical Instruction,* trans. Peter Martin (London: S. Highley, 1834), p. 2.
18. See S. Weir Mitchell, "An Early History of Instrumental Precision in Medicine," *Trans. Congr. Am. Phys. & Surg.* 2 (1891): 159–98; Kenneth D. Keele, *The Evolution of Clinical Methods in Medicine* (Springfield, Ill.: Charles C. Thomas, 1963).
19. "Employment of the Stethoscope in Practice," *Med. Recorder* 7 (1824): 432–33.

urine. By the mid-1860s the manual was appearing on the recommended reading lists of at least two medical schools, Harvard and Vermont.[20]

By the eve of the Civil War Austin Flint, probably the most prominent American internist of his generation, had become the leading exponent of teaching auscultation. For this his peers dubbed him "the American Laennec." Between 1850, when he published his first "Contributions to the Study of the Physical Diagnosis of Diseases of the Chest" in the *Buffalo Medical Journal*, and his death in 1884, Flint wrote seven major works dealing with physical diagnosis, including the first American classic on cardiac disease, a description of the murmur which bears his name, and a textbook that appeared in its ninth edition forty-one years after his death.[21]

By the end of the nineteenth century the technical methods of internal medicine had been developed. It was possible to examine a patient at the bedside and to learn from the outside much about what was occurring inside. But if physical examination made medicine more precise, it also made it more difficult. As James Jackson, Jr., wrote to his father from Paris, "If Laennec has added an important aid to our insufficient means of exploring diseases of the chest, he has, at the same time, rendered the study of those diseases more difficult, more laborious I would say, to the learner."[22]

Most American physicians who learned physical diagnosis did so on their own initiative, and it would be wrong to assume that the methods were in general use in the nineteenth century. More important, they were not consistently a part of undergraduate medical education in the United States until the twentieth century. Gerhard attributed this deficiency to "the small number of observers who [were] interested in prosecuting medicine as a science, with but a slender expectation of ultimate pecuniary reward." Describing what he called "the profitless pursuits of medical science," Gerhard predicted that such would always be the case in a society in which "commerce and manufactures offer large rewards for the employment of capital, and, indirectly, rather obstruct pursuits in which an immediate advantage is not presented."[23]

20. Thomas H. Tanner, *A Manual of Clinical Medicine and Physical Diagnosis* (Philadelphia: Blanchard and Lea, 1855). This book was among those recommended to students in the Harvard catalogue for 1867/68, and in the University of Vermont catalogue for 1866/67.

21. Austin Flint, *A Practical Treatise on the Diagnosis, Pathology and Treatment of Diseases of the Heart* (Philadelphia: Blanchard and Lea, 1859); Austin Flint, "On Cardiac Murmurs," *Am. J. Med. Sci.*, n.s., 44 (1862): 29–54; Austin Flint, *A Manual of Physical Diagnosis*, 9th ed. (Philadelphia and New York: Lea and Febiger, 1925).

22. James Jackson, *Memoir of James Jackson, Jr., M.D., Written by his Father, with Extracts from His Letters* . . . (Boston: Hilliard, Gray, 1836), p. 109.

23. Quoted in Lawrason Brown, *The Story of Clinical Pulmonary Tuberculosis* (Baltimore: Williams and Wilkins, 1941), p. 177.

Had Gerhard lived to the end of the nineteenth century, when the fruits of commerce and manufacturing began to benefit medical education in the form of endowments, he would have seen himself contradicted. With the subsidization of medical education, it became possible to provide the expensive individual instruction needed to train students in the use of the tools and techniques of internal medicine.

THE HOSPITAL: A CLINICIAN'S LABORATORY

Before the methods of bedside physical examination were available, the ambulatory medical apprenticeship had often provided satisfactory clinical experience, as William Beaumont, who later became famous for his studies of digestion, attested. Beaumont's preceptor in rural Vermont put his young apprentice in "charge of many of his patients during his calls elsewhere."[24] When it became necessary to master precise techniques like stethoscopy, however, the occasional and often solitary bedside experience of the apprentice, though it might stimulate self-reliance, could not provide proper instruction. The hospital, which brought together large groups of patients, made it possible to do many examinations sequentially and to repeat the examinations periodically. It also attracted to its staff those men who especially wanted to teach. The hospital provided the laboratory for systematic clinical training, and the appearance of this institution was one of the prerequisites to any major change in the clinical curriculum.

Teaching was, almost without exception, one of the reasons physicians gave for promoting hospitals.[25] But using the hospital for teaching was not always easy. Throughout most of the nineteenth century only the poor sought hospital care, and the attending physician offered his services free in return for the privilege of bringing medical students with him on his rounds.[26] Inevitably, conflicts arose regarding the rights of patients to competent care and personal privacy, the need to provide training for inexperienced students, and the effort to conserve public funds by accept-

24. Jesse S. Myer, *Life and Letters of Dr. William Beaumont* (St. Louis, Mo.: C. V. Mosby, 1912), p. 27.

25. Samuel Bard, *A Discourse on Medical Education* (New York: C. S. Van Winkle, 1819); Daniel Drake, *An Inaugural Discourse on Medical Education* (Cincinnati: Looker, Palmer and Reynolds, 1820); Connecticut Senate Committee Report in Pliny A. Jewett, *Semi-Centennial History of the Gen'l Hospital Society of Connecticut* (New Haven: Tuttle, Morehouse and Taylor, 1876), p. 29; James Jackson and John C. Warren, *Circular Letter to Benevolent Citizens of Boston, August 20, 1810,* rpt. in N. I. Bowditch, *A History of the Massachusetts General Hospital,* 2nd ed. (Boston, 1872), pp. 3–9n.

26. D. G. Thomas, "History of the Founding and Development of the First Hospitals of the United States," *Am. J. Insan.* 24 (1867): 130–54.

ing the free service of physicians. The emphasis usually fluctuated. In prosperous times politicians talked about the dignity of the poor, while in times of recession they were only too glad to allow teaching in return for free professional care. Misunderstandings between the professional staff, both physicians and students, and the hospital managers and administrators compounded the problem. None of the early hospitals was exempt.

When seeking tax funds, the promoters of the Massachusetts General Hospital found it necessary to reassure the legislature that there was no intention "to give to students in medicine an opportunity to experiment, at the expense of the feelings, health, and lives of the poor patients." A few years later the managers of the same institution announced that

> pupils are not to remain at the Hospital longer than is absolutely necessary for the visits. They are not to converse with the patients or nurses. During operations and while in the wards they are to abstain from conversation with each other; they are not to walk about; nor in any other way to disturb either the medical officer, or the patients. . . . In all cases, in which it will be proper for the pupils to make any personal examination of a patient, such as feeling the pulse, examining a tumor, etc. an intimation to that effect will be given them by the physician or surgeon. It must be obvious that the greatest inconveniences must arise, if such examinations were commonly made by the pupils.

This feeling apparently still existed in 1846 when the managers, responding to a proposal to move the medical school adjacent to the hospital, stated "that they cannot perceive any advantage to this institution to arise therefrom."[27]

In Philadelphia, the Guardians of the Almshouse at Blockley stated that their concern for medical teaching did "not predominate over the interest we feel in the discharge of duty towards the poor, as their legal Guardians," and they worried "whether it is consistent with our duty toward these unfortunate inmates of the Hospital to place them in [the] charge of mere novices who never had a case before entering its wards."[28]

In the seventy years before the Civil War this institution, later known simply as Blockley Hospital and generally considered the finest teaching

27. R. Sullivan, *Address Delivered Before the Governor and Council, Members of the Legislature and Other Patrons of the Massachusetts General Hospital at King's Chapel, Boston, June 3, 1819* (Boston: Wells and Lilly, 1819); T. F. Harrington, *The Harvard Medical School*, 3 vols (New York and Chicago: Lewis, 1905), 2:582–83; Bowditch, *A History of the Massachusetts General Hospital*, p. 197.

28. Quoted in William S. Middleton, "Clinical Teaching in Philadelphia Almshouse and Hospital," *Medical Life* 40 (1933): 191–200, 207–25; quotation on p. 215.

hospital of that day, was partially or entirely closed to student activity for more than one-third of the time as a result of these conflicts. On June 30, 1845, for example, a cockroach crawled onto the dining room table where the resident physicians were eating; the residents demanded to be served at the matron's table and, on being refused, walked out. The Board of Managers was only too happy to replace them all with one full-time resident physician at a salary of eighteen hundred dollars a year and three consultants—medical, surgical, and obstetrical—at one hundred dollars each. They abolished the entire teaching hierarchy of voluntary attending physicians, resident physicians and students, and Blockley ceased to function as a teaching hospital for nine years.[29] Commenting on this problem, one observer wrote that "very seldom, indeed, is there a cordial harmony between hospital managers and resident physicians. The exercise of power is as dear to the one as intolerance of it is natural to the other. The one lacks sympathy and the other humility."[30] This was later expressed even more strongly by another professor who wrote "that among the governors of the institution there must have been then, as there usually have been since, individuals who had attained the last possible degree in the way of being asses."[31]

Another problem was the disproportionate number of students to patients. As late as 1873, when the first hospital survey was made in the United States, there were fewer than 20,000 general hospital beds, many of which were not near a medical school.[32] At the same time there were 10,000 medical students in America. Though Blockley Hospital provided close to 8,000 patients a year in the 1850s for the 650 or so medical students in Philadelphia, the burden of clinical teaching fell upon the facilities of the Pennsylvania Hospital, with only 1,000 patients, during prolonged periods. Most other cities were even less fortunate. In the 1840s the Massachusetts General Hospital had only about 400 patients a year, while there were 90 medical students at Harvard.

It was physically impossible to provide individual clinical experience until the number of students was reduced, the number of patients increased, and more sympathetic administrators were appointed.[33] It is not surprising that in 1849 the American Medical Association's Committee on

29. W. S. Middleton, "Clinical Teaching," pp. 215–16; D. G. Thomas, "History of the Founding and Development," p. 113.

30. Alfred Stillé, quoted in W. S. Middleton, "Clinical Teaching," p. 215.

31. John Chalmers DaCosta, "The Old Blockley Hospital: Its Characters and Characteristics," in *Selections from the Papers and Speeches of John Chalmers DaCosta, M.D., LL.D.* (Philadelphia: W. B. Saunders, 1931), p. 159.

32. Joseph M. Toner, "Statistics of Regular Medical Associations and Hospitals of the United States," *Trans. AMA* 24 (1873): 285–333.

33. For comparison, today there are twenty-four thousand inpatients a year at the Uni-

Medical Education reported that only nine of thirty-five American medical schools required *any* hospital experience for a diploma.[34]

A few schools attempted to gain control of some nearby hospital beds or to establish hospitals of their own, but these efforts were generally unsuccessful.[35] In the late 1850s New York Medical College, founded in 1850 with a commitment to implement the educational reforms proposed by the American Medical Association, operated a charity ward of twenty-seven beds in the school building for the express purpose of teaching. But this experiment did not survive. It was not until later in the century that the University of Michigan (1869) and the University of Pennsylvania (1874) established clinical facilities under school control.[36]

In the meantime another solution, the college clinic, became popular. This was essentially a dispensary, similar to the later outpatient department or neighborhood health center. Philadelphia had a dispensary as early as 1786, and New York, Boston, and Charleston each established one in the early part of the nineteenth century. But even here there were frequent conflicts between physicians and managers over student activities. At the Boston Dispensary in 1827 the visiting physicians defended their action in allowing students to prescribe on the grounds that it was good practical experience and pointed out that student fees were the only recompense the physicians had for their professional services. They denied that students experimented on patients. The matter was resolved (and the real nature of the managers' concern clarified) when it was agreed that the apothecaries would instruct the students once a week to acquaint them "with the price of medicine."[37]

In spite of such difficulties, the medical profession defended the

---

versity of Rochester's Strong Memorial Hospital and two hundred medical students in the clinical classes, a 120 to 1 ratio. In addition, four other affiliated hospitals are used for teaching purposes.

34. "Report of the Committee on Medical Education," *Trans. AMA* 2 (1849): 257–352. The nine schools were Harvard, University of Pennsylvania, Jefferson, Pennsylvania College, University of Maryland, University of Louisville, Rush, St. Louis University, and the University of Louisiana—all schools in large cities where there were hospitals.

35. George W. Corner, *Two Centuries of Medicine* (Philadelphia: Lippincott, 1965), pp. 88–89; *Auburn (New York) Free Press*, January 21, 1829; *Deed of Trust from Lyne Starling to Robert W. McCoy and Others* . . . (Columbus, Ohio: William B. Thrall, 1847). This school was an ancestral component of Ohio State Medical School.

36. Abraham Jacobi, "The New York Medical College, 1782–1906," *Ann. Med. Hist.* 1 (Dec. 1917): 368–73; quotation on p. 371. Richard M. Doolen, "The Founding of the University of Michigan Hospital: An Innovation in Medical Education," *J. Med. Educ.* 39 (1964): 50–57.

37. *A History of the Boston Dispensary*, comp. by one of the Board of Managers (Boston: J. Wilson and Son, 1859), pp. 98, 106.

usefulness of dispensaries for teaching. In 1834 a physician at the Medical College of Ohio called service in a dispensary "a most desirable opportunity for acquiring a large fund of useful practical knowledge," but he was careful to emphasize the benefit the public might expect, especially in the case of "a dispensary maintained by the voluntary contributions of the poor, while in health," since this would reduce dependency among sick paupers.[38]

By the 1840s many medical schools were organizing their own dispensaries in order to avoid the problem of unsympathetic managers. In Philadelphia, "where hospital privileges had been so much restricted as to be of little service to the winter students," the popularity of dispensaries grew, especially after the more appealing name of "clinique" was substituted for "dispensary." A veritable "clinique epidemic" broke out and quickly spread to other cities.[39] In the winter of 1846, though there were six hundred to seven hundred medical students in New York City, one professor found the hospitals forsaken for the cliniques and reported that "it was a rare thing to see the face of a single student in any of [his] wards during the whole of [his] attendance." In his address to the students at the opening of the medical school session that year he pleaded for practical medical education in a hospital, stressing the liberality of the New York Hospital regarding the needs of students.[40] In Philadelphia the professors soon gave up the dispensaries and instead provided hospital tickets at their own expense for senior students.

The fundamental problem remained, however. Many schools offered no clinical opportunities, and those that did put little pressure on the students to make use of them. When Nathan Davis published his history of American medical education in 1851, he reported that only sixteen of the thirty-seven active medical colleges were near clinical facilities and that almost one-half of those who graduated from American schools had no "genuine bed-side instruction whatever."

> How many of the thousand students who annually congregate in Philadelphia, or of the seven hundred who spend their winter in New York, are daily found studying with care the most important of all subjects, viz.—clinical medicine and surgery, at the bed-side, in the capacious hospitals of those cities? I speak from personal obser-

38. Thomas D. Mitchell, *The Annual Oration of the Ohio Medical Lyceum* (Cincinnati: Truman, Smith, 1834), p. 15.

39. It was claimed by William H. Rideing, "Medical Education in New York," *Harpers Magazine* 65 (1882): 668–79 (quotation on p. 669), that Valentine Mott founded the first "clinique" in America at the medical department of the University of New York in the 1840s.

40. John Watson, *A Lecture on Practical Education in Medicine* (New York: J. and H. G. Langley, 1846).

vation, when I say that not one in twenty are found paying attention to these things.[41]

It was a problem of too many students, too few teachers, too little time, and too few patients.

Hospitals became more common in the latter half of the century, when large-scale urban poverty began to appear in small inland industrial cities and care of the sick poor became a serious problem. The need for the federal government to provide care for wounded or sick soldiers during and immediately after the Civil War created an even greater demand for hospital beds. With the coming of aseptic surgery at the end of the nineteenth century, hospital facilities increased rapidly and, as a result of the endowment of medical education by philanthropists, it became possible to reduce the size of medical school classes. At Johns Hopkins, for example, there were fewer than fifty students in a class and about thirty-four hundred patients hospitalized in 1897. During the first quarter of the twentieth century the number of hospital beds in the United States tripled while the number of medical students dropped by half. With an adequate setting in which to teach the new methods of internal medicine, an effective means of instructing undergraduates in clinical medicine finally evolved.

CLINICAL INSTRUCTION IN THE NINETEENTH CENTURY

The style of early American clinical teaching came from Scotland. Most American physicians who studied abroad in the late eighteenth century went to Edinburgh. Men like Benjamin Rush, William Shippen, Adam Kuhn, Caspar Wistar, Philip S. Physick, John Morgan and Samuel Bard were all products of the Scottish school, and it is not surprising that the traditions of that institution influenced the character of early collegiate education in the United States.[42]

The method of clinical teaching used at Edinburgh and in most English-speaking schools was the grand walking round, in which the professor, followed by an entourage of students, stopped successively at the bedsides of several patients. The professor questioned the patient in a loud voice, and a senior student chosen for the purpose repeated, in an equally loud voice, the patient's answers. The professor made appropriate

41. Nathan S. Davis, *History of Medical Education and Institutions in the United States* (Chicago: S. C. Griggs, 1851), pp. 166, 221, 217.

42. See Francis R. Packard, *History of Medicine in the United States*, 2 vols. (New York: Paul B. Hoeber, 1931); *Ann. Med. Hist.*, n.s., 4 (1932): 219–44. A more extensive bibliography appears in *Bull. Hist. Med.* 47 (1973): 40.

comments on diagnosis, prognosis, and treatment before moving to the next patient. Wrote a student of the period:

> It is no easy task; it requires an exertion almost stentorean to render this conversation between the physician and his patient audible by the more distant members of the class; while the impossibility of seeing the patient, obliges all who are not in his immediate vicinity to trust solely to their ears for information.[43]

Until the early nineteenth century, in Europe at least, the professor's remarks were rendered in what passed for Latin. The experience was hardly conducive to student participation or to acquiring proficiency in the care of patients.

An abundance of firsthand descriptions makes it clear that the few American schools with hospital facilities universally used this teaching method. Typical is Asa Fitch's account of his winter medical course in New York City. Each day he spent seven hours in lectures and one visiting the wards of New York Hospital with the attending physician. He reported that there were so many students on the round that it was "impossible to make any improvement by attending here. However I crowded around with the rest and saw all I could."[44] The typical student paid a fee of about ten dollars for a hospital ticket, which entitled him to attend the rounds, usually held twice a week. The proceeds went to the hospital, and in the early days most schools with hospital facilities required attendance.

When classes grew to several hundred students—the University of Pennsylvania had over four hundred by 1810 and Jefferson had over three hundred by the middle 1830s—it was necessary to substitute the clinical lecture in an amphitheatre for the walking round on the ward. Medical leaders touted the clinical lecture highly. Edward Delafield told medical students in 1837 that it "will prove to be the best possible means of preparing you by engaging yourselves in the treatment of disease."[45] Critics observed that this was making a virtue of necessity. "Except that

43. Robert J. Graves, "On Clinical Instruction; with a Comparative Estimate of the Mode in Which It Is Conducted in the British and Continental Schools," *Lond. Med. Gaz.* 10 (1832): 401–6; quotation on p. 403. This talk had been given by Graves in 1821 as an introductory lecture. Latin was abandoned at Dublin in the early 1830s.

44. Samuel Rezneck, "A Course of Medical Education in New York City in 1828–29: The Journal of Asa Fitch," *Bull. Hist. Med.* 42 (1968): 555–65; quotation on p. 559. See also William D. Hoyt, Jr., "A Young Physician Prepares to Practice Medicine, 1796–80," *Bull. Hist. Med.* 11 (1942): 582.

45. Edward Delafield, *Introductory Address to the Students in Medicine of the College of Physicians and Surgeons of the University of the State of New York* (New York: Scatcherd and Adams, 1837), p. 33.

the [clinical] lecture is made more imposing by the subject of it being present, and possibly the students' attention to the case being fastened by the display," said members of one unsympathetic hospital board, "we know of no benefit which can accrue from it which would not equally result from the case being lectured on in the absence of the patient, from the notes of the physician, which form, in reality, the basis of the lecture."[46] Even country schools could provide this type of experience by using ambulatory patients.

Some medical educators recognized the faults of the clinical lecture. Not only did the lecturer tend, then as now, to describe the unusual,[47] but also he provided no continuity to his instruction. "What idea has a man of typhus fever who has seen a case once and then only for the space of five minutes?" asked a professor in 1844, adding that there was "no hospital in America which furnishes a sufficient clinic to any other pupils than those which reside within its walls." The most important matter, he continued, is constant access to the bedside. "One case, however slight, thus studied, is worth a hundred seen at long intervals, and worth a thousand seen once from the benches of the amphitheatre, then sent away and never heard of more. The student should also be allowed to take part, from time to time, in the treatment of the sick."[48]

Despite these criticisms, the large clinical lecture prevailed as late as 1890 in most schools, including the country's most prestigious, the University of Pennsylvania. "The old type of lecture system was in full flower," recalled one student.

> We were lectured to from nine in the morning until six at night, [he wrote] although by four o'clock the saturation point had been reached and we were far too sleepy to comprehend what was said to us. . . . [We also had] what were called clinical lectures in the pit of a huge amphitheater. The patient would be brought in and the several hundred students on the benches could see him, but they learned very little in a practical way from that kind of exercise. It really made no difference what ailed the patient; the professor could use him as text for almost any disease and we would be none the wiser. Occasionally we were taken into the wards . . . but I cannot recall that I examined more than two or three cases in my entire course.[49]

46. Quoted in J. A. DaCosta, "The Old Blockley Hospital," pp. 159–60.
47. Robley Dunglison, *The Medical Student* (Philadelphia: Carey, Lea and Blanchard, 1837), p. 165.
48. Henry S. Patterson, *Lecture Introductory to the Course of Materia Medica and Pharmacy* (Philadelphia: W. S. Young, 1844).
49. David Riesman, "Clinical Teaching in America, with Some Remarks on Early Medical

A student who graduated from the College of Physicians and Surgeons in New York in 1890 had similar recollections. "During the last two years," he said, "we had a few clinical lectures in the Vanderbilt Clinic, but we never came within a mile of touching a patient." It was common for students to graduate from even the best schools without ever examining a patient.[50]

At first this was not a serious drawback since students were still expected to get their clinical experience during a three-year apprenticeship with a hometown preceptor. Since antiquity the apprenticeship had been the fundamental means of professional replication, and it was required by law in the early nineteenth century. The early American medical schools merely supplemented this training by providing lectures to cope with a rapidly expanding (as it seemed even then) body of knowledge.

Over the years emphasis on lectures grew, stimulated especially by state legislatures which, hoping to encourage attendance at the lectures, gave medical school diplomas equal legal status with the licenses hitherto issued exclusively by county medical societies. The societies, of course, were strict since each new licensee was a professional colleague and an economic competitor. The schools, whose fame and income came from large numbers, were lenient. It is not surprising that the apprenticeship dwindled and, with it, clinical training. Though the three-year apprenticeship remained a requirement of American medical schools until late in the nineteenth century, it had long since become a formality, often amounting to little more than the preceptor lending the student a few books and his name as sponsor. The student was left without clinical training, since the schools could not provide it; and undergraduate medical education became didactic and passive.

Significant clinical training for most American physicians came in one of two ways. Some went abroad for a year or two after graduating, and others, especially after the Civil War, served as house officers in a hospital, almshouse, or asylum. But for most, practical learning came by trial and error on their first patients. The reasons were simple: too many students, too few patients, too few teachers, too little time. Lectures were

Schools," *Trans. & Stud. Coll. Phys. Phila.*, 4th ser., 7 (1939–1940): 89–110; quotation on p. 100.

50. Lewis A. Conner, quoted in James A. Harrar, *The Story of the Lying-in Hospital of the City of New York* ([New York]: Society of the Lying-in Hospital, 1938), p. 75. Statements to this effect may be found in J. Marion Sims, *The Story of My Life* (New York: D. Appleton, 1884) p. 139, and Henry M. Thomas, "Some Memories of the Development of the Medical School and of Osler's Advent," *Johns Hopkins Hosp. Bull.* 30 (1919): 185–89; quotation on p. 187.

given from 9:00 to 12:30 and from 3:00 to 6:00, so that even where hospitals were available there was no time for bedside medicine. One solution, proposed in 1851 by Nathan Davis, was to lengthen the term from four months to nine or ten months, reduce fees so that more students could attend schools with hospital facilities, and limit lectures to four hours a day, leaving two hours for practical training, including dissection, clinical medicine, surgery, and, "of course, physical diagnosis."[51] In 1859 Davis experimented with two five-month graded terms at Lind University, but it was over three decades before Harvard adopted a four-year graded curriculum with terms of nine months.

Extending the medical course from a total of eight or nine months to thirty-six months had at least two important effects: it increased curriculum time fourfold, providing time for clinical teaching, and it segregated students into graded courses, reducing the size of classes. By the end of the nineteenth century the techniques of bedside clinical medicine had been developed, hospitals where these methods could be taught effectively had come into existence, and the course had been made sufficiently long to include clinical training. Further reduction of the number of students, provision of salaries for clinical teachers, and collegiate control of hospitals were yet to be established.

THE STUDENT TOUCHES THE PATIENT

It was not until the twentieth century that undergraduate medical students in America had much personal contact with patients. Bedside instruction of individual students existed in Hippocratic times and during the Renaissance at Padua, but it did not survive or spread from there. Its modern ancestry can be traced to the University of Leyden, where in 1630 students were required to examine patients and commit themselves to a diagnosis and plan of treatment. Pupils of Hermann Boerhaave carried this tradition to Vienna and later to Germany.[52]

At the University of Berlin in the early nineteenth century the professor of clinical medicine held daily teaching clinics in which students examined ambulant patients while their classmates sat around a large table.

51. Nathan S. Davis, *History of Medical Education and Institutions*, pp. 218–19, 225.
52. Theodor Puschmann, *A History of Medical Education* (1891; reprint ed., New York: Hafner, 1966), pp. 410–12. Theodor Billroth, *The Medical Sciences in the German Universities* (New York: Macmillan, 1924), p. 32. A more detailed examination of the Dutch origins of bedside instruction appears in Evert C. Van Leersum, "Contribution to the History of the Clinical Instruction in the Netherlands," *Janus* 30–31 (1926–1927): 133–51.

The examining pupil declared aloud, in Latin, "his diagnostic, prognostic, and *methodus curandi*," after which the professor questioned him further and the student prepared a prescription, which his instructor signed. The patient returned daily "to be examined in the same way by the same pupil, until the cure be completed." If the patient was unable to attend, the student made a house call. This experience was required for graduation.[53] At another Berlin institution the patient was put under the immediate management of a fourth-year "out-door pupil" who interrogated and examined him and decided upon a diagnosis and treatment.[54]

Robert Graves of Dublin introduced this German system to the English-speaking world. He had travelled on the continent for three years prior to his appointment in 1821 as professor of medicine and physician at the Meath Hospital. In his first lecture as professor the twenty-four-year-old Graves proposed to replace the Edinburgh grand round system of clinical education, then used at Dublin, with the German clinical clerkship method. Said Graves to the students:

> You come here to convert theoretical into practical knowledge. . . . The human mind is so constituted, that in practical knowledge its improvement must be gradual. Some become masters of mathematics, and of other abstract sciences, with such facility, that in one year they outstrip those who have laboured during many. It is so, likewise, in the theoretical parts of medicine; but the very notion of practical knowledge implies observation of nature; nature requires time for her operations; and he who wishes to observe their development will in vain endeavor to substitute genius or industry for time . . . therefore . . . a certain portion of each day should be devoted to attendance at a hospital. . . . Students should aim not at seeing many diseases every day . . . no, their object should be constantly to study a few cases with diligence and attention; they should anxiously cultivate the habit of making accurate observations.[55]

53. T. F. Andrews, "An Account of the Medical Institutions of Berlin," *Am. Med. Record* 6 (1823): 471–86; quotation on p. 475.

54. Ibid., p. 479; Joseph Leo-Wolf, "Medical Education in Germany," *Am. Med. Record* 13 (1828): 481–90.

55. R. J. Graves, "On Clinical Instruction," pp. 401–3. One of America's early clinical professors, Dr. Thomas Bond of the Pennsylvania Hospital, made similar observations fifty years before this. "Language & Books alone," he said at the start of his lectures in the hospital, "can never give him [the student] Adequate Ideas of Diseases. . . . For which reasons Infirmaries are Justly reputed the Grand Theatres of Medical Knowledge. There, the Clinical professor comes in to the Aid of Speculation & demonstrates the Truth of Theory by Facts" (quoted in Thomas G. Morton, *The History of the Pennsylvania Hospital*, rev. ed [Philadelphia: Times Printing House, 1897], p. 463).

After a decade of experience with the clerkship method Graves was able "strongly to recommend the method of instruction pursued in Germany," regretting only that it had not become more generally accepted.

By the 1830s even Americans were commenting on the German system.[56] Reynell Coates, speaking in Philadelphia about 1835 on the defects of American 'medical education, noted that "clinical instruction [is] regarded as a thing of almost no importance!" Hospital rules were designed to exclude students "except for two short hours upon two mornings in the week!" Coates felt that only in Germany was the student properly taught. Who in America, he asked, excluding the trivial number of house pupils, "has enjoyed the privilege of genuine, thorough observation, upon a single case within their wards, before he sallies forth, with licence to commence his medical career and claim the confidence of the public?"[57]

Another professor, James Conquest Cross of Louisville, proposed that the term be 50 percent longer, that not just one, but all professors give clinical instruction, and that classes be divided into small groups so that

> every student would . . . be enabled, to hear and see all that he could wish. . . . At every visit the professor should spend two or three hours, and even longer if necessary. The student must be taught the "use of his eyes, his ears, and his hands." . . . Every pupil should be presented with a stethoscope . . . and the professor should patiently stand by the bedside while he is listening.[58]

A few undergraduate students received clinical experience as institutional residents, apprenticed to hospitals instead of to individual physicians and instructed by the attending physicians. However, hospitals soon showed a preference for more experienced help, and after 1814 at New York Hospital and 1824 at Pennsylvania Hospital, for example, such "house physicians" were always graduates.[59] Only a few institutions, such as the Baltimore Infirmary, opened in 1823, continued to have under-

56. T. F. Andrews, "An Account of the Medical Institutions"; Reynell Coates, *Oration on the Defects in the Present System of Medical Education in the United States* (Philadelphia: James Kay, jun. and Brother, [1835?]).

57. Coates, *Oration on the Defects*, p. 24.

58. James Conquest Cross, *Thoughts on the Policy of Establishing a School of Medicine in Louisville* (Lexington: N. L. Finnell, 1834), pp. 90, 91.

59. At the Massachusetts General Hospital "house pupils," as they were known, were graduates of the Harvard Medical School from the time the hospital opened in 1821. See *128th Annual Report of the Society of the New York Hospital* (New York and Albany: Wynkoop Hallenbeck Crawford, 1899); George Bacon Wood, *An Address on the Occasion of the Centennial Celebration of the Founding of the Pennsylvania Hospital* (Philadelphia: T. K. and P. G. Collins, 1851); Grace W. Myers, *History of the Massachusetts General Hospital* (Boston, [1929?]).

graduates as resident pupils. In this infirmary, five students were personally responsible for patients. The attending physician

> is to be present at all important operations of surgery and if he does not operate himself, assigns the cases to the students, viz: obstetrical cases alternately, commencing with the senior student; at which only two students shall be present. In difficult cases, the attending physician is to direct in presence of all the students,[60] all other surgical operations alternately—the senior taking always the first of each class of such operation.

Patients were assigned in rotation to the students, who cared for them "until the case is decided."[61]

By the 1840s some schools were beginning to provide individual clinical experience. One of these, at least for a while, was the Medical College of Ohio in Cincinnati. During the session of 1841/42 the faculty included a professor of physical diagnosis and pathological anatomy, fresh from a year in the hospitals of Paris, who attended at the hospital each morning for one hour before lectures began and gave practical bedside instruction to groups of ten students.[62]

By the middle 1840s Harvard was offering students "an opportunity of visiting all the cases, and of observing and learning the symptoms and treatment of each case, and particularly of the exploration of the body, for the PHYSICAL SIGNS of disease, by *palpation, auscultation* and *percussion.*" By 1857 it was possible for students to "investigate disease for themselves, and study it minutely." After 1846 the older students at Harvard met "once a week for the reading of cases and for criticisms thereupon" as a Society for Medical Observation, modelled after the one founded twenty-five years earlier in Paris.[63]

About half of the students at Harvard also attended the private Tremont

60. Such training in midwifery was rare, at least in the North. When introduced by Dr. James P. White at Buffalo Medical College in 1851, it led to public consternation and a lawsuit. See Oliver P. Jones, "A Bench Mark for the Obstetric History of the United States," *Obst. & Gynec.* 43 (1974): 784–91.

61. *Report of a Committee Appointed by the Guardians for the Relief and Employment of the Poor of Philadelphia, etc., To Visit the Almshouses of Baltimore, New York, Boston, and Salem, Nov., 1833* (Philadelphia: W. F. Geddes, 1834), p. 11.

62. *Annual Catalogue of the Officers and Students of the Medical College of Ohio: Session 1841–42* (Cincinnati: L'Hommedieu, 1842), with an additional circular appended, p. 5.

63. Harvard University, *Catalogue of Students Attending Medical Lectures in Boston, 1844–45, with a Circular of the Faculty* (Boston: D. Clapp, Jr., 1845), p. 12; Harvard University, Medical Department, *Announcement of the Medical Course, Commencing on the First Wednesday in November, 1857* (Boston: David Clapp, 1857), p. 8; Harvard University, Medical Department, *Announcement of the Medical Course, Commencing on the First Wednesday in November, 1861* (Boston: David Clapp, 1861), p. 6.

Street Medical School, which provided instruction from March until November when the medical college was not in session. From its start in 1838 until 1858, when Harvard formally recognized it as the second or summer semester of an extended curriculum, the school was in reality part of that institution. The official medical school announcement for 1855/56 even promoted it. Tremont was, in effect, a group preceptorial run by members of the Harvard faculty who took their private students into the wards of the Massachusetts General Hospital in the summer as they did all Harvard students in the winter. Particular attention was paid "to auscultation, percussion and all physical signs in connection with diseases of the chest and abdomen." Students also learned chemical and microscopic analysis of blood and urine.[64] At least three other private schools in the Boston area offered similar instruction. At the United States Marine Hospital in Chelsea, where Henry I. Bowditch taught, students were permitted "to examine and make records of all the cases."[65]

Such extramural training was common in many cities, though perhaps not as comprehensive as in Boston. Many professors had large groups of students to whom they gave private instruction, in addition to their public lectures in the medical school. In these smaller groups a more active experience was possible for the student.[66]

At the University of Michigan in the late 1850s a "full two hours each day (except Sundays) were spent by the students in examining, immediately under the direction of their instructors, the patients in the hospital." These students had learned the normal sounds by practicing on each other, and were expected to learn about the evolution of physical changes by reexamining patients periodically.[67]

Despite these early efforts, it was Erasmus Darwin Fenner, professor of medicine, dean, and leading light of the New Orleans School of Medicine,[68] who really introduced the clinical clerkship to America. In his introductory address at the opening of the new school in November

64. *Catalogue of the Past and Present Students of the Tremont Street Medical School* (Boston: David Clapp, 1855), p. 9.

65. Advertisement in the *Boston Med. & Surg. J.* 22 (1840): 308.

66. See, for example, Douglas Guthrie, *Extramural Medical Education in Edinburgh* (Edinburgh and London: E. and S. Livingstone, 1965); William Williams Keen, "The History of the Philadelphia School of Anatomy and Its Relation to Medical Teaching," in *Addresses and Other Papers* (Philadelphia and London: W. B. Saunders, 1905); James A. Harrar, *The Story of the Lying-in Hospital*, p. 30.

67. Letter from Alonzo B. Palmer to Zina Pitcher, 7 Dec. 1857, *Peninsular J. of Med. & Col. Sci.* 5 (1858): 400–402; "Report of a Clinical Lecture by Dr. Palmer to the Clinical Class at St. Mary's Hospital—Tuberculosis," ibid. 5 (1857): 225–32.

68. Not to be confused with the older University of Louisiana Medical Department, later

1856, Fenner cited Graves's statement that a student should observe patients daily throughout the course of their illnesses and should do so during the whole period of pupilage. This could be done only in a hospital, and the new school was directly opposite the Charity Hospital. *Every one* of the seven professors on the faculty was to give clinical instruction there daily until 10:30 A.M., when lectures began.[69]

The next year Fenner published a detailed description of the New Orleans Plan.

> The course of qualification preparatory to entering upon the practice of medicine hitherto pursued by nine-tenths of the medical students in this country, has been, to read a textbook on each of the different branches, to hear two courses of lectures, occasionally walk through the wards of a hospital, where he may see a Professor prescribe for a number of patients or perform a surgical operation, then be able, when questioned, to repeat a respectable amount of what he has read in books or been told by his teachers, and he obtains his diploma. Under such a system of instruction, experience is only to be acquired at a considerable expense of human life. . . . I think I may safely say that previous to the present day, nothing like a systematic course or plan of clinical instruction has been adopted by any of the Medical Colleges in the United States.[70]

At New Orleans the student received a printed ticket containing spaces to record data identifying the patient by location, name, age, nativity, vocation, diagnosis, duration, and outcome. This he pasted in his notebook. In addition, he was given a list of questions to ask regarding the duration of the illness, symptoms, course, previous therapy, and present state including a review of systems. He was also to record the patient's appearance and any abnormal findings on physical examination: "Note the Chest symptoms—breathing, cough, pain[,] physical signs. Note the Heart, sounds of. Note the Pulse, number and character of." From these data the student was expected to write a "connected narrative," to be read to the professor on rounds. If the patient died, an autopsy was performed before the class after the professor predicted what the findings would be.[71]

Several factors were essential to the success of this innovation. The faculty, which soon grew from seven to ten men, *all* gave bedside instruc-

---

Tulane, this school boasted a remarkable faculty which included Austin Flint.

69. E. D. Fenner, "Introductory Lecture," *New Orleans Med. News & Hosp. Gaz.* 3 (1856): 577–600; quotation on pp. 598–99.

70. E. D. Fenner, "Remarks on Clinical Medicine," *New Orleans Med. News & Hosp. Gaz.* 4 (1857): 458–72; quotations on pp. 458, 467.

71. Ibid., pp. 468–69.

tion. The term was lengthened from four to five months so there were fewer lectures per day and more time for clinical activities, and the school was adjacent both to a dispensary and to Charity Hospital, which cared for 15,634 patients in 1849. With well over two thousand deaths a year and the most liberal autopsy laws in the United States, New Orleans had clear advantages for training physicians.

Where did Fenner get the idea? In his introductory address he said that the faculty had "adopted a course of clinical instruction very much like that pursued in Germany, where this branch is taught better than anywhere in the world."[72] The next year he stated that the plan was "much the same as that pursued in the General Hospital of Vienna, which was introduced into the Meath Hospital, of Dublin, by Dr. Graves, in 1821, and has been continued there ever since, with entire satisfaction."[73] Possibly it was through contact with his friend John Y. Bassett, who had studied in Dublin and who was a regular contributor to a journal edited by Fenner, that the idea came.[74]

Such clinical instruction proved popular and the New Orleans School of Medicine prospered until closed by the Civil War. Its enrollment increased from 76 to 216 in the first four years, at the end of which it was the seventh largest school in America. The school reopened after the war, but it soon fell victim to bad times, made worse by Fenner's death in 1866.[75]

Though more than two decades passed before William Osler successfully established a clinical clerkship program at Johns Hopkins, individual clinical instruction became more common during the 1870s and 1880s. The Syracuse catalogue stated that "students will be required to examine

72. E. D. Fenner, "Introductory Lecture," p. 599.
73. E. D. Fenner, "Remarks on Clinical Medicine," p. 470. The announcement of the school the year before stated that "the plan [of clinical instruction to be] adopted will be that which has been found so eminently successful in the hospitals of Paris. This is founded on the great truth: that observation in medicine, to be profitable, must be complete . . ." (see Harold Cummins, "Formal Medical Education in New Orleans, 1834–," *Bull. Med. Libr. Assoc.* 30 (1941–1942): 300–308; quotation on p. 307). Members of the Paris School, especially Louis, used the same techniques as in Berlin and Dublin, but only graduate students were exposed to them.
74. David Riesman, "The Dublin Medical School and Its Influence upon Medicine in America," *Ann. Med. Hist.* 4 (1922): 86–96. Riesman found records of only four Americans who studied with Graves and Stokes in Dublin. The first was John Y. Bassett. Fenner published *Southern Medical Reports* (1849–1851), which included several papers by Bassett, and it was these papers which later stimulated Osler to write his famous biographical essay, "An Alabama Student." See William D. Postell, "Erasmus Darwin Fenner and the Beginnings of Medical Literature in Louisiana," *Ann. Med. Hist.*, 3rd ser., 3 (1941): 297–305. See also David C. Elkin, ed., *The Medical Reports of John Y. Bassett, M.D., the Alabama Student* (Springfield: C. C. Thomas, 1941), p. 69.
75. A. E. Fossier, "History of Medical Education in New Orleans from Its Birth to the Civil War," Part II, n.s., *Ann. Med. Hist.* 6 (1934): 427–47.

cases and report them before the class." Rush Medical College offered individual clinical instruction in 1879, and students were "specially drilled in the methodical examination of patients [and] the taking of histories." At the Chicago Medical School, predecessor of Northwestern, a distinguishing feature was individual bedside instruction in small groups and student contact with patients.[76]

But none of these experiments was the same as the experience at New Orleans or Hopkins. Osler, like Fenner, had been influenced by the methods of the European medical schools. His first preceptor in medicine, James Bovell, had been a student of Graves and of William Stokes,[77] as were three of his teachers at McGill in the early 1870s. The bedside instruction at the Montreal General Hospital at that time, Osler later recalled, "was excellent and the clerking a serious business." Later, while studying physiology in London, he was impressed by "the admirable English system, with the ward work done by the student himself the essential feature." Afterward, when he went to Berlin, he saw the students examine, explain, and follow—"day by day"—the cases to which they were assigned.[78]

Osler became professor of medicine at the University of Pennsylvania in 1884, but it was not until he reached Hopkins that he found his classes small enough to establish a clerkship system at an American school. At Pennsylvania in 1890, a clinical class had around 130 students, at Hopkins about 25. It was for this clerkship that Osler wished especially to be remembered, saying, "I desire no other epitaph . . . than the statement that I taught medical students in the wards, as I regard this as by far the most useful and important work I have been called upon to do."[79]

76. *Fourth Annual Announcement of the College of Medicine of Syracuse University 1875–76* (Syracuse: William L. Rose, 1875), p. 8; *Thirty-Seventh Annual Announcement of Rush Medical College, Chicago, for the Session of 1879–80* (Chicago: Bulletin Printing Co., 1879), p. 11; *Twenty-Fourth Annual Announcement of the Chicago Medical College, Session of 1882–83* (Chicago, 1882), p. 5. The medical department of the University of California provided a similar, if less detailed, experience in the early 1870s. "A patient is placed in charge of a senior student, and by him examined, a diagnosis and prognosis given, together with his views of treatment, in the presence of the class. . . . Every student, thus detailed, is expected to keep a complete history of the case" (*Biennial Report of the Regents of the University of California for the Years 1873–75*, p. 94). I am indebted to Dr. Gert Brieger for bringing this evidence to my attention.

77. See *Dictionary of Canadian Biography*, Vol. 10, ed. Marc LaTerreur (n.p.: University of Toronto Press, 1972), pp. 83–84.

78. William Osler, "An Address on the Medical Clinic: A Retrospect and Forecast, Delivered before the Abernethian Society, St. Bartholomew's Hospital, London, Dec. 4th, 1913," *Brit. Med. J.* 1 (1914): 10–16; quotations on p. 10.

79. William Osler, *Aequanimitas*, 3rd ed. (Philadelphia: Blackiston, 1943), p. 390.

The plan established at Hopkins in the middle 1890s—and adopted by most schools in the twentieth century—included wardwork, "in which the students, acting as clinical clerks, will be assigned beds and take the histories of new cases as admitted, and be responsible (under the direction of the house physician and the first assistant) for the ward notes. . . . The student will make the visit with Professor Osler on three days of the week at 9:00 A.M., and in this way will be enabled to study in a routine manner the progress of the cases."[80] During the third year the twenty-two students "arranged their chairs informally in a semicircle around a rattan couch for the patient and a plain deal table with Osler sitting beside it." One of the students made the examination. Osler stressed order and thoroughness, emphasizing inspection, and then proceeding to palpation, percussion, and auscultation. Students recalled that "until we had gained all the information possible by one method, we were forbidden to pass on to the next." Like the great Louis, Osler also emphasized the careful recording of data.[81]

Though the clinical clerkship may not have been Osler's idea, it was he who established it firmly in the American scene. That he was able to do so was a consequence of his times. Medical school endowments made it possible to pay professors, restrict class size, and establish clinical facilities under faculty control. Johns Hopkins was the first school to do all these things.

Other schools gradually followed suit.[82] The experience at Western Reserve, one of the first to do so, gives some idea of the trend. The school offered its first clinical clerkships in 1901. By 1907 the class was being assigned to wards in small groups. Between 1910 and 1923 the total amount of formal instruction rose from 1,052 to 1,788 hours with the didactic portion declining from 32 percent to 6 percent. Perhaps most striking was the threefold increase in the time for clinical clerkships, from 250 hours in 1913/14 to 800 hours in 1916/17.[83] At the thirty-seventh annual meeting of the Association of American Medical Colleges in 1926, it was reported that "ward clerkships . . . have been instituted in all

---

80. Alan M. Chesney, *The Johns Hopkins Hospital and Johns Hopkins University School of Medicine: A Chronicle*, 3 vols. (Baltimore: Johns Hopkins Press, 1943–63), 2:130.
81. Ibid., pp. 127–29. Recollections of Walter R. Steiner, Joseph H. Pratt, and Percy M. Dawson. See also Lewellys F. Barker, "The Teaching of Clinical Medicine," *Proc. AAMC*, 26th Annual Mtg., Chicago, Feb. 8, 1916, pp. 43–57.
82. Harvard instituted clerkships in 1913. See James Howard Means, "The Teaching of Medicine in the Massachusetts General Hospital," *Harvard Med. Alumni Bull.* (October 1934): 1–5.
83. Frederick C. Waite, *Western Reserve University Centennial History of the School of Medicine* (Cleveland: Western Reserve University Press, 1946), pp. 393–94.

medical schools."[84] Only two years later Northwestern claimed to be the first school to appoint a supervisor of clinical clerks.[85]

As the nineteenth century progressed, individual bedside experience—laboratory experience in the clinical sciences, so to speak—became a necessity. The need to take a careful systematic history of a patient's illness, to examine his body, and to draw diagnostic and prognostic conclusions by relating the data collected to the practice of medicine could not be avoided. No amount of talent or inspiration could replace time and practice in acquiring this ability.

The hospital provided an ideal clinical arena. But until the number of beds increased and the number of medical students decreased, it was impossible for each student to have an active experience. Without financial subsidies it was not practical to limit class size or to have sufficient faculty to supervise the student at the bedside and adequately to protect the rights and safety of the patient.

GOODBYE, DR. OSLER

The clinical clerkship was almost universally established by the 1930s and became the fundamental way of teaching internal medicine.[86] At first, the lecture continued to be the principal mode of conveying information. On the wards the student was not welcomed but tolerated, partly for his service as a paramedical domestic who did "scut" work; he was hardly an integral part of the "team." In the 1930s at Columbia-Presbyterian Hospital in New York, for example, clerks were not allowed on the wards during rest hours from noon until two o'clock or after eight o'clock in the evening. Gradually, after 1950, lectures and other non-ward activities became fewer, the clerk's responsibility for his assigned patients became greater, and his place in patient care became more secure.

Changes have occurred in the past fifty years, some intentional, but many of the most important ones not. Most medical schools introduced curricular variations, such as changes in the timing and duration of the clinical clerkships, including contact with patients in the first two years, but these modifications had limited effect, their extent often restricted by the "territorial imperatives" of other medical school disciplines.[87] Preclin-

84. John W. Moore, "Clinical Clerkships in Medicine: Student Unit System," *Bull. AAMC* 2 (1927): 136–39; quotation on p. 136.

85. Fred C. Zapffe, "The Clinical Clerk System at Northwestern University Medical School," *Bull. AAMC* 3 (1928): 41–46.

86. Council on Medical Education and Hospitals, *Medical Education in the United States, 1934–1939* (Chicago: American Medical Association, 1940), pp. 173–74.

87. A good summary of curricular changes may be found in Vernon W. Lippard, *A*

ical departments usually resisted encroachments on any time that had become established as part of a sacred progression, raising in their defense the specter of the scientifically illiterate student of the nineteenth century who, in fact, had become almost extinct among medical school matriculants.

Attempts to design interdisciplinary courses, whether on a cellular, regional, or social level, were often unsuccessful, partly because of the departmental political structure of medical schools. Also, while it became increasingly common for clinicians to be conversant with basic science, the lack of comparable clinical sophistication among the full-time basic science teachers put them at a disadvantage.

The growing demands of inpatient service all but smothered efforts to provide or maintain effective experience with ambulatory patients, whether of a comprehensive or a limited type. While there was greater emphasis on the psychosocial aspects of illness in many schools, the ambulatory patient who sought care in clinics used for teaching students frequently had disabling social problems which could be neither disentangled from the medical sickness nor resolved in a brief visit by pharmacologic means. The clinic patient was unreliable in keeping his appointments, and was often less observant and less able to convey to the physician what might have been apparent if seen in the home setting. The hospitalized patient offered easy continuity and a more efficient use of professional time and became the focus of teaching medicine.

Probably the most significant intentional change in the undergraduate clinical curriculum was the introduction of electives. This innovation was an attempt to alleviate curricular rigidity. The Commission on Medical Education, which functioned in the late 1920s, urged such flexibility, at the same time warning against "the dangers of superficial, undisciplined training, lack of unity in courses, dissipation of energy, and too early endeavors towards specialization," which would occur if the student was unaccustomed to independence or lacked adequate guidance.[88] As late as 1950, however, a survey of medical education found only four schools that had introduced substantial amounts of elective time into the clinical years.[89] At Harvard, for example, there was no elective time in the third year and only one to three months in the fourth year.

This situation changed drastically in the 1960s and 1970s, partly in

Half-Century of American Medical Education: 1920–1970 (New York: Josiah Macy, Jr., Foundation, 1974), pp. 8–27.

88. *Final Report of the Commission on Medical Education* (New York: Office of the Director of the Study, 1932), p. 230.

89. John E. Deitrick and Robert C. Berson, *Medical Schools in the United States at Mid-Century* (New York: McGraw-Hill, 1953), pp. 235–36, 242–43.

response to student demands and partly in recognition of the fact that students were entering medical school well—but variously—prepared. However, the effect of electives on clinical training was different from their effect on instruction in the laboratory sciences. It was one thing to offer the student choices and exemptions in theoretical laboratory courses in which he might already have had considerable experience, but quite another to do so in the practical clinical years for which he had no previous training. Furthermore, as subspecialization in medicine developed, an increasing proportion of clinical electives were of a specialized type which often failed to provide the undergraduate adequate supervision by house officers or comprehensive involvement with patients. The commission's fear was realized.

The most fundamental changes in undergraduate clinical instruction were unintentional and occurred quite independently of curricular manipulation. They involved the relationships between student, patient, and teacher and resulted mainly from the increasing complexity of diagnostic and therapeutic technology, and the expansion of hospital facilities and financial support for medical education, to say nothing of broad changes in society generally. Universities and medical schools established control over major teaching hospitals. These institutions became sophisticated laboratories rather than infirmaries with nurses, as the hospitals of the nineteenth and early twentieth centuries had been. Technicians instead of physicians and students increasingly filled diagnostic and therapeutic functions. Full-time teacher-investigators replaced practitioners as clinical teachers. As an increasing proportion of the population had hospital insurance, it became necessary to use private patients for teaching. The patient was sicker but usually stayed a shorter time. Frequently, his problems were so complicated that the junior student was unable to have significant involvement in his care. Consequently the student often had a briefer and more superficial relationship with the patient, had less personal responsibility for him, and had less opportunity to perfect his own abilities.

As the twentieth century progressed and technology became more complicated, specialized postdoctoral training became more important. Consequently, the student shared the patient and the experienced teacher with a growing number of house officers, trainees, fellows, and junior faculty specialists, to say nothing of paramedical students such as nurse practitioners. On the medical service of the University of Rochester's Strong Memorial Hospital, for example, the patient-intern ratio fell from 18:1 to 12:1 and the patient–assistant resident ratio from 25:1 to 12:1 between 1955 and 1975. The number of senior residents, trainees, and fellows more than doubled in a dozen years, and the number of medical students in a class rose from seventy-two to ninety-seven. Yet the number of hospital beds remained the same, partly as a result of community planning efforts to control rising hospital costs.

Diagnostic and therapeutic tests that were performed away from the patient's room and by people other than the student occupied an increasing portion of the patient's hospital stay and further limited the student's involvement with the patient. In five years since 1970 the total number of radiographic, nuclear, and electrodiagnostic examinations (excluding electrocardiograms) at Strong Memorial Hospital increased 33 percent. Academic expectations, fear of litigation, high fixed costs of maintaining complex technical appliances, and the incentive of a procedure-oriented insurance system encouraged maximum use of tests and drowned out pleas for restraint. Such tests added about 30 percent to the patient's hospital bill, and were a substantial source of income to hospitals.[90]

The most important change in undergraduate teaching of clinical medicine was the gradual replacement of the practitioner by the specialized full-time investigator as the student's professional model. When William Osler left Johns Hopkins Medical School in 1905 he predicted that the full-time system would soon include the clinical faculty as it did already the preclinical teacher. He was strong in his opposition to this. "The primary work of a professor of medicine in a medical school is in the wards . . . to turn out men who know how to handle the sick," wrote Osler.[91] The new system, he thought, would produce "a set of clinical prigs."[92] Though his judgment seems harsh, there is no doubt that the present teachers of medicine are quite different from those of the past, partly because of new and more complicated therapeutic techniques such as cardiac surgery, renal dialysis, assisted ventilation, musculoskeletal reconstruction, and cancer chemotherapy, all of which require subspecialization.

Though the full-time teacher had an established position prior to World War II, the teaching role of the practitioner did not diminish drastically until after the war. The full-time teacher of preclinical subjects became increasingly common toward the end of the nineteenth century, especially after Johns Hopkins put its entire preclinical faculty on salary in

90. Paul F. Griner and Benjamin Lipzin, "Use of the Laboratory in a Teaching Hospital: Implications for Patient Care, Education and Hospital Costs," *Ann. Int. Med.* 75 (1971): 157–63. By 1976 several states were refusing to accept automatic rises of per diem patient costs, thus limiting the profit from increased laboratory utilization.

91. William Osler, "The Coming of Age of Internal Medicine in America," *Internat. Clinics*, 25th ser., 4 (1915): 4.

92. William Osler to Ira Remsen, quoted in Alan M. Chesney, *The Johns Hopkins Hospital*, 3:180.

1893. But the full-time clinical teacher did not begin to appear until the time of the First World War at that same institution. Serious doubts that the nonpractitioner could teach the practice of medicine and the economic realities of the Depression initially checked the early proliferation of the full-time faculty member. After the Second World War full-time clinical faculties expanded rapidly under the stimulus of federal support to research. Between 1955 and 1975 the full-time senior faculty in the Department of Medicine at the University of Rochester increased from fourteen to sixty-seven physicians. During the same period the percentage of practitioners on the part-time faculty who served annually as attending physicians on the wards of that school's medical service declined from fifty to less than fifteen. The practitioner of medicine gradually played a smaller role as teacher, and medical education itself became a medical specialty.

The centripetal force of modern technology made inevitable the loss of the practitioner as a model for the student and has tended to drive the teacher from the bedside to the chalkboard.[93] At the end of the nineteenth century the physician himself was able to perform virtually all of the diagnostic techniques at the bedside. By the middle of the twentieth century this was no longer true and was rapidly becoming less so.

Other factors further diminished the influence of the practitioner as a teacher. After the 1960s students and house officers were less dependent on the hospital. Often married, they spent less time within the walls, ate fewer meals in the cafeteria, and were less interested in older physicians for social contact with the outside world. Another major educational experience was lost as a result of this. By 1975 undergraduate and house officer contact was largely restricted to the full-time clinical specialist while he made his daily ward round with an entourage of junior colleagues who themselves tended to isolate the senior man from direct student contact.

Though clinical medicine has changed considerably in recent decades, the clinical clerkship remains the most satisfactory method of instruction. In the words of one observer, "It is never behind the times."[94] It requires much smaller classes than instruction by lecture, it requires a substantial number of patients who are sick but not too sick, it requires teachers who are comfortable at the bedside and who have the time and knack for teaching. Each of these prerequisites is to some degree in jeopardy today. The demand for more physicians has led to larger classes, the patients in

93. Anne R. Somers, "Conflict, Accommodation, and Progress: Some Socioeconomic Observations of Medical Education and the Practicing Profession," *J. Med. Educ.* 38 (1963): 466–78.
94. Lippard, *A Half-Century of American Medical Education*, p. 11.

teaching hospitals are often sicker and dependent on complicated technological devices for survival, the clinical teacher is required to practice medicine increasingly as a means of support so that he is, in effect, again being called upon to subsidize clinical medical education as he was throughout the nineteenth century. Nevertheless, the clerkship seems secure in the foreseeable future.

Surgery

GERT H. BRIEGER

THE teaching of surgery, like the craft itself, has a long and honorable history. The Roman medical writer Celsus, in the introduction to the surgical books of his *De medicina* around 30 A.D., pointed out that four centuries earlier in the time of Hippocrates the art of surgery began to be much practiced. "Later," Celsus claimed, "it was separated from the rest of medicine, and began to have its own professors. . . ."[1] From antiquity to the eighteenth century and the beginnings of medical education in America, surgery was taught by surgeons, some of whom were famous professors and others of whom were fathers or preceptors passing on the knowledge of their craft to a son or apprentice. It is the teaching of surgery in America, its methods, organization, and relationship to medical education as a whole, that will be the focus of this chapter.

Surgery, since ancient times, has been taught and learned by precept. The early history of surgical education in this country, like that of medical education in general, is a spotty one. In many areas of early nineteenth-century America most of those practicing medicine did not hold degrees, hence had little, if any, formal surgical education. In pioneer Ohio, for

1. A. Celsus, *De medicina*, 3 vols., Loeb Library Edition (Cambridge: Harvard University Press, 1961), 3:295.

instance, Frederick C. Waite has estimated that in the first decade considerably less than 10 percent of the practicing physicians held medical degrees. By 1835 it was probably no more than 20 percent.[2] This by no means meant that the young physicians of the day learned no surgery. The apprenticeship system is particularly well suited to the teaching of surgery, and is, after all, still the way much of the surgical craft is learned. As Waite has also pointed out, however, the preceptor system was less efficient in the frontier states because the quality of preceptors was lower and the supply of books and journals available to their students was limited. Depending upon the extent of the preceptor's practice, the student had the opportunity of learning much about the basic skills needed by the surgeon. Bandaging, dressing changes, and care of skin lesions all presented opportunities for the apprentice to learn.

As an increasing number of medical schools came into existence, surgery assumed its place as one of the seven basic medical subjects. Taught by lecture, demonstration, and occasionally by direct contact with the patient and his operation, most medical students learned at least a modicum of surgery. Because it is a complex and far from uniform educational pattern, only some aspects of the story can be highlighted in a single chapter.

The material for a history of surgical teaching in the medical schools is vast, much of it overlapping in many respects. The medical literature of the nineteenth century is filled with professorial pontification in the form of inaugural lectures, commencement addresses, annual discourses, and medical society discussions, some of which concerned surgery. Not until the decade of the 1890s does one find any number of papers or meetings devoted to the teaching of surgery. Since that time there has been no dearth, and the discussions seem to continue in our own time.

In addition to the rich medical periodical literature, many physicians have written memoirs, often describing in some detail their educational or teaching experiences. Biographies as well are on occasion a fruitful source of information. Far more valuable, however, for the historian of surgery are the many feet of surgical texts that line the library shelves and the annual medical school catalogues that may be found in profusion as well.

Two further points by way of introduction are necessary. First, the history of surgical education has, at least since the turn of the century, come to refer primarily to what we today call residency training. This is

---

2. Frederick C. Waite, "The Professional Education of Pioneer Ohio Physicians," *Ohio St. Arch. & Hist. Q.* 48 (1939): 189–97.

postgraduate in time, though perhaps not in substance, but in any case is well beyond our present scope. Second, as one reads about and evaluates the literature on medical education of the last two hundred years in America, one naturally tends to do so from the vantage point of medicine and its development, theoretical as well as practical. Equally important are concurrent societal and economic conditions and the status of higher education as a whole. Before condemning medical students and their teachers too harshly, one must also look at what was happening in the colleges and then the universities, themselves only slowly and painfully reformed. Admission practices, curriculum, course content, and teaching methods of American medical schools look much better if viewed in this broader light.[3]

I

Fruitful as it might be to trace the professorship of surgery in its historical development in a number of representative American medical schools, the documentation for most would be very scanty. For one school and its department of surgery the effort is well worth while, however, since others have already written about it, thus making the task easier. The reason that the University of Pennsylvania has found its several historians, but especially the noteworthy George Corner, is that it was the first true American school of medicine.[4] It was blessed with a succession of eminent surgeons who would naturally figure in any story of surgery and surgical education in America. Furthermore, the University of Pennsylvania's John Rhea Barton Chair of Surgery is claimed to be one of the oldest fully endowed surgical professorships in the United States.[5]

Formal medical education began in Philadelphia with the advent of the medical school at the College of Philadelphia beginning in 1765. At the inaugural ceremonies Dr. John Morgan delivered his oft-quoted two-day lecture. In this discourse Morgan spoke of the economic advantages of specialization. If surgeons and physicians each had a specific province

3. I have been unable in this chapter to consider the teaching of the surgical specialties. They do, of course, deserve more attention. Articles on this subject may be found in the medical literature. See, e.g., Ernest M. Seydell, "The Development of the Teaching of Otology in Europe and America," *Laryngoscope* 52 (1942): 453–57; Eugene M. Blake, "Historical Review of the Teaching of Ophthalmology at the School of Medicine, Yale University," *Yale J. Biol. Med.* 15 (1942–43): 755–61.

4. George W. Corner, *Two Centuries of Medicine: A History of the School of Medicine, University of Pennsylvania* (Philadelphia: Lippincott, 1965).

5. William A. Damon, "A Brief History of the John Rhea Barton Chair of Surgery," *Trans. & Stud. Coll. Phys. Phila.* 23 (1955): 94–104.

assigned, his argument went, each would become more skillful and dextrous in his respective parts.[6] This was much the same line of reasoning Adam Smith was to take in the first book of *The Wealth of Nations* in 1776 when he discussed the advantages of a division of labor in the manufacture of pins.

Surgery, Morgan said in 1765, called for special skills, different powers and qualifications that should not be blended with those of the apothecary. According to Morgan the various branches of knowledge which compose the science of medicine were anatomy, materia medica, physiology, chemistry, botany, pathology and the theory and practice of physic. Conspicuously absent from this list was surgery, though Morgan did stress the necessity of anatomical knowledge for the surgeon.[7] Thus Morgan hoped to bring to the colonies the separation of medicine and surgery as well as the separation of the compounding of drugs, as he had observed in Europe, from where he had recently returned.

Morgan, while he wished to separate surgery from medicine, nevertheless stressed that surgeons too should acquire a good education. Both medicine and surgery he believed to be necessary to progress in the healing arts. Surgery was not relegated to a lower caste, yet to him it was definitely an irksome task. To be proficient in surgery and to acquire the necessary dexterity required frequent practice at operating. This, Morgan claimed, was inconsistent with the occupation of a physician who needed time to study his patients and their illnesses.

William Shippen, Morgan's colleague and rival on the first faculty of the Medical College of Philadelphia, carried the duties of teaching anatomy, surgery, and midwifery. Not until 1805 was there to be a separate professorship of surgery. As George Corner has pointed out, Edinburgh, where the first faculty of the school had received their own training, did not separate the chair of surgery from anatomy until 1831.[8] Philip Syng Physick, a graduate of the University of Pennsylvania with an A.B. degree who then became a favorite pupil of the eminent London teacher of surgeons, John Hunter, was elected in 1805 as professor of surgery at his alma mater. Two years later he asked the trustees to appoint as adjunct professor of surgery his nephew and former apprentice, John Syng Dorsey, to share the teaching duties. The ill-fated Dorsey died of a fever in 1818.

From surviving notes of students in Physick's classes one can see that

6. John Morgan, *A Discourse Upon the Institution of Medical Schools in America* (Philadelphia, 1765; reprint ed., Baltimore: Johns Hopkins Press, 1937), p. xv.

7. Ibid., p. xvi.

8. Corner, *Two Centuries of Medicine*, p. 51.

this early professor of surgery was a thoughtful teacher. "Surgery is that branch of medical science," Physick proclaimed, "which teaches us the proper exhibition of remedies by instruments and external applications. . . ."[9] The first subject to master was inflammation. "Every surgeon who is desirous of excelling in his profession ought to make himself acquainted with inflammation. Indeed this is naturally the first subject for consideration as local inflammation is of so frequent occurrence, that there is [sic] few chirurgical diseases in which it is not considered as a cause, symptom or consequence."[10] Much of the discussion about various forms of inflammation was based on surgical pathology. Much to one student auditor's interest, Physick spoke about John Hunter's studies on the frozen ear of a rabbit. This was an early example of experimental pathology, and throughout the surviving lectures Physick's own teacher, John Hunter, loomed large. Yet the lectures were not merely theoretical. They contained much practical information as well. Physick told his students when and where to incise or to bleed. "Abscesses," he said, "ought to be opened when they are situated on the thorax, abdomen, face or knee joint, before the matter bursts inwards occasioning death."[11]

Dr. Physick, who of course is quoted at great length in these beautifully written notes, was certainly no cut-and-slash, rough-and-ready surgeon. There are numerous remarks to the effect, "I always tell my patients," or "I warn the patient," and "I suggest to the patient." John Syng Dorsey seems to have learned and practiced a similarly gentle approach. In discussing amputations, Dorsey began his lecture by urging his students to be cautious: "Before proceeding to this operation, gentlemen, recollect that it is an extremely painful one and that by it you place the patient in a mutilated state for life: on this account you should take the advice of several practitioners if possible before having recourse to it."[12]

In 1819, the year after Dorsey's death and after some complex faculty maneuverings, William Gibson, a pupil of John Bell of Edinburgh and Sir Charles Bell of London, two of Britain's greatest surgeons, was appointed to the professorship in Philadelphia. Succeeding Physick at the age of thirty-three, Gibson was already a seasoned veteran, having been the first professor of surgery at the University of Maryland since the age of

9. "Notes on Surgery from the Lectures of Dr. Physick, 1812–13," *Bull. Am. Coll. Surg.* 26 (1941): 285–87; quotation on p. 285.

10. Lee Griggs, "Notes on Surgery, Lectures by Philip S. Physick and John S. Dorsey," 3 vols., 1811 and 1812, MS in Trent Collection, Duke University Medical Center Library. Dr. Lee Griggs is identified by address only, which he wrote in the third notebook as Charlestown, Jefferson Co., Virginia.

11. Ibid., 1:9.

12. Ibid., 3:51.

twenty-three. For nearly thirty years he taught in Philadelphia, and his textbook, *The Institutes and Practice of Surgery*, better known as "Gibson's Surgery," carried his fame and his teaching far beyond the bounds of his city.

In the preface to the third edition of 1831, Gibson proudly proclaimed that his book had been called by hypercritics "a book on the practice of medicine." "A greater compliment could not have been paid to it," he exulted, because in America the physician had to be both physician and surgeon.[13] Gibson's two-volume text covered general principles in the first and diseases of specific parts of the body in the second. The first course (volume) of lectures was deliberately styled to fit with the concurrent anatomical lectures the students were attending at the time, and covered inflammatory diseases and bone and joint disorders.

In 1847 the University of Pennsylvania created a chair of clinical surgery to be held by one of the surgeons at the Pennsylvania Hospital. The chair was first held by Jacob Randolph, who was succeeded by George W. Norris a year later. When the latter vacated the position in 1857, clinical teaching at the Pennsylvania Hospital had become well established, so that no one was designated to the position again until 1870, when D. Hayes Agnew, who had already been lecturing to University of Pennsylvania students at the hospital for several years, assumed the title. It was Agnew then, in 1878, who became the first John Rhea Barton Professor of Surgery.[14]

Barton, himself a University of Pennsylvania medical graduate in 1818, had learned surgery from Philip Physick and his nephew John Dorsey. He had practiced medicine and surgery in Philadelphia until his retirement in 1840. Though having no further formal connection with the university, he had been widely known for his advances in orthopedic surgery, especially the head bandage named after him, and for his description of the technique of arthroplasty or joint reconstruction.[15]

Barton had lived for thirty years beyond the date of his retirement. Six years after his death in 1871, his widow had given to the University of Pennsylvania fifty thousand dollars, the income of which was to provide a salary for a professor of surgery to hold the chair named in honor of her

13. William Gibson, *The Institutes and Practice of Surgery*, 4th ed., 2 vols. (Philadelphia: Carey, Lea, and Blanchard, 1835), 1:xi. The preface to the 1831 edition was reprinted in the 4th edition.

14. J. Howe Adams, *History of the Life of D. Hayes Agnew, M.D., LL.D.* (Philadelphia: Davis, 1892), is the most complete source for information on Agnew.

15. Damon, "The John Rhea Barton Chair," and Kelly and Burrage, *Dictionary of American Medical Biography* (New York: D. Appleton, 1928), for data on Barton.

husband. In 1878 the first designated John Rhea Barton Professor was the eminent D. Hayes Agnew. Agnew, as was to be the case for all succeeding Barton professors as well, was a graduate of the school of medicine. This exceptional line of men, including such well-known names as John Ashhurst, John B. Deaver, and Isidore S. Ravdin, certainly are proof that so-called inbreeding is not an inherent evil.

David Hayes Agnew was a Pennsylvanian by birth, the son of a physician. When Agnew entered the medical department of the University of Pennsylvania in 1836 he encountered one of the best faculties in America. Nathaniel Chapman taught the practice of physick, the brilliant Samuel Jackson had just been appointed professor of the institutes of medicine, William Gibson was the surgeon, and William Horner, whose popular textbook of anatomy was very widely used in American medical schools, was the dean and professor of anatomy. Much of what Agnew and his classmates learned was from didactic lectures and some clinical conferences. In surgery the students were particularly fortunate because in addition to auditing Gibson's remarkably clear lectures, they attended clinics at the Pennsylvania Hospital and at the almshouse. There they could hear and watch some of the other great Philadelphia surgeons of the day, including Joseph Pancoast, Thomas Hewson, George Norris, and John Rhea Barton.

After graduation Agnew joined his father and for some years was a country practitioner. In 1848 he began practicing in Philadelphia and became actively involved in the Philadelphia School of Anatomy. Not until 1871 did he become professor of surgery at his school. This position, amounting to the chief of surgery, enabled him very quickly to add members to the faculty, thereby fashioning what today we would call a true department of surgery. An associate clinical professor and four demonstrators in surgery were soon at work, thereby enlarging the scope of teaching.[16] Agnew's own experience in practice and teaching was now put into effect, so that first-year students learned not only anatomy but bandaging and fracture dressing as well.

Agnew took his teaching responsibilities seriously. According to his biographer, he lectured three times a week and on Wednesday noon he held a surgical clinic at the new university hospital. This scene has been well captured in the famous *Agnew Clinic*, a painting by Thomas Eakins. Here one can see Agnew lecturing, knife in hand, as he momentarily stepped back from the operating table. His *Principles and Practice of Surgery* further enlarged his audience. Its three volumes, a total of three

16. Adams, *Agnew*.

thousand pages, appeared between 1878 and 1883. He was equally in demand as a consultant and, along with Dr. Frank H. Hamilton of New York, was one of two surgical consultants called to advise on the treatment of President James Garfield in the summer of 1881.

While to Philadelphia goes the credit for the first medical school in the American colonies, it was New York that could claim the first true professor of surgery. William Shippen in Philadelphia did encompass the subject, but concentrated his efforts on anatomy and midwifery more than on surgery. Meanwhile, at King's College Samuel Clossy in his lectures on anatomy and especially John Jones, the professor of surgery, discoursed on surgical topics.

John Jones was perhaps the most famous surgeon of his time in the colonies. His manual of military surgery, published in 1775, is usually accorded pride of place as the first American textbook of surgery. Born into a family of physicians on Long Island in 1729, Jones studied medicine as an apprentice in Philadelphia, attended lectures of William Hunter in London, and learned surgery from Percival Pott and the French surgeons, Jean-Louis Petit and Henri-François Le Dran. He earned the M.D. degree in Rheims in 1751. After his return to the colonies he made his reputation as a surgeon, widely in demand as a skillful and rapid lithotomist.

It is not his surgical skill and accomplishments that interest us here, but rather his surgical teaching. There are doubtless many extant records of his lectures, but one at least has been printed. Surgery, in Jones's opinion, was a broad field indeed. Presaging views of today's surgical leaders, Jones told his students two hundred years ago that surgery was both medical and manual. "The first, comprehends, an infinite variety of diseases, which require the assistance of both internal and external applications. . . . the last, is confined to those cases, which admit of relief from the hand alone, or assisted with instruments. Hence it will appear very evident, how necessary it is for the student in surgery to make himself thoroughly acquainted with all those branches of medicine, which are requisite to form the most accomplished Physician. . . ."[17]

A good knowledge of anatomy acquired by careful dissection as well as experience acquired from practice were both necessary to achieve perfection as a surgeon, according to Jones. Only continual study would bring this about. And, interestingly enough, Jones in the mid-eighteenth century stressed what his successors in the mid-nineteenth as well as those in

17. W. B. McDaniel II, "John Jones' Introduction Lecture to His Course in Surgery (1769), King's College, Printed from the Author's Manuscript," *Trans. & Stud. Coll. Phys. Phila.*, 4th ser., 8 (1940): 180–90; quotation on p. 183.

the mid-twentieth also held up to their students: the rapid progress of medicine and surgery. Men in each age firmly believe they are living in a time of great change and a burgeoning of medical knowledge. "Though surgery is one of those sciences which have been cultivated with the utmost industry and attention, and its progress, particularly during the present century, has been very rapid, new lights having been thrown upon it, by a variety of different discoveries, yet none but very superficial minds can imagine, that the limits of our present knowledge are the limits of the art," claimed Jones.[18] He further stressed to his students that surgery was a science, that operations alone were but one part of the treatment, and that a firm knowledge of anatomy and "the animal economy" were equally necessary. The lectures following the introduction with its exhortations were such as one would expect: on inflammation, tumors, hernia, wounds, ulcers, and fistulae.

II

Typical, and probably a bit more colorful than some of the many printed lectures to medical students by American professors of surgery, were those by Frank H. Hamilton of New York. Born in Vermont but educated in upstate New York, Hamilton had an illustrious career as surgical teacher, author, and practitioner. That he was one of two outside consultants (the other was D. Hayes Agnew of Philadelphia) called into the case of President James Garfield's wound from an assassin's bullet in the summer of 1881 attests to his national stature.[19]

Hamilton's own medical training, so typical of the 1830s, included a preceptorship, a course of lectures at the medical college in Fairfield, New York, in 1831, practice with a license granted by the Cayuga County Medical Censors, and a second course leading to the M.D. degree from the University of Pennsylvania in 1835. Soon thereafter he began teaching, first in Fairfield, then in Geneva, in Buffalo, and finally, from its inception in 1861 until 1875, at the Bellevue Hospital Medical College in New York City.

Hamilton was best known for his book on fractures, which went through eight editions between 1860 and 1891, though he always taught general surgery as well. His lectures usually stressed the knowledge of

---

18. Ibid., p. 184.
19. For biographical data on Hamilton, in addition to Kelly and Burrage, *Dictionary of American Medical Biography*, see the *Dictionary of American Biography* and Samuel W. Francis, *Biographical Sketches of Distinguished Living New York Surgeons* (New York: Bradburn, 1866), pp. 59–74.

anatomy as the first requisite for the properly trained surgeon. "It is not sufficient, gentlemen," he told a class of private students in Auburn, New York, in 1837, "that a surgeon acquaint himself with the number and order of the bones—the names and situation of the viscera; these are but the grand divisions, the continents and the mountain ranges. . . . Such an anatomical acquirement might indeed enable him to carve and disjoint a turkey or canvass-back with sufficient skill, but would never qualify him to carry the scalpel through the gory wound amid the mazy structure of muscles, tendons, and ligaments. . . ."[20] Of equal importance was the study of pathological anatomy. A firm knowledge of normal and abnormal anatomy, he stressed to his students, was the only basis for correct theory and, by implication, correct therapy.

It is difficult to assess the quality and scope of this private instruction Hamilton gave in Auburn prior to his affiliation with the various formal schools of medicine. In his privately printed lecture of 1837, the only additional information is that there were forty-three students. Since this was "an introductory lecture," one may assume a series followed. Most of the class were probably apprentices in Hamilton's office at the time.

A few years later, when Hamilton gave the introductory surgical lecture to the class of the Geneva Medical College, he repeated many of the same points. In addition, to these students formally enrolled in a medical school, he stressed the fact that in America surgery and medicine were closely associated. They had to learn both. "You, gentlemen, are to become surgeon-physicians, and wherever in these states, or on this continent you may locate, you must cut as well as cure. . . ."[21] There was no way the physician could escape the responsibilities of the surgeon. "It is this miserable error, more than all else, which exposes us daily to legal prosecution, and our profession to disgrace."[22]

Just how much surgery the average nineteenth-century American medical student learned during his medical school years is, of course, the question at hand. Obviously the variables were the student, the professor, and the facilities of the medical school in question. Asa Fitch, a student at the Castleton Medical School, subsequently had a career combining entomology and medicine. With these interests, then, one would not necessarily expect him to have devoted much attention to the study of surgery.[23]

20. Frank H. Hamilton, *Introductory Address on Anatomy and Surgery* (Auburn, 1837), p. 5.
21. Frank H. Hamilton, *Introductory Lecture before the Surgical Class of Geneva Medical College* (Geneva: Merrel, 1840), p. 7.
22. Ibid.
23. Samuel Reznek, "The Study of Medicine at the Vermont Academy of Medicine (1827–29) As Revealed in the Journal of Asa Fitch," *J. Hist. Med.* 24 (1969): 416–29.

As the end of his second year of study at Castleton approached, Fitch remembered that he had to race in order to finish his work, because he was deficient in many fields. He had never read on surgery or midwifery and would not do so as he finished the term at Castleton. In 1828, between his two courses at Castleton, Fitch went to the Rutgers Medical School for one term. Here he seems to have seen more anatomy and certainly more surgery. He described several operations he watched. Like many students, it was not pure joy of learning that he experienced: "But, oh, how my feelings recoiled at the sight [of an amputation]. To behold the keen shining knife drawn around the leg severing the integuments, while the unhappy subject of the operation uttered the most heart-rending screams in his agony and torment . . . to hear the saw working its way through the bone, produced an impression I never can forget."[24]

William W. Mayo, the founder of the medical dynasty, began his medical education at the Indiana Medical College in LaPorte in the 1849/50 term. This was typical of the mid-century proprietary schools. The teaching consisted almost entirely of lectures with very little clinical instruction. LaPorte had no hospital and the medical school did not provide an ambulatory clinic either. The student's practical bedside experience was gained entirely through his work with his preceptor. Occasionally the professor of surgery did demonstrate an operation in the amphitheatre before the medical class. This was reported in all its gory detail in the next day's local newspaper.[25]

Even thirty years later, when the young William Mayo was attending one of the country's best schools at the University of Michigan, surgical learning was acquired at a distance. The more junior the student, the farther he was from the patient in the amphitheatre or the operating theatre. Certainly, however, some value from observing surgical procedures was to be realized. Charles Mayo, who began his medical studies in Chicago in 1885, is reputed to have been a keen observer at the operations of Doctors Nicholas Senn, Edmund Andrews, and Christian Fenger. He could, it seems, describe to his friends and roommate every move made by the operator.[26]

Surgery at Harvard in the 1870s was taught by lectures and clinics held by Dr. Henry J. Bigelow, professor of surgery, and Dr. David W.

24. Samuel Reznek, "A Course of Medical Education in New York City in 1828–29: The Journal of Asa Fitch," *Bull. Hist. Med.* 42 (1968): 555–65; quotation on pp. 560–61.

25. Helen Clapesattle, *The Doctors Mayo* (Garden City, New York: Garden City, 1943), pp. 20–21.

26. Ibid., p. 191.

Cheever, professor of clinical surgery. Two young instructors who in future years would become eminent professors in their own right were Charles B. Porter and J. Collins Warren.[27] Bigelow taught and worked at the Massachusetts General Hospital while Cheever was surgical chief at the Boston City Hospital. Each lectured at the medical school as well. At least once a week each man made rounds on his hospital service in company with medical students. In the 1870s, John B. Wheeler recalled, this was not very satisfactory because it was difficult for forty or fifty men to gather around one bed. As third year students, each member of the class had the occasion to be assigned to at least one surgical patient who was followed closely throughout his or her hospitalization.[28]

The study of medicine has, since the time of the original founding of the medical school in Pennsylvania, been divided into two parts. The first part has dealt with the so-called preclinical sciences, the second with experience in the clinical fields. Whether surgery was taught at the operating table, at the bedside, or in the didactic lecture period, it has always formed a part of so-called clinical teaching. Henry J. Bigelow wrote about this extensively. "Clinical study is bed study," he claimed. "Here the student closes and grapples with the malady of whose Protean forms he has as yet only read. Here he learns at once the language of disease and the language of suffering humanity; and if his scientific sense is educated, his kindlier feelings are also developed."[29]

It is quite obvious that in this lecture Bigelow, the professor of surgery, is discussing the broad field that is medicine. The doctor must learn to understand disease. He then must form a medical opinion. This is as true for the surgeon as it is for the non-operating physician. Both must learn to formulate a diagnosis. Here clinical instruction plays its important role. The skillful surgeon will make diagnoses and detect disorders of the body not because he is more sensitive but because his knowledge will lead him to the correct conclusions.

Operative surgery, Bigelow told his students, was the direct province of the surgeon. It is with operative surgery that the public associates the surgeon, and his fame is directly related to the number and the magnitude of the operations he performs. Bigelow warned his students that

27. Edward D. Churchill, ed., *To Work in the Vineyard of Surgery: The Reminiscences of J. Collins Warren (1842–1927)* (Cambridge: Harvard University Press, 1958), is a fine source for surgical education at Harvard over many decades. See also Henry K. Beecher and Mark D. Altschule, *Medicine at Harvard: The First Three Hundred Years* (Hanover: The University Press of New England, 1977), passim.

28. John B. Wheeler, *Memoirs of a Small-Town Surgeon* (New York: Stokes, 1935), p. 43.

29. Henry J. Bigelow, *Introductory Lecture, Delivered at the Massachusetts Medical College, November 6, 1849* (Boston: Mussey, 1850), p. 11.

the public has an undue appreciation of surgery and that this was both useful and dangerous to them. "Much of this spirit of exaggeration still invests the science. Why is the amphitheatre crowded to the roof, by adepts as well as students, on the occasion of some great operation, while the silent working of some well-directed drug excites comparatively little comment? Mark the hushed breath, the fearful intensity of silence, when the blade pierces the tissues, and the blood of the unhappy sufferer wells up to the surface. Animal sense is always fascinated by the presence of animal suffering."[30] The surgeon, Bigelow warned, is all too prone to foster and to encourage the mystique and the undue appreciation. Speaking as his father's son, Bigelow told his students that "nature is the great surgeon, and art is at best but an assistant."[31]

By the first decade of the twentieth century the surgical teaching at Harvard had changed somewhat. Lectures and clinics continued, but more was done in small groups. A course on surgical technique was taught to second-year students. Consisting of six hours of lectures to the entire class and twelve two-hour laboratory exercises, the course covered bandaging and surgical dressings. In addition, the students learned to give hypodermic injections and enemas, techniques now only a part of the nursing curriculum.[32]

According to Francis M. Rackemann, after the large third-year teaching clinics that were held on most mornings, the class was disbursed to section assignments. Fourth-year surgery left a deep impression on Rackemann and his fellow student George R. Minot. The highlight of the fourth-year surgical course was following Dr. Maurice Richardson, Moseley Professor of Surgery, on his rounds for a whole day. This privilege was granted to only two students at a time and was indeed a memorable occasion that included a ride in a Pierce Arrow. Richardson too seemed to enjoy this form of teaching and made the most of it, as Rackemann remembers: "Whenever the car was moving, Dr. Richardson would turn around and talk to us about the patient we had just seen, and

30. Ibid., p. 21.
31. Ibid., p. 25. H. J. Bigelow's father, Jacob, was a proponent of rational medicine, one that stressed the healing power of nature. In 1835 he had written his widely quoted paper "On Self-Limited Diseases."
32. "The Department of Surgery," in *The Harvard Medical School, 1782–1906* (n.p., n.d.), pp. 49–62. Bandaging courses were taught in many medical schools until about the time of World War II. For an informative survey of what courses were taught in schools in 1900 and what their content was, see the survey by Herbert L. Burrell, "The Teaching of Surgery," *Boston Med. & Surg. J.* 147 (1902): 449–53, 477–80. This paper also appeared in the *Trans. Am. Surg. Assoc.* 20 (1902): 86–103, followed by a long discussion. For the way the homeopaths taught surgery in their schools see William B. Van Lennep, "The Teaching of Surgery in Our Colleges," *Trans. Am. Inst. Homeo.* 2 (1906): 169–78.

about other cases too. He had the facility of sharing his enthusiasm, as well as his knowledge, with us. He liked to teach, probably because he liked people. He was a real doctor with a capital 'D'."[33]

One must remember that the observation of actual surgery was not necessarily a daily occurrence. In spite of what many students have said about the limitations of this method of teaching and learning, it doubtless proved of some stimulus to those students who themselves wished to become like their teachers and wished to develop an ability with knife, forceps, and ligature. But even as late as 1890, the major teaching hospitals did fewer than one operation per day. Of 6,083 admissions to Charity Hospital in New Orleans in 1890, for instance, only 291 had what Rudolph Matas called important or major operations.[34] Statistics for teaching hospitals elsewhere were similar. So the opportunity to observe, whether closely or at a distance, was in the first place limited by the development of surgery itself.

At the Massachusetts General Hospital, Saturday morning was known as "Operating Day," a tradition that continued well into the 1920s. The first decade or two of the twentieth century saw the heyday of showmanship in operative surgery. The two surgical services of the Massachusetts General Hospital, the East and the West, vied with each other in trying to stage the better show. The operations were usually well attended by both medical students and practitioners.[35]

J. Collins Warren left his native Boston, where his family name was preeminent in medicine, to serve as a medical cadet in 1863 and to attend medical school in Philadelphia. The Jefferson Medical School in the midnineteenth century was outstanding in surgery because two of the most prominent surgeons of the country were on its faculty. Samuel D. Gross was professor of surgery and Joseph Pancoast was professor of anatomy. Warren has left a graphic description of Samuel Gross's class:

> The lecture room was a large, well shaped amphitheatre into which the class poured tumultuously; it held four or five hundred students and was always well filled. A most painstaking instructor, Gross hammered on the rudiments of surgery with a clearness and force

33. Francis M. Rackemann, *The Inquisitive Physician: The Life and Times of George Richards Minot* (Cambridge: Harvard University Press, 1956), pp. 50–52; quotation on p. 52.

34. Rudolph Matas, *Am. J. Surg.* 82 (1951): 111–21; p. 121. One of the most widely quoted papers on surgical education is William Halsted's "The Training of a Surgeon," *Bull. Johns Hopkins Hosp.* 15 (1904): 267–75. That, however, is mostly concerned with post-M.D. training, hence not pertinent for this chapter. Halsted did include good statistics of the numbers of operations performed in various leading hospitals.

35. Churchill, *To Work in the Vineyard of Surgery,* p. 30.

which commanded the attention of the class and left an impression never to be forgotten. Instinctively he selected the small details of rudimentary knowledge for which the student mind was craving and dwelt upon them with patient care, somewhat to the detriment of the brilliant discourse which he was quite capable of delivering. By understanding how to keep on the level of his audience, he kept his lectures both popular and instructive. This was in strong contrast to the many prominent medical lecturers of the day who conversed easily and eloquently with the class but left behind, at least to a beginner like myself, a sense that many difficulties stood in the way of a proper comprehension of their themes.[36]

Warren seems to have had a distinctly superior undergraduate surgical education. He tells us that both Gross and Pancoast gave him every opportunity to see their surgical cases and on occasion they allowed him to assist at surgical operations. Warren was, therefore, one of the few nineteenth-century surgeons in whose memoirs one finds reference to satisfactory medical school surgical experiences.

The New York Hospital in the latter half of the nineteenth century was one of the clinical centers for medical education in New York City. Only a handful of the attending surgeons, however, actually gave instruction to a few medical students on the wards. The students followed their teachers on their rounds, often brief, generally once a week. As Robert F. Weir recalled, "When a case required an operation, a notice was sent, if time permitted, but not regularly to the then existing medical colleges, to be posted on their bulletin boards. Unless the operation was of especial importance not many students appeared, except on Saturday, when as there were no lectures given in the afternoon, they could more readily attend hospital clinics."[37]

There was in the early 1860s, partly from the exigencies of the Civil War, a revival of the purely clinical or practical schools of medicine that were more prevalent in Europe. In New York in 1860 and 1861 the Long Island College Hospital and the Bellevue Hospital Medical College both hoped to emulate the great hospital medical schools of London.[38] Many physicians in the 1850s had bemoaned the lack of hospital experience obtained in the average school. New York, with several fine hospitals, was a case in point.

One of the surgeons on the Bellevue faculty, Stephen Smith, cited what

36. Ibid., p. 50.
37. Robert F. Weir, *Personal Reminiscences of the New York Hospital from 1856–1900* (n.p., n.d.), pp. 21–22.
38. William F. Norwood, *Medical Education in the United States before the Civil War* (Philadelphia: University of Pennsylvania Press, 1944; reprint ed., 1971), pp. 143–48.

he called only feeble attempts to correct the deficiencies of an excessively didactic medical curriculum. Instead of moving the medical colleges to the hospitals, the teachers invited the sick to the classroom. Here the student and the patient were not brought into direct contact. The student learned, if at all, by proxy. Such schools, Smith told an audience at the opening of the school year at Bellevue in 1863, were the theoretical schools of the ancients. "They teach theories and systems, but they do not teach practical medicine. They educate the brain, but leave the hand palsied, the eye blind, and the ear deaf. Their graduates go forth to practical life like full fledged eaglets deprived of wings."[39]

In the memoirs of those physicians and surgeons who have recorded them, one often finds an isolated lecture or demonstration of an operation that was particularly impressive to the student. Thus Dr. Ernest V. Smith's days at the University of Minnesota College of Medicine and Surgery from 1903 to 1907 seemed to have been quite typical. He especially remembered the consultation by Dr. William J. Mayo, who was unheard of by Smith, a fourth-year student, until the surgeon's appearance before the class with a patient suffering from gastric cancer. "The effect produced upon the entire class by Dr. William J. Mayo was electrical. He captured and held the attention of every student. . . ."[40] By implication, of course, one can assume that the everyday teaching of surgery was somewhat less than attention producing. It is also of interest that Smith, a subsequently well-trained and successful surgeon, said nothing else about his surgical education as an undergraduate.

Dr. J. M. T. Finney, on the other hand, remembered his medical school days in the mid 1880s at Harvard somewhat differently. "As I was always particularly interested in surgery rather than medicine, it followed naturally the members of the faculty who impressed me most were connected with the surgical specialties. As that was the era of the didactic lecture, most of the teaching consisted of lectures, either clinical or didactic."[41] Finney remembered particularly the beautifully illustrated lectures of Dr. Maurice Richardson. What particularly impressed students, apparently, was Dr. Richardson's ambidextrous style. Finney also had a social relationship with Dr. C. B. Porter, another well-known Harvard surgeon, and was asked to assist in surgical cases on some of Porter's private patients.

Dr. Hugh Young, a future Hopkins colleague of Finney, had a some-

39. Stephen Smith, "Union of Didactic and Clinical Instruction," *Am. Med. Times* 9 (1864): 119–22; quotation on p. 121.
40. Ernest V. Smith, *The Making of a Surgeon* (Fond du Lac, Wis.: Berndt, 1942), p. 120.
41. J. M. T. Finney, *A Surgeon's Life* (New York: Putnam's, 1940), p. 57.

what less satisfying medical school experience. Young went to the University of Virginia where two nine-month sessions were taught by full-time men in the preclinical sciences. The clinical sciences were not as well taught as the basic sciences, according to Young. "At the university we had no hospital—only a small dispensary for out-patients—and the only surgery I saw was performed by Dr. William C. Dabney. . . . Although Dr. Dabney was professor of medicine, he was also an excellent surgeon, but had to do his work in the homes of his patients. I was invited to see a few of his operations. When I got my degree, although crammed full of science and booklearning, I knew next to nothing about the practice of surgery."[42]

Until very late in the nineteenth century, surgical teaching, even in the best medical schools, often kept students, especially junior students, at a distance from the patient in the amphitheatre or on the operating table. Even when a student was part of the operating team, as the junior member he was often relegated to holding the ether cone over the patient's face, thus having to stretch mightily to observe the surgery in the lower portions of the body.

Abraham Flexner in his 1910 report on medical education also observed the dangers of surgical teaching from a distance when he wrote that "in general, the less a school has to offer in the way of clinical facilities, the more heavily is surgery overweighted. Its pedagogical value is relatively slight; for operations are performed in large amphitheaters in which the surgeon and his assistants surround the patient, to whom they give their whole mind, in practical disregard of the students, who loll in their seats without an inkling of what is happening below. Most of the students see only the patient's feet and the surgeon's head."[43]

It is a well-known fact that American medical students from colonial times until at least World War I frequently completed their medical education in the schools and hospitals of Europe. Thomas N. Bonner has estimated that between 1870 and 1914 nearly fifteen thousand American physicians went to German schools alone to study.[44] Many surgeons subsequently wrote about their European experiences. One of the typical German travel memoirs comes from Arthur D. Bevan, himself a very important figure in the reform of American medical education early in the twentieth century.

42. Hugh Young, *A Surgeon's Autobiography* (New York: Harcourt, Brace, 1940), pp. 45–46.
43. Abraham Flexner, *Medical Education in the United States and Canada* (New York: Carnegie Foundation for the Advancement of Teaching, 1910), p. 116.
44. Thomas N. Bonner, *American Doctors and German Universities* (Lincoln: University of Nebraska Press, 1963), p. 23.

Bevan began the study of medicine in Chicago in 1880. He was much influenced by Moses Gunn, professor of surgery at Rush Medical College. Bevan later recalled that the kind of operations Gunn and other surgeons were performing in 1880 were amputations, removal of tumors, cutting for stone, operating on hemorrhoids, opening abscesses, setting fractures, reducing dislocations, occasionally ligating large blood vessels for aneurysm, draining empyema, trephining for depressed fracture of the skull, dilating urethral strictures, and occasionally removing tonsils. Bevan did not feel that his own education was sufficiently complete at graduation and so went to Europe to further his medical experience. One of the places he visited for some time was Vienna, where Theodor Billroth was the leading surgical teacher. Billroth trained his students very thoroughly in anatomy, physiology and pathology. Bevan recalled the teaching was done in the outpatient dispensary, the hospital, and the surgical clinic. The student was an apprentice who learned by helping the master and seeing how surgical operations were performed. As Bevan put it, "He taught his students surgery as a successful football coach teaches his squad football, by training them in the actual work itself. He would have had very little patience with some of the modern makers of medical curricula, who take the position that the student is to be given a cadaver and a book or a patient and some books and be left to educate himself."[45] This latter was a snipe at Franklin P. Mall, professor of anatomy at Hopkins, who was known to favor this nondirected approach. The experience of Bevan is of interest because Mall and his generation of medical faculty members were profoundly influenced by their German experiences as well, but with an emphasis on *Lernfreiheit* and *Lehrfreiheit*. It was Billroth who discussed these concepts in his influential 1876 book on the German medical schools.[46] Thus depending on their own educational philosophy and preferences, physicians gleaned from the European experience what they were seeking.

III

It is very difficult to generalize about the surgical curriculum in nineteenth-century schools of medicine. The medical school catalogues, while useful guides, are misleading in several ways. Promises went unfulfilled and thus actual quality is difficult to measure. An additional

45. Arthur D. Bevan, "The Study and Teaching and the Practice of Surgery," *Ann. Surg.* 98 (1933): 481–94; quotation on p. 486.
46. Theodor Billroth, *The Medical Sciences in the German Universities* (New York: Macmillan, 1924). This was the English translation of the book that appeared originally a half century earlier.

problem for the historian trying to draw together a composite picture is that schools varied greatly. Even the so-called best schools, F. P. Mall showed in 1899, had variations in the number of hours assigned to the various subjects reaching 1,000 percent. In the six schools whose names he does not identify, but which are designated as "leading medical schools," the hours allotted to surgery were 470, 390, 385, 570, 670, and 660. The first three schools gave more time to medicine, while in the latter three the departments of surgery had the greater number of hours. [47]

Catalogues are an obvious and fairly useful source of data about surgical teaching in many American medical schools of the nineteenth and twentieth centuries. They listed the professors and the course titles. Occasionally the course content was described in the nineteenth century and much more explicitly in recent decades, and they are in general helpful guides because they served as both advertisement and information for the medical students of their time. All this is obvious. What is not quite so obvious is that, as is true for any historical document, the catalogues too must be used with caution. One of the most vivid examples of criticism of promises held out by a catalogue with subsequent failure in actual performance was chronicled by Andrew Boardman, an 1839 graduate of the Geneva Medical College.

There were several students in his class, Boardman claimed, who had paid for the various class tickets as required for graduation but seldom, if ever in fact, attended. Even more serious, Boardman charged, was that students had to pay for a private course in anatomy so that they might actually learn the subject. Boardman listed several additional unfulfilled promises made in the catalogue: the course on chemistry was to be delivered by a doctor of medicine, but in fact was taught by a doctor of divinity who was ill prepared at that; there was to be a course on physiology but none was ever offered; specimens were to be available for dissection, but not a single subject was provided; clinical instruction, including surgery, was promised at the Western Hospital, but in fact, the so-called hospital consisted of the second floor of an old building labelled Geneva Shoe Store and was devoid of patients save one surgical case. [48]

Clinical teaching in America is as old as the preceptorship method. In addition, many American medical schools advertised in their catalogues

---

47. Franklin P. Mall, "Liberty in Medical Education," in R. M. Pearce, ed., *Medical Research and Education* (New York: Science Press, 1913), pp. 211–22; quotation on p. 216.

48. Andrew Boardman, *An Essay on the Means of Improving Medical Education and Elevating the Medical Character* (Philadelphia: Haswell, 1840), reprinted for the most part in G. H. Brieger, ed., *Medical America in the Nineteenth Century* (Baltimore: Johns Hopkins Press, 1972), pp. 25–36.

that the students spent some time with faculty in hospital work. The extent of surgical training in the hospital setting, of course, varied greatly, depending upon the hospital, the number of operations performed, and, perhaps most of all, upon the teachers. Not all hospital settings were conducive to much surgical learning. Witness, for instance, the ruling of the managers of the Massachusetts General Hospital of May 1824:

> The pupils are not to remain at the Hospital longer than is abso-
> lutely necessary for the visits. They are not to converse with the
> patients or nurses. During operations and while in the wards they
> are to abstain from conversation with each other; they are not to
> walk about; nor in any other way to disturb either the medical
> officer, or the patients. . . . In all cases, in which it will be proper
> for the pupil to make any personal examination of a patient, such as
> feeling the pulse, examining a tumor, etc. an intimation to that
> effect will be given them by the physician or surgeon. It must be
> obvious that the greatest inconveniences must arise, if such exam-
> inations were commonly made by the pupils.[49]

The College of Medicine and Surgery of the University of Michigan, according to Dr. David Riesman, faced this issue squarely. "Clinical instruction," read the Michigan catalogue, "it is believed, is far better imparted in the walks of private practice, especially in that section of the country where the student intends to locate himself, than can be done even in the best regulated hospitals. The hasty walk through the wards of a hospital furnishes at best but a sorry substitute for the close and accurate study of cases as they occur in the professional rounds of the private practitioner."[50]

Dr. Riesman, recalling his own medical school days at the University of Pennsylvania around the turn of the century, claimed that he had to spend very long days in the lecture room. Occasionally the students were given what were called clinical lectures in the huge amphitheatre. The patient would be brought in and the large class of students would be told about the course of the disease. Dr. Riesman believed they learned very little of a practical nature from this exercise. He also recalled that "occasionally we were taken into the wards of the Philadelphia General Hospital or the University Hospital, but I cannot recall that I examined more than two or three cases in my entire course."[51]

This kind of testimony is in conflict with the reports of other physicians

49. Thomas F. Harrington, *The Harvard Medical School*, 3 vols. (New York: Lewis, 1905), 2:582–83.
50. David Riesman, "Clinical Teaching in America, with Some Remarks on Early Medical Schools," *Trans. & Stud. Coll. Phys. Phila.* 6 (1938–39): 89–110; quotation on p. 106.
51. Ibid., p. 109.

and with the reports of British observers such as Dr. Norman Walker of Edinburgh. Walker, reporting to his Scottish colleagues his observations during an American trip in 1890, claimed that the clinical teaching he saw in America was often very good. He extolled the Johns Hopkins Hospital and paid a particular tribute to the University of Pennsylvania, to which he gave "the first place among the teaching schools of America."[52] At Harvard he reported, "A student is given a case. Without any assistance he is supposed to take the history of this case and describe its course. This case he reads before the class, and his fellow students then proceed to ask questions, criticize, and pick holes generally in his report."[53] And a final example comes from the biennial report of the regents of the University of California for the years 1873 to 1875. Here one reads the astonishing statement that in the medical school clinical instruction was carried out as follows: "A patient is placed in charge of a senior student, and by him examined, a diagnosis and prognosis given, together with his views of treatment, in the presence of the class; after which, all errors of investigation, conclusion, or suggestion in the treatment are corrected, with such remarks upon the subject as may be pertinent to practical medicine, etc. Every student, thus detailed, is expected to keep a complete history of the case, in due form, for his own and lecturer's use."[54] Despite the fact that the evidence for such an advanced idea comes from an official university report, it shows nevertheless that the clinical or bedside teaching turned into a routine by William Osler and William Halsted was already being discussed and probably carried out in other parts of the country a full two decades before Johns Hopkins opened its doors to medical students.

Surgical teaching at the Cooper Medical College in San Francisco in the 1880s is representative of the better methods of the time. At this, the oldest and certainly one of the best medical schools on the Pacific Coast, a degree was awarded after a three-year graded course of study. Surgery was taught by lecture and clinical demonstration. Professor L. C. Lane, president of the college and nephew of Eli Cooper, the founder, arranged his surgical lectures in such a manner, the catalogue claimed, so as to give the student, by the end of three years, a set of notes incorporating a "complete system of surgery derived from American, English, French, and German sources."[55]

52. Norman Walker, "The Medical Profession in the United States," *Edinburgh Med. J.* 37 (1891–92): 135–42; 239–49; quotation on p. 140.

53. Ibid., p. 142.

54. *Biennial Report of the Regents of the University of Calif. for the Years 1873–75*, p. 94.

55. *Annual Announcement, Cooper Medical College Session of 1884* (San Francisco, 1884).

The school used the 450-bed City and County Hospital of San Francisco and the Morse Dispensary in the college building to hold clinical teaching sessions. The students relying on the Morse Clinic for surgical experience were limited, however, by the relative paucity of patients. In 1883, for instance, the surgical clinic reported seeing only 252 patients, 48 of whom had operations. These figures do not include 537 patients and 20 operations reported by the eye, ear, nose and throat clinics.[56]

A decade later, in the 1894 catalogue, the Morse Clinic reported 634 patients and 161 operations for the previous year in the surgical department. Eye, ear, nose and throat patients had, meanwhile, increased to 1,149, with 260 operations.[57] Not only did numbers of patients and operative procedures increase here as well as elsewhere, but the size of faculty increased accordingly. By 1904 Cooper Medical College had a separate department of surgery of nine faculty members, the largest single department in the school. This is the more impressive when one considers that urology and EENT were separate departments, each with three faculty members who must also, of course, be considered as surgeons. The annual report for 1894 of Cooper Medical College tells us that the total number of operations performed before the class in the college clinic and the City and County Hospital of San Francisco during the previous year was 150.[58]

In addition to catalogues, the numerous and voluminous textbooks of surgery published with increasing frequency and bulk after the middle of the nineteenth century indicate much of what was taught to students in their surgical courses.[59] The historian of surgery can profitably follow the advances of the craft and its increasingly scientific nature in the progressive editions of the major European and American texts. One of the most popular of the latter group was authored by Samuel D. Gross of Philadel-

56. Ibid.

57. *Annual Announcement, Cooper Medical College Session of 1894–95* (San Francisco, 1894).

58. *Annual Report for 1894 of the Clinics Conducted Under the Auspices of the Cooper Medical College* (San Francisco, 1895), p. 7.

59. In addition to catalogues, notes, and texts, a fruitful source for determining what was taught as well as what was expected of medical students in the nineteenth century (or at any other time for that matter) may be seen in the questions they were asked on board examinations or when they went into the military. *Trans. Med. Soc. St. N.Y.* (1862), pp. 388–89, e.g., printed questions submitted to applicants for positions as military surgeons. Candidates were expected to describe the course of various blood vessels and nerves, to describe operations such as thigh amputation, to describe appropriate dressings for a variety of wounds, to know the chemical constituents of various common drugs, and to describe the constitutional disturbances caused by burns. Any young medical graduate who passed this examination, and many did, had learned some surgery!

phia, certainly one of the medical world's most indefatigable writers. Begun in 1859 as a single volume, it soon grew so that the fifth edition of 1872, for instance, was two stout tomes of 1,098 and 1,170 pages, respectively. Dedicated to his numerous pupils who had attended his lectures for thirty-odd years, Gross's work covered the principles of surgical pathology and all operative procedures.

General words about surgery, philosophy, history, aims, and limitations, were, by comparison to technical matter, relatively few. Less than two pages in the edition of 1872, for instance, were devoted to the qualifications of a surgeon. But these few paragraphs did stress that operative surgery was a progressive art, that its limits had not been reached, and that only the well-qualified and properly trained should perform surgery. Courage, Gross believed, was the first requisite, though it might be disguised in bravado that led to knivesmanship. A reprehensible few surgeons still lacked caution and good sense, those who operated more for the benefit of the surgeon than for that of the patient.

"A most thorough knowledge of anatomy" was the other prime requisite. Not only long and patient study and dissection, but cadaver surgery as well should be taught to the student. Gross believed that "no man can become an accomplished operator unless he practices constantly on the dead subject. Dexterity, grace, and elegance are to be acquired only by long and patient exercise. From what I have seen of our students, they are lamentably deficient in the use of the knife. Many of them, indeed, engage in the active duties of their profession without ever having performed a solitary operation on the cadaver, and hence it is not surprising that failure and disgrace should so often attend their early trials on the living subject."[60] All schools, Gross repeatedly stressed, should have such courses.

The fifth edition, greatly enlarged and revised according to the claims of its title page, no longer, however, carried two very interesting pages found in the earlier editions. These began the text and were called "preliminary observations." For a long time, Gross pointed out in his second edition of 1862, surgery was regarded "merely as a kind of handicraft, fit to be exercised only by men of inferior attainment, ability and skill." The surgeon was thought to be the mere servant of the physician. "His task was completed when he had made his incisions, spilt a certain quantity of blood. . . . his occupation was a mere mechanical one. . . ." But this surgery of the past and its contrast to the surgery of 1862, Gross observed

60. Samuel D. Gross, *A System of Surgery*, 5th ed., 2 vols. (Philadelphia: Lea, 1872), 1:494.

enthusiastically, formed one of the brightest pages in the history of human progress and achievement. Surgery was no longer a handicraft, but a science and an art. Surgery, Gross believed, could no longer be set apart from medicine.[61]

Surgery was separated by some writers into two parts: principles and operations. But for Gross, the two had to proceed hand in hand and should be so taught. "A work on surgery, or, indeed, on any subject, without principles, may be compared to a vessel at sea without helm or rudder to guide it to its place of destination."[62] Let the student learn principles, Gross taught, and what is merely operative will be more justly appreciated.

The study of surgery is more than the mastery of diagnosis and of operative technique; it is also the understanding of disease processes. Surgical pathology has played an important role in the training of surgeons since the time of the Paris School early in the nineteenth century. Many American students read James Paget's lectures on surgical pathology, delivered at the Royal College of Surgeons in the years 1847 to 1852 and first published in a single volume in 1854. It was Paget's intent to "illustrate the general pathology of the principal surgical diseases, in conformity with the larger and more exact doctrines of physiology."[63] Beginning with nutrition and ending with tuberculous disease, Paget's 699-page text is a wonderful compilation of current knowledge of structure, function, and dysfunction of the human body. Loaded with references and very well indexed, it extensively covered the principles of surgery. An earlier pathology text by Samuel Gross was also very popular among students in the decades before Paget's book was available.[64]

One of America's foremost exponents of surgical pathology was Christian Fenger, a Dane, who taught medicine for many years in Chicago. Arthur Hertzler, himself a future surgeon, recalled that during his student days at Northwestern, Fenger preached that the only way to learn surgery was to beat a path from the operating room to the laboratory. Fenger's insistence on the value of studying surgical pathology systematically, Hertzler believed, was one of the most valuable lessons he learned from any of his teachers.[65]

61. Ibid., 2nd ed. (1862), 1:35–36.

62. Ibid., p. 36.

63. James Paget, *Lectures on Surgical Pathology* (Philadelphia: Lindsay and Blakiston, 1854), p. vii.

64. Samuel D. Gross, *Elements of Pathological Anatomy* (Philadelphia: Blanchard and Lea, 1839), and subsequent editions.

65. Arthur E. Hertzler, *The Horse and Buggy Doctor* (New York: Harper, 1938), p. 49. For Chicago surgery see also Thomas N. Bonner, *Medicine in Chicago, 1850–1950* (Madi-

IV

By the first decade of the twentieth century medical school departments of surgery were beginning to take on an appearance we would easily recognize today. Instead of having one professor of surgery, perhaps another of clinical surgery, and a third surgeon teaching anatomy, the departments began to have a senior and junior faculty, often amounting to four or six men. From its inception Johns Hopkins Medical School, for instance, appointed the surgeon in chief of the hospital as professor of surgery in the school of medicine. By 1908 this person was backed by four associate professors, some concentrating on a surgical specialty such as neurosurgery; urology; or ear, nose and throat. In addition, there were four or five assistants, whom we would today probably call instructors. This senior staff, assisted by a junior staff of house officers, taught the students.

The surgical teaching at Hopkins as well as at many other schools was carried out in the dispensary, on the wards, in the operating rooms, and in the Hunterian Laboratory. Although Dr. Halsted did hold a clinic once a week, often giving a clinical lecture with demonstrations of several cases, at Hopkins there were no systematic lectures in medicine or in surgery. There were systematic sessions, however, in surgical pathology. As one observer noted in the *Scottish Medical and Surgical Journal*, "One cannot but be struck with the thoroughness with which the principles of operative surgery are thus instilled into the students in the way that he is not likely to forget."[66]

It is well known that in 1910 Abraham Flexner held up to the country the Johns Hopkins as a model medical school. As such it is worth describing its methods of teaching surgery. It is very difficult, however, to judge how many other medical students across the country were taught surgery in a similar way. Though the Hopkins method may have been among the best publicized, by its own faculty and students as well as by outside observers, Harvard, Michigan, Columbia, Pennsylvania, and other schools had by 1910 probably equally improved their surgical teaching. One feature that does seem to be principally a Hopkins contribution to the teaching of surgery was a course given in the Hunterian Laboratory of experimental medicine. This course allowed students to perform opera-

son: American History Research Center, 1957); C. Frederick Kittle, "The Development of Academic Surgery in Chicago," *Surgery* 62 (1967): 1–11; and George Rosen, "Christian Fenger, Medical Immigrant," *Bull. Hist. Med.* 48 (1974): 129–45.

66. E. Scott Carmichael, "The Surgical Department and Teaching of Surgery in the Johns Hopkins Hospital," *Scottish M. & S. J.* 22 (1908): 513–17.

tions on anesthetized dogs using the techniques of strict asepsis. It was described in detail by Harvey Cushing in 1906.[67]

As Cushing properly pointed out, medical degrees, in theory at least, included medicine and surgery. Prior to Joseph Lister and to anesthesia, the surgeon had to have a detailed knowledge of anatomy, because without anesthesia speed was of paramount importance. But in the nineteenth century surgery was increasingly based on physiological principles as well. "Hence much more than before, the surgeon's requirements of ready information have become those of the physician—he has become an operating physician. . . ."[68]

But when it comes to treating the surgical patient, seeing and hearing is not enough. "A student may read surgery, may hear and see surgery; and yet, without having himself practiced operations and those on the living body, he remains totally incapable of carrying out those measures which alone distinguish this branch of medicine. One would not expect to play the violin after a course of lectures on music and merely by watching a performer for a few semesters."[69] Observing surgery is really only beneficial to those who have already performed operations themselves. This was the theory behind the cadaver course which had been taught at medical schools for some decades. Cushing credits this teaching innovation to the German surgeon Bernhard von Langenbeck. On the cadaver, however, the operations were performed in the most unsurgical surroundings.

With the advent of the twentieth century, a distinctly new way of teaching surgery was introduced to the third-year students at the Johns Hopkins University School of Medicine. Credit for this innovation properly goes both to William Halsted and probably in much greater measure to his young associate, Harvey Cushing. Ironically, this course of comparative surgery, popularly known as dog surgery, came into being and flowered because Cushing did not have a firm position at Hopkins when he returned from a European study trip in 1901.

J. M. T. Finney had been teaching a cadaver course in surgery, and it was he who suggested that Cushing take it over. Cushing decided to use dogs instead. When the course first started, he used a ground-floor room in the anatomy building until the Hunterian Laboratory was built and opened in 1905. The course began on Friday mornings at eleven o'clock

67. Harvey Cushing, "Instruction in Operative Medicine," *Bull. Johns Hopkins Hosp.* 17 (1906): 123–34. According to Emile Holman, dog surgery was incorporated into the medical curriculum of the first Pacific Coast school, the Cooper Medical College, in 1858 ("Our Surgical Heritage," in *Stanford University School of Medicine: The First Hundred Years* [n.p., n.d.], pp. 49–55; quotation on p. 49).

68. Ibid., p. 125.

69. Ibid., p. 127.

and lasted until late in the afternoon. It proved to be very popular. Most of the surgery that the small groups of students performed was gastrointestinal surgery, but some amputations and laminectomies were also done. This was the time when the antivivisection movement was at its height in Baltimore. Cushing was able to win over the most militant woman in the movement when he removed a tumor from her poodle. In fact, the laboratory did quite a bit of veterinary surgery.[70]

Cushing was very pleased with the results of this course and later wrote: "I feel that this third year Friday afternoon exercise carried on in the old Hunterian from 1905 to 1912 was by far the most satisfactory and profitable source of contact between student and teacher that I have experienced."[71] The animal surgery course was important because it taught students things that the cadaver course could not teach. When working on living, anesthetized animals, the students had to learn and to observe the principles of surgical cleanliness. They had to develop an ability to dissect and gently manipulate living tissues without damaging them. And also they had to learn proper control of hemorrhage. After participating in such a course, the students were more useful as assistants in the operating room, and they learned more from watching surgical procedures. Additional benefits, Cushing pointed out, were that students learned to keep proper records and to appreciate the risks of anesthesia. "I am far from claiming that this method will make more surgeons out of a body of students," Cushing observed, "but it will, I believe, make the future physician more appreciative of the surgical point of view; more capable of understanding when handicraft may with propriety be called for, and the only safe methods of applying it; able too in case of need, to put his own hands to the work."[72]

V

Surgical teaching is in part dependent upon the prevalence of surgical diseases. With the changing patterns of disease, as seen most dramatically in thoracic surgery, old standby procedures became less and less used

70. C. M. Faris, H. C. Thacher, J. F. Ortschild, and F. C. Beall, "Comparative Surgery," *Bull. Johns Hopkins Hosp.* 16 (1905): 179–80. For details of Cushing's role in the course see John F. Fulton, *Harvey Cushing* (Springfield: Thomas, 1946), pp. 204, 217–22.
71. Fulton, *Cushing*, p. 220.
72. Cushing, "Instruction in Operative Medicine," p. 132. By the late 1930s an AMA survey revealed that half the medical schools offered courses in animal or cadaver surgery. Those who did not question the advisability of such courses, fearing that they could lead to an unjustified confidence of the students to undertake operative procedures upon their patients (*Medical Education in the U.S., 1934–39* [Chicago: Council on Med. Educ. and Hosp. AMA], p. 182).

while new techniques came to the fore. Chest surgery early in the century, after the problems of negative intrathoracic pressure were overcome, was usually indicated in chronic infections, such as empyema, bronchiectasis, or tuberculosis. After Evarts Graham's demonstration in 1934 that total pneumonectamy was possible, thoracic surgeons began to operate more and more in cases of cancer of the lungs and bronchi as well. In the years right after World War II antibacterial therapy was used to treat lung infections. It proved to be so effective that these disorders were more often treated on medical wards than on the surgical service. Thoracic surgeons then became cardiovascular surgeons, attacking the problems of congenital heart lesions especially. When, by the late 1960s, much of the backlog of these operable cases had been cleared, coronary artery disease and other occlusive vascular lesions became important to the thoracic surgeon.

Much of what students are exposed to in the future, especially those students going to medical schools with large and active departments of surgery, will likewise depend to a large extent on disease patterns, on available technology, and in part also on surgical fads and fashions. Owen Wangensteen has summarized this aptly: "The medical student attending surgical wards today is confronted with a sight quite different than that of intern days in 1921–22. More than one third of the patients admitted to Gillette Hospital in St. Paul then came because of tuberculosis of lymph nodes and bones. Today none are to be seen there. A decade later, one of the important activities of our Surgical Service was treatment of pulmonary tuberculosis, first by thoracoplasty and later by lobectomy and segmental excision. These, too, have disappeared."[73] Not only have surgical diseases changed over time, but the place of the student in the operating room has thereby also been affected. With the emphasis on cardiac surgery, often requiring copious blood, much equipment, and a large team, the student's place at the scene of surgery could be easily usurped.

These trends and other changes in the teaching of surgery had already become evident by the third and fourth decades of the twentieth century, by which time surgery had assumed its modern dress. That is, it had become thoroughly scientific, was based on physiological principles, and was becoming increasingly specialized. Surgical educators in the 1920s were already taking it for granted that the surgeon was really trained in the postgraduate residency programs. It was the business of the medical schools, as Hugh Cabot, chairman of the Committee on Undergraduate

73. Owen Wangensteen, "Department of Surgery," in J. Arthur Myers, *Masters of Medicine: An Historical Sketch of the College of Medical Science, University of Minnesota 1888–1966* (St. Louis: Green, 1968), p. 403.

Teaching of Surgery of the American Association of Medical Colleges, concluded in 1921, not to train either physicians or surgeons but to turn out young men trained comprehensively with the broadest possible understanding of disease and therapy. "It is not desirable," Cabot continued, "to attempt to teach undergraduate students to be operating surgeons. With the complexity of modern surgery this is obviously impossible and has long since been pushed out of the medical curriculum into the part of medical education given to hospital interns."[74] The technique of surgery, therefore, belonged to postgraduate training, the committee believed. What the medical schools should do was to turn out students who were well versed in the principles of surgery and who were properly impressed with the axioms of surgery regarding bleeding vessels, manipulation of tissues, and the avoidance of shock.

In most phases of medical school teaching, but especially in the surgical specialties, the medical school curriculum has become more general as specialty training has improved and slowly grown longer.[75] As specialization increased after World War II and as the technical paraphernalia surrounding much major surgery became increasingly complicated, more of the operative aspects of surgery have been left to the postgraduate or residency years. Elliot Cutler of Harvard spoke of this trend over forty years ago.[76] In 1935 he believed that much less technical surgery was being taught in the medical schools than in 1915. Yet licensing was and continues to be structured in such a way as to give every physician the permission to operate. This has long been seen as an anomalous situation, and the American College of Surgeons has pressed for proper qualifications for all operating physicians.

All medical educators recognized, however, that many physicians, especially those in general practice, had to treat disorders for which minor surgery was the chief therapeutic agent. Thus, as Cutler outlined it in 1935, "Every medical school must provide its students with teaching and experience in the elements and principles of surgery and particularly in the care of individuals suffering from injury and infection."[77] In more

74. Hugh Cabot, "Undergraduate Teaching of Surgery and Surgical Specialties," *Proc. AAMC* 31 (1921): 44–62; quotation on p. 53.

75. Surgical educators continue to reevaluate their role in the undergraduate medical curriculum. See, e.g., Michael Hume, "Changes in the Surgical Clerkship: Renewal or Revolution," *J. Med. Educ.* 39 (1964): 1090–95; and C. Rollins Hanlon, "Surgical Specialties in the Medical Curriculum, Their Pertinent and Impertinent Purposes," *J. AMA* 202 (1967): 113–15; and C. G. Child III, "Surgical Clerkship, Milestone or Millstone?," *J. AMA* 202 (1967): 108–12.

76. Elliot C. Cutler, "Undergraduate Teaching of Surgery," *Ann. Surg.* 102 (1935): 497–506.

77. Ibid., p. 498.

recent times leading professors of surgery have used a similar line of argument. Dr. Francis D. Moore has pointed to the surgical part of the medical school curriculum that "opens one door to wide vistas in human biology not seen elsewhere in the hospital."[78] Thus it is on surgical services that the student will have a major experience in the care and treatment of cancer patients, that he will be able to study and understand shock, hemorrhage, burns, fractures, and other common ills to which the human flesh is heir.

In a similar vein Dr. J. Engelbert Dunphy has written about "Surgery's Relevance to an Understanding of Basic Biology," especially through the process of wound healing.[79] In an extremely thoughtful paper in 1965 Dr. Dunphy has also defended the place of surgery in the medical curriculum.[80] This question has received wide attention in the last dozen or so years. Some surgical teachers have come to believe that the core surgical clerkships should be shortened and that the real teaching should come at the postdoctoral level. But Dr. Dunphy claims that "the diseases most common to Western man, in one way or another, sooner or later are treated surgically." Further, he has argued that "the point at issue here is not what does the student learn about surgery but what does he learn about medicine, about the care of the sick, about life and death, and disability, and the impact on a man and his family of being snatched from death and restored to life." The surgical portion of the undergraduate curriculum, Dr. Dunphy maintains, becomes therefore an "integrating" as well as a "humanizing" force in the medical school.[81]

I cannot further define nor argue this point here. Suffice it to say that in many American medical schools today some of the highest student evaluations for teaching go to their surgical professors, much as has been true for two hundred years. Surgical technique and surgical thinking—in other words, the entire surgical point of view—is what all physicians, properly educated, should be exposed to in medical school. Thus the courses in surgery have become increasingly important for the future internist or pediatrician. The future surgeon learns much of his craft in postgraduate training, but his appreciation for surgery has always developed during his medical school years.

78. Francis D. Moore, "Surgical Teaching in the Development of Clinical Competence," *J. AMA* 202 (1967): 104–7.
79. J. Englebert Dunphy, "Surgery's Relevance to an Understanding of Basic Biology," *J. AMA* 202 (1967): 16–17.
80. J. Englebert Dunphy, "The Role of Surgery in the General Education of the Physician," *Am. J. Surg.* 110 (1965): 100–104; quotation on p. 100.
81. Ibid., p. 101.

Obstetrics and Gynecology

LAWRENCE D. LONGO

O N January 31, 1765, the *Pennsylvania Gazette* carried the following notice:

DOCTOR SHIPPEN, JUNIOR,

Proposes to begin his first course on Midwifery as soon as a number of pupils sufficient to defray the necessary expense shall apply. A course will consist of about twenty lectures, in which he will treat of that part of the anatomy which is necessary to understand that branch, explain all cases in midwifery—natural, difficult, and preternatural—and give directions how to treat them with safety to the mother and child; describe the diseases incident to women and children in the month, and direct to proper remedies; will take occasion during the course to explain and apply these curious anatomical plates and casts of the gravid uterus at the Hospital, and conclude the whole with necessary cautions against the dangerous and cruel use of instruments.

This study was supported in part by USPHS HD 03807. Lawrence D. Longo is the recipient of USPHS Research Career Development Award 2–K4 HD 23,676.

In order to make the course more perfect, a convenient lodging is provided for the accommodation of a few poor women, who otherwise might suffer for want of the common necessaries on these occasions, to be under the care of a sober, honest matron, well acquainted with lying in women, employed by the Doctor for that purpose. Each pupil to attend two courses at least, for which he is to pay five guineas. Perpetual pupils to pay ten guineas.

The female pupils to be taught privately, and assisted at any of their private labors when necessary. The Doctor may be spoke with at his house, in Front Street, every morning between the hours of six and nine; or at his office in Letitia Court every evening.[1]

Thus were announced the first formal lectures on midwifery in the American colonies.

William Shippen, Jr. (1736–1808), son of a prominent Philadelphia physician, had spent the years 1759 to 1762 in Great Britain, much of the time studying under William Hunter in London. Inspired by his mentor, Shippen focussed his interests on anatomy and midwifery. Upon returning to his native city, he immediately began lecturing on anatomy, but postponed giving obstetrical lectures for several years because of prejudice against man-midwifery.

By 1765, however, Shippen decided that he must do something about the appalling care given by local midwives. He described the situation as follows:

The poor women having suffered extremely, and their innocent little ones being entirely destroyed, whose lives might have been easily saved by proper management, and being informed of several desperate cases in the different neighborhoods which had proved fatal to the mothers as to the infants and were attended with the most painful circumstances too dismal to be related, he thought it his duty immediately to begin his intended courses in Midwifery, and has prepared a proper apparatus for that purpose, in order to instruct those women who have virtue enough to own their ignorance and apply for instructions, as well as those young gentlemen now engaged in the study of that useful and necessary branch of surgery who are taking pains to qualify themselves to practice in different parts of the country with safety and advantage to their fellow citizens.[2]

His course constituted the first formal clinical teaching of obstetrics in

1. *Pennsylvania Gazette*, 31 January 1765.
2. Ibid.

America, although he had included some midwifery instruction in his earlier anatomy lectures.

Apparently, ten students, including Benjamin Rush, attended Shippen's midwinter lectures in 1765.[3] They heard a fairly systematic series of presentations covering pelvic architecture, anatomy of female and male generative organs, the uterus and its changes during pregnancy, the placenta, fetal circulation and nutrition, symptoms and signs of pregnancy, menstruation, *fluor albus* (lochia), the cause of natural labor, preternatural (abnormal) labor, and the use of obstetrical instruments. Lectures on the diseases of women and children and instruction on the care and diet of infants concluded the series.[4]

According to one student's notes from Shippen's lecture on the fetus in 1766, the doctor raised a number of thoughtful questions:

> How does the placenta adhere to the uterus? How is the foetus nourished? is it by the mouth, the umbilical vein, or by both together? Does red blood go immediately from the uterine vessels of the mother through the placenta to the foetus or visa versa? From whence comes the liquor of the amnion?[5]

To what extent Shippen answered these questions remains unknown. Some of his lectures, however, were identical to those of his teacher, Hunter.

Little is known of Shippen's pedagogic methods, except that he employed both patients and manikins for demonstrations and used drawings and casts supplied by John Fothergill, a Quaker physician in London.[6] Caspar Wistar, a student during the 1790s, recalled that Shippen

> went through the substance of each proceeding lecture by interrogation, instead of recapitulation, this fixing the attention of the students—and his manner was so happy that this grave process proceeded like a piece of amusement. His irony was of a delicate kind and so blended with humor that he could repress forwardness and take notice of negligence so as to admonish his class without too much exposing the defaulter.[7]

3. Betsy Copping Corner, *William Shippen, Jr.: Pioneer in American Medical Education* (Philadelphia: American Philosophical Society, 1951), p. 102.
4. G. W. Norris, *The Early History of Medicine in Philadelphia* (Philadelphia: W. F. Norris, 1886), pp. 36–46.
5. William Shippen, "Notes Taken from the Lecture on the Fetus of Dr. William Shippen by Johnathan Elmer, 1766" (National Library of Medicine, Bethesda, Md.).
6. Corner, *William Shippen*, p. 98.
7. William Shippen, "Notes Taken from the Anatomical Lectures of Drs. William Shippen and Caspar Wistar by William Darlington, Student in Medicine, November 1802–1803,

Wistar also noted that "there was no lecture in which he [Shippen] shone so much, as in his introductory one on midwifery, upon the subject of address and deportment."[8]

For textbooks Shippen used those British works that he had studied as a student: William Smellie's *Treatise on the Theory and Practice of Midwifery* (1752) and *Sett of Anatomical Tables* (1754). In 1786 an American abridgment of Smellie appeared. This was not only the nation's first obstetrical book, but its first medical work containing illustrations. After 1774 Shippen was also able to use Hunter's magnificent folio, *Anatomia Uteri Humani Gravidi Tabulis Illustrata*.

Shippen was, of course, not the only teacher of midwifery during the eighteenth century. Others included John Van Brugh Tennant (1737–1770) and Samuel Bard (1742–1821) of New York, and James Lloyd (1728–1810) of Boston. Valentine Seaman (1770–1817) lectured on midwifery exclusively to women at the New York Almshouse and in 1800 published the first American manual for midwives, *The Midwives Monitor, and Mothers' Mirror*, a modest work of little merit. In Baltimore, George Buchanan (1763–1808), one of Shippen's students, lectured on diseases of women and children in 1789 and added midwifery the next year. By the close of the century the United States had ten medical schools, but only two of them included obstetrics in their curricula and its role was relatively minor.

During the first half of the nineteenth century, midwifery continued to be taught with gynecology and pediatrics in American medical schools. The two most important developments during this period were the establishment of chairs of obstetrics in medical schools and the publication of the first American textbooks of obstetrics and diseases of women.

In 1807 (or possibly 1808) Samuel Bard, professor of midwifery at King's College, published America's first textbook of obstetrics. Although the edification of midwives was a stated objective, Bard's text also was useful to physicians. In a rather lengthy introduction Bard admonished "every young person engaging in the study of midwifery, not to trust wholly to the information he may derive from books, in an art in which so much depends on that which is to be obtained only from practice." He also advised students

---

Followed by Notes of William Shippen's Lecture on Midwifery," MS 7635 (Osler Library, McGill University, Montreal, Canada).

8. Caspar Wistar, "Eulogium on William Shippen, M.D. . . . Delivered before the College of Physicians of Philadelphia, March 1809," *Phila. J. Med. & Phys. Sci.* 5 (1822): 173–88.

to spend at least one or two seasons, under the professor of this branch of medical learning, at one of the colleges, where he may have the opportunity to add experience to theory, and while he is learning the rules, see their application in actual practice; for as is the case in every other mechanical operation, so in those of midwifery; although the manner of performing them may be described in words, and the principles on which that depends may be acquired by study, practice alone can give the coolness and dexterity which are necessary to ensure success.[9]

Caspar Wistar (1761–1818), Shippen's successor to the chair of anatomy, midwifery and surgery at the University of Pennsylvania, cared little for obstetrics and in 1808 urged the trustees to establish separate chairs of anatomy and midwifery. In 1810 the trustees finally acceded to his request, but stipulated that "it shall not be necessary in order to obtain the degree of Doctor of Medicine, that the students shall attend the Professor of Midwifery." Despite the optional nature of the course, a large number of students attended it.[10] In 1813 the trustees finally legitimized obstetrics by passing a resolution

> that hereafter the Professor of Midwifery shall be a member of the medical faculty, and shall have all the power, authority, and privileges belonging to a professorship in the said Faculty, and that no person shall be admitted hereafter as a candidate for the degree of Doctor of Medicine in this University, unless he shall have regularly attended the lectures of said Professor for two years.[11]

In addition to its insecure standing in the medical curriculum, the chair of midwifery had other liabilities. It is reported, for example, that Thomas Chalky James (1766–1835), the professor at Pennsylvania, was often embarrassed by his subject: "His cheeks would be mantled by blushes while engaging in demonstrating some pelvic viscus, or discussing topics not mentionable in ordinary conversation. It was often painful to witness his embarrassment."[12] On occasion, he would turn over the lectures on the female organs of generation to his assistant, William Edmonds Horner

<hr>

9. Samuel Bard, *A Compendium of the Theory and Practice of Midwifery, Containing Practical Instructions for the Management of Women During Pregnancy, in Labour, and in Childbed; Calculated to Correct the Errors, and to Improve the Practice of Midwives; As Well as to Serve as an Introduction to the Study of This Art, for Students and Young Practitioners* (New York: Collins, 1807), p. 11.

10. H. L. Hodge, "Biography of Thomas C. James, M.D.," *Am. J. Med. Sci.* 6 (1843): 91–106.

11. Ibid., p. 103.

12. A. Haller Gross and Samuel W. Gross, eds., *Autobiography of Samuel D. Gross, M.D.*, 2 vols. (Philadelphia: George Barrie, 1887), 2:239–40.

(1793–1853). In 1833 he withdrew from the major teaching duties, and the following year William Potts Dewees (1768–1841) succeeded him as professor of midwifery.

Among his other accomplishments Dewees authored the first definitive and original American textbook on obstetrics. His 602-page *Compendious System of Midwifery*, which appeared in 1824, presented principles modelled after Jean Louis Baudeloque and the French School, rather than the traditional English teachings that had been so influential in America. Although he retired from the professorship after only one year, he made a lasting impression on the teaching of obstetrics in America, both because of his voluminous writings and the number of students that he taught. According to Hugh Lennox Hodge, "Drs. James and Dewees should be regarded as the fathers of obstetric science in America; the former, erudite and polished, gave currency to teachings of the British school; the latter, more vigorous and energetic, exemplified theoretically and practically the doctrines of French obstetricians."[13]

At Harvard Medical School there was apparently no provision for teaching obstetrics until 1815, when Walter Channing (1786–1876) became lecturer. Perhaps one of his greatest contributions to obstetrical instruction was to assist in the organization of the Boston Lying-In Hospital, one of the country's earliest institutions wholly devoted to the practice and teaching of obstetrics. Channing was one of America's great teachers of obstetrics and an eloquent speaker. He also emphasized practical obstetrics. According to one of his students,

> Once or twice during the course we were treated to a little practical midwifery. A female pelvis was placed on the table. The head of a rag baby was thrust into it. It was our duty to ascertain the presentations, and to deliver with the forceps.[14]

Despite increased attention to obstetrics in the training of physicians, advances were slow and midwives continued to deliver almost all but the upper middle classes in Philadelphia, New York, and Boston. Passions against the meddlesome midwifery of physicians and the immorality of employing men in the lying-in chamber continued unabated. For instance, as late as 1848 Samuel Gregory, a Boston pamphleteer, inveighed strongly against the growing influence of accoucheurs.[15] To a certain ex-

13. Hugh L. Hodge, *An Eulogium on William P. Dewees, M.D., Delivered Before the Medical Students of the University of Pennsylvania, November 5, 1842* (Philadelphia: Merrihew and Thompson, 1842).

14. William W. Wellington, *Biographical Sketches of Deceased Members of the Obstetrical Society of Boston; with an Outline of the Earlier Obstetrical History of Boston and Vicinity* (Boston: David Clapp and Son, 1881), pp. 35–73.

15. Samuel Gregory, *Man-Midwifery Exposed and Corrected: Or the Employment of*

tent, this undoubtedly reflected the rugged individualism and anti-intellectualism of the Jacksonian era. But it also probably reflected a disillusionment with regular physicians and the excesses of Benjamin Rush's "heroic" medicine, a disillusionment which gave rise to various irregular schools like homeopathy, hydropathy, and Thomsonianism.[16]

The half century from about 1840 to 1890 witnessed epochal achievements in the practice of obstetrics, including the use of anesthesia in childbirth and the elucidation of the physician's role in transmitting puerperal sepsis. In the teaching of obstetrics, however, neither of these developments had as profound an effect as the introduction of demonstrative midwifery. Although Shippen's students participated in a delivery, this mode of teaching never gained widespread acceptance, and students generally had only a theoretical knowledge of obstetrics. Student clinical instruction during obstetric labor and delivery first occurred at the University of Buffalo Medical College in 1850. James Platt White (1811–1881), one of the founders of the school and its professor of midwifery, flew in the face of tradition on 18 January 1850 when he demonstrated a normal labor and delivery to the senior class of twenty students. The patient, a single twenty-six-year-old woman, had delivered previously. When she was a few days from term, White persuaded her to move from the Erie County Almshouse to the Medical College. There, each of the students examined her, auscultating the fetal heart tones in White's presence. When labor commenced, the class gathered in another room and then singly examined the patient, performing a vaginal examination under White's direction. Finally, during the actual delivery, the students crowded into the room. Attempting to preserve the patient's modesty, White draped her so that only the emerging head of the child was visible. With a napkin in each hand, White carefully supported the perineum, one of the main points of his demonstration.

This educational innovation elicited both praise and condemnation. Austin Flint, editor of the *Buffalo Medical Journal*, published a note from the college:

> The illustration of labor with the living subject is, doubtless, a novelty in this country. We are not aware that it has ever before been attempted. It enters, however, into the instruction of some

---

Men to Attend Women in Childbirth, and in Other Delicate Circumstances, Shown to be Modern Innovation, Unnecessary, Unnatural, and Injurious to the Physicial Welfare of the Community, and Pernicious in Its Influence . . . (Boston: George Gregory, 1848).

16. John B. Blake, "Health Reform," in Edwin S. Gaustad, ed., *The Rise of Adventism: Religion and Society in Mid-Nineteenth-Century America* (New York: Harper and Row, 1974), pp. 30–49.

foreign schools, constituting one of the features in which the latter are supposed to possess advantages over our domestic institutions. Whatever may be the sentiments on the subject entertained by a portion of the community at large (were it to be submitted to them), the plan must, we think, commend itself to the cordial approbation of the medical profession; and, indeed, as it seems to us, the more intelligent members of any community, not excepting the female portion, must appreciate not alone the motives and the object, but its propriety in view of better preparing those soon to become practitioners of medicine, for the responsible duties of the accoucheur. It should be stated that, during the demonstration, every regard was had for delicacy, the patient being entirely concealed from observation, except in so far as was requisite for the illustration. The privilege of being present was restricted to candidates for graduation, and medical gentlemen in attendance on the course of lectures; all of whom exhibited that degree of decorum so proper to the occasion.[17]

Others, however, were not so charitable. Scathing indictments of White, signed only by "L," appeared in the *Buffalo Daily Courier* and the *Buffalo Medical Journal*, the latter accompanied by a testimonial signed by seventeen Buffalo "medical gentlemen" denouncing White. Angered at this response, White and his colleagues induced the county attorney to sue a local physician, Horatio N. Loomis, for libel. The trial began on 24 June and lasted five days. The arguments used by the defense attorney reflected the false modesty of the day. Amazingly, fifteen physicians testified that obstetrical demonstrations were neither necessary nor proper, that they were offensive to the moral sense of the community and would lower respect for physicians, and, finally, that students could learn the necessary obstetrical operations from illustrations and manikins. A Dr. Bryant Burwell testified that students could learn midwifery by studying the comparative anatomy and delivery of animals. The prosecution countered with numerous medical witnesses of its own, including some who had observed such live demonstrations at leading European medical schools. However, because the prosecution could not prove that Loomis actually had written the letter in question, he was acquitted.[18]

White's trials, however, continued. A Philadelphia physician, Caspar Morris (1805–1884), wrote in the *American Journal of the Medical Sciences:*

17. [Austin Flint], Editorial, *Buffalo Med. J.* 5 (1850): 564. See also Carl T. Javert, "James Platt White: A Pioneer in American Obstetrics and Gynecology," *J. Hist. Med.* 3 (1948): 489–506.

18. *Report of the Trial: The People vs. Dr. Horatio N. Loomis, For Libel. Tried at the Erie County Oyer and Terminer, June 24, 1850* (Buffalo, New York, 1850).

Some of our medical colleges resorted to efforts to allure classes by specious exhibitions miscalled "clinical instruction" and adapted rather to attract students by their novelty than to furnish them with solid information . . . when, however, we came to be apprised that the improvement consisted in subjecting the process of parturition to ocular inspection in one of its stages, our surprise at the excitement yielded to astonishment that any teacher of the obstetric art should suppose that it could be made the subject of the sense of vision, and mortification that the medical profession should have been placed in a position so well calculated to array public feeling in hostility to it.[19]

Even the recently created American Medical Association attacked White. In 1851 its Committee on Education held that while his practice was neither immoral nor wrong, it was entirely unnecessary for purposes of instruction.[20] Undaunted by his critics, White continued his demonstrations, but few others followed his lead. As late as 1877, in his address as chairman of the AMA's section on obstetrics, White noted that clinical instruction remained neglected in most schools. Thus, "the neophyte is still obliged to gain his first experience at the bedside of his own patient, without the guidance of a preceptor."[21] In most places, vaginal examination—"touching"—was resorted to only on urgent indications, and even then it was performed under protective covering to spare the genitals from the examiner's eyes.

Despite lay and professional hostility, demonstrative midwifery gradually won acceptance. In 1874, for example, Thaddeus Asbury Reamy (1829–1909), professor of obstetrics, clinical midwifery and diseases of children in the Medical College of Ohio (Cincinnati), established a small hospital of two or three rooms in the rear of his amphitheater, the first women's hospital west of the Allegheny Mountains. Here pregnant women were delivered. Apparently, Reamy allowed students to observe labor and delivery in the amphitheater, a practice that outraged the citizens of Cincinnati—and not a few physicians. Some local obstetricians argued that since they had learned this branch of medicine from lectures and reading, such training was sufficient.[22]

19. [Caspar Morris], "Letter—Report of the Trial: 'The People v. Dr. Horatio N. Loomis for Libel,' " *Am. J. Med. Sci.*, n.s., 20 (1851): 441–51.

20. W. Hooker, Chairman, T. W. Blatchford, J. R. Wood, and N. S. Davis, "Report of the Committee on Medical Education in Relation to 'Demonstrative Midwifery,' " *Trans. AMA* 4 (1851): 436–41.

21. James P. White, "Address in Obstetrics and Diseases of Women and Children," *Trans. AMA* 28 (1877): 293–318.

22. Arthur G. King, *The Cincinnati Obstetrical and Gynecological Society, 1876–1976* (Cincinnati: privately printed, 1976).

As middle-class Westerners followed their Eastern sisters in calling for accoucheurs, the demand for obstetricians outstripped the available supply and resistance to clinical instruction slackened. Nevertheless, it was years before most schools required student attendance at a delivery. The University of Michigan Medical School, for instance, did not do so until 1890.[23]

The year 1850 also saw the establishment of what was apparently the first regular obstetric clinic in America. While White was introducing demonstrative midwifery in Buffalo, Gunning S. Bedford (1796–1872), professor of obstetrics and diseases of women and children at the University Medical College in New York, was beginning a weekly Monday clinic for students, in which he would lecture on various clinical problems observed in the clinic. For instance, Bedford gave short case reports of emergencies such as convulsions or hemorrhage during pregnancy, discussing the management in detail.[24] The clinic provided Bedford's students with exposure to a wide variety of gynecologic problems, but also created a local furor. Physicians and laymen alike severely criticized Bedford as indecent for using a vaginal speculum in demonstrating cervical pathology to his students.[25]

The latter half of the nineteenth century also saw increased interest in gynecology, which emerged as a separate specialty in many medical schools. During the first half of the century, teaching had focussed almost exclusively on obstetrics. In contrast, gynecologic practice consisted of little more than topical treatment of cervical erosions and leukorrhea, and inserting or replacing various pessaries for uterine prolapse.

Several mid-century developments changed this. One was the gradual acceptance of ovariotomy as a legitimate surgical procedure. Although Ephraim McDowell had pioneered this operation in the early decades of the century, few practiced or taught this procedure until the Atlee brothers, John Light Atlee (1799–1885) and Washington Lemuel Atlee (1808–1878) of Lancaster, Pennsylvania, began to popularize it in the 1840s. They showed that despite a mortality rate of 15 to 30 percent the operation was worthwhile. Although he held an academic chair for a relatively short time (professor of medical chemistry in the Pennsylvania College from 1844 to 1852), Washington Atlee influenced a generation of students to adopt this procedure.[26]

23. Richard W. Stander and Warren H. Pearse, *Obstetrics, Gynecology, and the University of Michigan* (Ann Arbor: privately printed, 1968).

24. Gunning S. Bedford, *Clinical Lectures on the Diseases of Women and Children* (New York: W. Wood, 1855).

25. C. E. Heaton, "Obstetrics at the New York Almshouse and at Bellevue Hospital," *Bull. N.Y. Acad. Med.* 16 (1940): 38–47.

26. W. L. Atlee, *A Retrospect of the Struggles and Triumphs of Ovariotomy in Philadel-*

Even more influential for the emergence of gynecology as a specialty was the successful repair of vesico-vaginal fistulae, developed by James Marion Sims (1813–1883). In 1855 Sims opened the Women's Hospital in New York City, the first institution in the world devoted exclusively to the treatment of gynecologic disorders. Its primary purpose was to serve as a center for instruction in gynecology, a vehicle for the diffusion of medical knowledge.[27] Unfortunately, Sims himself was a poor teacher, who operated with such rapidity that few students could learn much by observing him. He did, however, write an influential book that, although prepared for clinicians, was used by many students as a text. Under the influence of Sims's associates, Thomas Addis Emmet (1828–1919), Edmund Randolph Peaslee (1814–1878), and Theodore Gaillard Thomas (1831–1903), the Women's Hospital trained many students. These professors would invite the entire senior class to observe surgical clinics at the hospital, until the operating room became so crowded the number of observers had to be limited to fifteen. In addition, the New York example influenced cities such as Philadelphia, Boston and Chicago to establish similar institutions.

Within a decade of Sims's work, separate professorships of gynecology became commonplace in American medical schools. In 1870 the AMA passed a resolution urging the establishment of separate departments of gynecology,[28] and by the following year at least seven medical colleges had independent chairs: Dartmouth, Albany, Long Island, the St. Louis College of Physicians and Surgeons, the University of Louisville, the Medical College of Ohio, the University of Pennsylvania, and Detroit Medical College. Eight other schools had a combined professorship of gynecology and diseases of children.[29] In 1879 the College of Physicians and Surgeons in New York City divided its department of obstetrics and diseases of women and children, with Thomas occupying the chair of gynecology, James Wood McLane the chair of obstetrics, and Abraham Jacobi (1830–1919) the chair of diseases of children. This arrangement set the pattern for many medical schools. It was not until the turn of the century that pediatrics became a distinct specialty in most medical schools, and even much later before gynecology reunited with obstetrics.

Despite these institutional beginnings, progress in gynecology was

phia, *with Some Additional Remarks on Allied Subjects. The Annual Address Before the Philadelphia County Medical Society* (Philadelphia: Collins, 1875).

27. James Pratt Marr, *Pioneer Surgeons of the Woman's Hospital: The Lives of Sims, Emmett, Peaslee, and Thomas* (Philadelphia: F. A. Davis, 1957), p. 40.

28. "Resolution of the American Medical Association," *Trans. AMA* 21 (1870): 64.

29. Edward D. Jenks, "Historical Sketch of American Gynecology," in Matthew D. Mann, ed., *A System of Gynecology*, 2 vols. (Philadelphia: Lea Brothers, 1887), 1:17–67.

slow. In an address to the AMA in 1888 Ely Van de Warker (1841–1910), chairman of the section on obstetrics, bemoaned the deficiencies in gynecologic education. He observed that in 66 of 109 medical colleges gynecology either was taught by an ill-trained obstetrician or not taught at all. Although gynecology was an American specialty, American medical students scarcely encountered it. The graduate leaves his alma mater, said Van de Warker, "with his mind like virgin soil so far as this great branch is concerned. . . . "[30]

Conditions were not much better in obstetrics. Following a period of rapid development between 1840 and 1860, the field became relatively sterile. This was partly because the empirical basis of obstetrics— describing the mechanism of labor, employing anesthesia, and developing the concept of puerperal infection—had gone about as far as it could without cellular pathology and bacteriology. The teaching of obstetrics, as reflected in the late nineteenth century, presented few innovations.

Despite White's introduction of demonstrative midwifery in 1850, few medical schools adopted this mode of instruction, and in most institutions the teaching of obstetrics consisted of little more than didactic lectures. In 1888 George S. Englemann wrote that

> whilst theoretical teaching is all that can be desired in the United
> States, practical instruction is but limited, notwithstanding the
> noble efforts of James P. White, the pioneer in obstetric teaching,
> who braved the wrath of his colleagues and his fellow citizens when
> he established the first obstetric clinic in the United States in his
> home in Buffalo, N.Y. The student is taught the management of
> pathological cases, but how to guard his patient against their occur-
> rence, the practical management of simple labor, examination, and
> manipulation, he must learn by experience; and not, until the
> proper guidance in normal labor, a physiological, prophylactic, and
> antiseptic obstetrics, is thoroughly taught, practically and theoreti-
> cally, will the results of private obstetrics practice equal those of the
> hospital, which are far better under circumstances far worse. The
> efforts of the obstetric teacher must now be directed to practical
> instruction in the lying-in room, to the perfection of the manage-
> ment of normal labor, and the introduction of antiseptic methods
> into private practice as they have been received in the hospital.[31]

In an effort to improve obstetric education, some obstetricians devoted considerable attention to developing manikins and other teaching aids. J.

30. Ely Van De Warker, "How Gynecology Is Taught," *J. AMA* 11 (1888): 181–85.
31. George J. Engelmann, "History of Obstetrics," in B. C. Hirst, ed., *A System of Obstetrics*, 2 vols. (Philadelphia: Lea Brothers, 1888), 1:65.

Clifton Edgar (1859–1939) of New York developed models from paper-mache, plastic, wax, leather, and metal that not only illustrated various pelvic forms, the uterus, and the mechanism of labor, but lacerations and other injuries of the genital tract as well. With Theophilis Parvin, he invented the ultimate obstetric manikin, a life-sized female doll that could be placed in any desired position, and on which almost any conceivable obstetric procedure could be carried out.[32]

Some teachers used manikins to great advantage. Richard Alexander Fullerton Penrose (1827–1908), professor of obstetrics at Pennsylvania, dramatically illustrated the management of childbirth with the aid of a manikin. With fullest gesture, he acted out every movement and procedure of the accoucheur, carrying on a running conversation with "Mrs. O'Flaherty," as if the manikin were a living patient. According to contemporary reports, he staged the drama of birth and all its emergencies with a realism that thrilled the inexperienced students and clothed his precepts with unforgettable poignancy.[33]

An even more significant contribution to the teaching of obstetrics was the use of lying-in hospitals for the training of physicians. In 1881 William Lambert Richardson (1842–1932) reopened the Boston Lying-In Hospital for teaching Harvard students home deliveries, but America's first large lying-in hospital did not appear until 1888, when the Sloane Maternity Hospital opened in New York City with accommodations for twenty-eight patients.[34] Similar institutions soon appeared elsewhere, sometimes in response to student demands. For instance, in 1888 the senior class at the University of Michigan Medical School petitioned the faculty to establish a lying-in ward for clinical instruction, and shortly thereafter a small unit was built for this purpose.[35]

The opening of the Johns Hopkins Medical School in the early 1890s contributed greatly to a scientific basis of medical education. Howard Atwood Kelly (1858–1943), professor of gynecology, established the first true residency training in gynecology, and many of his residents matured to become the gynecologic leaders in American medical schools. Nevertheless, Kelly expressed concern about the quality of undergraduate instruction, observing in 1900 that

> gynecology is, as a rule, very badly taught, and the medical student gains but little from this part of his course. This fact would be

32. J. Clifton Edgar, "The Manikin in the Teaching of Practical Obstetrics," *N.Y. Med. J.* 52 (1890): 701–9.
33. Corner, *Two Centuries of Medicine*, p. 122.
34. Harold Speert, *The Sloane Hospital Chronicle* (Philadelphia: F. A. Davis, 1963).
35. Stander and Pearse, *Obstetrics, Gynecology, and the University of Michigan*, p. 21.

evident at once to anyone familiar with thorough scientific methods of teaching employed in other departments; but, unfortunately, the object-lessons of this sort in America are still few and far between.[36]

Surprisingly, Kelly thought that too much attention was given to gynecology in many schools. Since few students ever became gynecologists, he considered it "a waste of valuable time to treat the whole class as if they were working with this end in view." The ideal plan would have students studying gynecology from three to four hours a week throughout their senior year. Instruction would be divided as follows: (1) history-taking and ward work, attending to dressings and removing sutures, and studying the sequels of operations, the convalescence; (2) a touch course once a week in which gynecological diagnosis would be taught, with the patient preferably under anesthesia; (3) an hour a week in the pathological laboratory studying scrapings and cultures and examining gross specimens; (4) watching gynecological operations, the class divided into small sections; (5) lectures.

> I think the day for teaching gynecology by performing operations in an amphitheater before a large class of students has long since gone by. The students see practically nothing of what is going on, absolutely nothing in a deep, abdominal, or vaginal operation, and their very presence is a serious menace to the life of a patient. . . . The history-taking, the ward work, the touch-course, all of which demand personal instruction, are the most valuable methods, bringing student and patient together, as they must meet in the natural course of events after graduation, and carrying the student up to the point beyond which he will not be apt to go, that is, up to the point of deciding upon the line of surgical treatment to be followed.[37]

In his own classes Kelly taught mainly from patients in the clinics and on the wards, using clinical demonstrations and examinations. When lecturing, he often used lantern slides to illustrate interesting pathologic specimens and operations.

In 1899 Kelly, a surgeon with little interest in obstetrics, turned over obstetrics to a junior colleague, John Whitridge Williams (1866–1931). Williams had spent several years in the great clinics of Europe and was appalled by the lack of scientific standards in America. In the late 1890s he observed that

> there are very few institutions in which it is attempted, in connection with the obstetric course, to give practical laboratory instruc-

36. H. A. Kelly, "Methods of Teaching Gynecology," *Phila. Med. J.* 6 (1900): 391.
37. Ibid., p. 392.

tion upon the anatomy and pathology of the female generative organs, and of the various diseases which may complicate the pregnant, parturient, and puerperal condition, by which the student may gain an intelligent idea concerning the structure of the organs with which he has to deal, and of the morbid changes in the various diseases, which he may be called upon to treat. Unless such practical instruction is added to the theoretical teaching and the practical work in the lying-in ward, we cannot consider that the student has received a well-rounded course. And it will not be until our schools equip laboratories that we can expect our students to have an accurate conception of many of the conditions with which they have to deal.[38]

In his opinion, the ideal obstetric course would include not only the customary lectures and practical work, but study in the laboratory as well.

Williams emphasized the importance of practical demonstrations:

Exercise upon the manikin should form an integral part of the obstetric course; but their scope should depend, to a great extent, upon the amount of material which is available for clinical instruction . . . if the clinical material is limited in amount, we consider it advisable that the students be taught the rudiments of palpation, touch, and pelvimetry upon the manikin, so that they will know exactly what they are to do when they examine the patients in the wards, whereby clinical material is economized, and the patients saved considerable annoyance. . . . The main object of the manikin is to teach the various operative procedures, and each student should be obliged to perform all possible operations upon the manikin at least once during the session.[39]

He also thought students learned from such objects as "frozen sections of the fetus and young children of various ages for demonstrating the fetal and infantile pelvis and the relations of the generative organs, series of ova at various periods of development, placental diseases and abnormalities, and many other anatomic and pathologic specimens." At Johns Hopkins, Williams continued White's pioneering efforts to have students participate in actual deliveries, recommending that

a small number of students, preferably two, but certainly not more than four, should be called to the ward to see every case of confinement. They should be required to examine the patient, both internally and externally, once during the first and again during the second stage of labor. In uncomplicated cases, one of the group

38. J. W. Williams, "Teaching Obstetrics," *Bull. Am. Acad. Med.* 3 (1897–1898): 409.
39. Ibid., p. 411.

should deliver the woman himself, under the guidance of a competent assistant.

A much larger number of students may be called to operative cases as onlookers. Each student should be required to see at least five cases delivered in the lying-in ward; for it is only there that he can learn the ideal method of conducting a labor case. . . .[40]

By the turn of the century home deliveries by students were accepted as part of the medical curriculum. Most schools, however, sent their students alone to attend women during labor and delivery. Williams disapproved of the practice, arguing that students should receive instruction and supervision. A graduate physician and nurse accompanied his pupils, even though the latter was directly responsible for the delivery. His students also wrote reports of their work and recorded their findings at subsequent postpartum visits.

In addition, Williams had students participate in weekly clinical case conferences. During the fourth year, he wrote,

> there should be a weekly meeting of the class, in which most of the teaching should be done by the students themselves. Here the interesting cases which have been observed by the students are discussed. A student, who has lately seen an interesting case . . . should read a concise history of the case, and then perform upon the manikin the operation which may have been required. The case is then discussed by the instructor, and the class questioned concerning more or less cognate cases.
>
> At another meeting, a dead born child and its placenta may be exhibited. Two students may be called upon to perform an autopsy upon the child and to ascertain its cause of death; to a third student the placenta may be given, with instructions to tease out some villi, examine them under the microscope, and ascertain if they present syphilitic lesions. . . . Then the diagnoses are called for, and the history read by the student, who observed the case, and it is attempted to bring the clinical history into accord with the anatomic findings and *vice versa*. . . .
>
> Another very practical manner of spending the hours is to take three deformed pelves and give each one to a group of students with a pelvimeter and a piece of paper. Allow them 15 minutes to measure each pelvis. Then call upon one student in each group for the diagnosis, his reasons for making it, and the measurements upon which it is based. And ask the other how he would diagnose a similar pelvis in the living woman, and what procedures he would adopt to deliver her, etc.[41]

40. Ibid., p. 417.
41. Ibid., pp. 418–19.

Unfortunately, few American medical schools came up to the standards set by Kelly and Williams at Johns Hopkins. In his report of the dismal picture of American medical education in 1910, Abraham Flexner observed that "the very worst showing is made in the matter of obstetrics." Didactic lectures and manikin work often constituted the sole means of instruction and many students seldom, if ever, saw a live delivery:

> The hospitals of Atlanta and Los Angeles exclude students from the obstetrical ward, at Burlington there is no obstetrical ward; but the "students see more or less"; at Denver, a "small amount of material is claimed"; at Birmingham it is "very scarce"; at Chattanooga there are "about ten cases a year", to which students are "summoned", how or by whom is far from clear. At the Hahnemann Medical College (Chicago) students "look on at interns who do the work"; a committee of the Missouri state board reports of the College of Physicians and Surgeons of St. Louis that it could find only incomplete records of 21 cases for a senior class of 57; at Augusta, Georgia, the cases "always come at night when you can't get students"; at Charlotte 15 cases were available from September 15 to February 4; the medical department of Lincoln Memorial University (Knoxville) has no out-patient department, but alleges "a few deliveries before the class"; Vanderbilt relies on out-patient work mostly.[42]

And so the story went, from the Carolinas to California.

Two years after the publication of Flexner's report, Williams surveyed 120 obstetric departments in the United States, receiving responses from 31 of the 61 schools the AMA rated "acceptable," from 11 of the 59 "non-acceptable" schools, and from one in Canada.[43] He reported a series of startling findings, such as the fact that more than one-third of the professors, including four in "high standard" schools, were not specialists. Many had no specialty training at all. One professor even confessed that he had never seen an actual delivery prior to assuming his professorship, and many others had participated in few deliveries. Six schools had no connection with a lying-in hospital, and only nine had adequate facilities. On the basis of his survey Williams calculated that the average medical student in America witnessed only one live delivery and that only eight schools in the nation provided students with a satisfactory number of deliveries.

In only thirteen schools were the departments of obstetrics and gynecology closely allied, and many chairmen frankly admitted their

---

42. Abraham Flexner, *Medical Education in the United States and Canada* (New York: Carnegie Foundation for the Advancement of Teaching, 1910), pp. 117–18.
43. J. W. Williams, "Medical Education and the Midwife Problem in the United States," *J. AMA* 58 (1912): 1–7.

deficiencies as surgeons. Several confessed, for instance, that they were unable to perform cesarean section, and about one-half replied that they could not cope with operative complications such as a ruptured uterus or ectopic pregnancy. Perhaps most surprising of all, one quarter of the professors surveyed admitted that their graduates were incompentent to practice obstetrics, and the better the school, the higher the incidence of such responses. The replies clearly indicated

> that most of the medical schools included in this report are inadequately equipped for their work, and are each year turning loose on the community hundreds of young men whom they have failed to prepare properly for the practice of obstetrics, and whose lack of training is responsible for unnecessary deaths of many women and infants, not to speak of a much larger number, more or less permanently injured by improper treatment, or lack of treatment. Moreover, the spontaneous admission of most of the respondents that poor training of medical men is responsible for many unnecessary deaths in childbirth, forces us to acknowledge that improvement in the status of the midwife alone will not materially aid in solving the problem [of maternal and infant deaths].
>
> A *priori*, the replies seem to indicate that women in labor are as safe in the hands of admittedly ignorant midwives as in those of poorly educated medical men. . . .
>
> The fault lies primarily in poor medical schools, in the low ideals maintained by inadequately trained professors, and in the ignorance of the long-suffering general public. [44]

Williams concluded that only one unidentified American school—not Johns Hopkins—was properly equipped to teach obstetrics along the lines of the German *Frauenklinik*.

Williams's solution to the problem consisted in part of combining departments of obstetrics and gynecology and staffing them with full-time medical scientists. [45] But even at Hopkins Williams failed to unify the departments of obstetrics and gynecology; he did, however, succeed in creating (by 1919) the first full-time department of obstetrics in America. The significance of Williams's department lay not only in its attempt to instill scientific precepts into obstetric education, but in the wide influence it had on academic obstetrics by training the professors who most influenced teaching in other schools.

The quarter century beginning in 1920 was marked by a gradual diffusion and acceptance of the principles of medical education and specialty

44. Ibid., p. 6.
45. Ibid., pp. 3, 7.

training first laid down at Johns Hopkins. To a large extent, this occurred because Williams continued his crusade for better clinical care in obstetrics through better teaching. He linked the poor practice of obstetrics[46] and the abuse of cesarean section[47] to deficiencies in the medical education of most doctors. Williams also observed that the general public was partially at fault, because although few patients would consent to having an appendectomy performed by an untrained person, they had scarcely any qualms about being delivered, a procedure of about equal difficulty and risk, by a poorly trained physician.

Another factor accounting for improved education in obstetrics and gynecology during the later 1920s and 1930s was the coterie of Hopkins-trained academicians who helped develop departments at other institutions similiar to that at Johns Hopkins. Also, during this period many of the medical specialty boards were established, including obstetrics and gynecology in 1930. This board helped codify what constituted training in the specialty, and indirectly influenced the undergraduate curriculum.

In the half-century following the Flexner and Williams reports the amount of time devoted to the teaching of obstetrics and gynecology remained more or less constant—roughly 10 percent of the clinical instruction time—but varied somewhat from institution to institution. In a few centers instruction stressed the newer concepts of basic reproductive biology, maternal and fetal physiology, and endocrinology. However, most programs continued to teach obstetrics from a quasi-mechanical approach and gynecology as applied pathology.

Despite numerous improvements and some excellent teaching in a few places, instruction in obstetrics and gynecology remained uneven. In 1926 Williams observed that most American medical schools still remained a half-century behind those in Germany.[48] An example of this state of affairs a decade later was Rushmore's analysis[49] of responses to a question given by the Massachusetts Board of Registration in Medicine, which 73 percent of the candidates (182 of 250) failed. Answers to the question "Give in detail your treatment of a patient in whom there appeared no sign of separation of the placenta twenty minutes after the birth of the child" varied widely and included: waiting indefinitely for its delivery, twisting the cord, massaging the uterus *à la Credé*, administering

46. J. W. Williams, "Why Is the Art of Obstetrics So Poorly Practiced?," *Long Island Med. J.* 11 (1917): 169–78.
47. J. W. Williams, "The Abuse of Caesarean Section," *Surg. Gynec. & Obstet.* 25 (1917): 194–201.
48. J. W. Williams, "The Functions of a Woman's Clinic," *Science* 64 (1926): 581–86.
49. Stephen Rushmore, "A Note on the Teaching of Obstetrics," *N. Eng. J. Med.* 217 (1937): 731–32.

ergot or pituitary extract, manually removing the placenta, applying hot fomentations to the abdomen, uterine curettage, and immediate hysterectomy. Rushmore observed that the candidates either had not read the question or they were really as ignorant of current teaching and practice as they appeared to be. He concluded that a reduction in maternal mortality could hardly be expected until more graduates understood the fundamental principles of obstetrics.

One of the problems of medical education in obstetrics and gynecology was that its objectives never had been explicitly formulated. Was the goal of undergraduate obstetrics, for instance, to prepare a student to handle every obstetrical problem? If not, what obstetrical problems should a family practitioner be trained to care for? Should teaching be oriented towards technical aspects, or should it emphasize a physiologic and endocrinologic understanding of the reproductive process? Should the fundamental physiologic mechanisms be taught during the first two years of basic science instruction and the more clinical aspects be deferred until the third or fourth year, or should they be combined? In an already overcrowded schedule, what was the optimal amount of time to devote to the teaching of this field?

A study in 1961 by the American Gynecological Society[50] addressed itself to several of these problems. It noted that the number of hours devoted to obstetrics and gynecology varied from 150 to 1,050 in the forty-four schools visited. While a few schools introduced students to gynecology during the first or second year, the didactic lectures usually were presented during the third or fourth year. In about half the departments, generally those with Ph.D.'s or full-time M.D.'s, students engaged in some research project, usually during elective time. Most schools, the survey revealed, operated on the assumption that all students must possess clinical competence to practice obstetrics and gynecology. In addition, state and national board licensure pressured the schools to maintain uniformity, which limited innovation and experimentation in the curriculum. This resulted in rather superficial training. The study noted that rather than presenting underlying principles and basic physiologic mechanisms, the mechanical and technical aspects were stressed, with obstetrics too often consisting of a how-to-do-it course. By ignoring new developments in perinatology, gynecologic endocrinology, and other challenging areas, the field of gynecology was failing to attract some of the more gifted medical students.

50. Howard C. Taylor, Jr., ed., *The Recruitment of Talent for a Medical Specialty: A Report to the American Gynecological Society* . . . (St. Louis: C. V. Mosby, 1961).

In conclusion, during the colonial period and for some time after, the teaching of obstetrics, like that of other branches of medicine, proceeded by preceptorship. With the emergence of medical schools during the latter eighteenth and early nineteenth centuries, formalized didactic lectures presented the subject of obstetrics and a modicum of information on gynecology and pediatrics. Practical clinical demonstrations in obstetrics were introduced first in the mid-nineteenth century, but were not generally included in the curriculum until early in the twentieth century. During the late nineteenth century gynecology and pediatrics emerged as distinct specialties; pediatrics remained a separate discipline, but the fate of gynecology depended on the institutional setting. Between the First and Second World Wars departments of gynecology gradually reunited with obstetrics.

The years since World War II have witnessed an almost dizzying proliferation of activities associated with obstetric and gynecologic education. Too often the result has been to minimize the educational function, so that teaching per se has become almost incidental to the overall activities of a department of gynecology. As the teaching of gynecology and obstetrics has responded to the pressures of society, the dilemmas in instruction have increased. To the basic medical core of obstetrics and gynecology have been added ethical and moral questions regarding abortion, the rights of the fetus as a person, and the whole subject of human sexuality. Departments have expanded to include subspecialists able to teach reproductive biology, gynecologic endocrinology, infertility, gynecologic oncology, perinatology, sexuality, and other areas. While this fragmentation has presented problems in instruction and practice, it also has been a strength. For in broadening their horizons and perspectives, obstetrics and gynecology have matured. Not only have they strengthened their scientific base, but they have become more socially responsible. Slowly, they have achieved John Whitridge Williams's goal: a field taught by broadly trained persons who combine a thorough understanding of scientific principles with clinical practice. Teaching in obstetrics and gynecology has thus evolved from a presentation of pelvic anatomy and pathology to an understanding of reproductive medicine in its broadest sense.

Neurology and Psychiatry

JEANNE L. BRAND

NEUROLOGY as a medical specialty is dated from Jean-Martin Charcot's appointment in 1882 as the first professor of neurology at the Faculty
of Medicine, University of Paris.[1] Training in clinical neurology had
commenced in a few American medical schools by the late 1860s.
Psychiatry, although subsequently to be linked with neurology in lectures
on "neuropsychiatry" and joint professional appointments in "mental and
nervous disorders," can be viewed as a practicing specialty from the late
colonial period. Both fields, since their entry into American medicine,

The author is indebted to Dr. George Mora, Medical Director and Director of the
Psychiatric Residency Programs, Astor Home and Child Guidance Clinics, Rhinebeck, New
York, and Zigmond M. Lebensohn, M.D., Clinical Professor of Psychiatry, Georgetown
University Medical School, Washington, D.C., for a number of helpful suggestions and for
reviewing this chapter in draft.

1. Lawrence C. McHenry, Jr., *Garrison's History of Neurology, Revised and Enlarged
with a Bibliography of Classical, Original and Standard Works in Neurology* (Springfield,
Ill.: Charles C. Thomas, 1969), p. 271. The first separate work on neurology was John
Cooke's *A Treatise on Nervous Disease*, 2 vols. (London: Longman, Hurst, Rees, Orme,
and Brown, 1820–1823). Moritz Romberg (1795–1873) of Berlin is credited with being the
first man to "bring order and system to neurology," and Guillaume-Benjamin A. Duchenne
of Boulogne (1806–1875) is termed the founder of French neurology (ibid., pp. 271–82).

have undergone profound changes directly reflected in the development of training programs. Not only has the scientific content mushroomed to encompass many new fields and patient populations; both psychiatry and neurology have altered in their relationships with each other, with other medical fields, with the establishment of professional standards, and with changing expectations of the American public. Recognized today as related but separate medical specialties, they are linked by the requirements of one certifying authority—the American Board of Psychiatry and Neurology.

PSYCHIATRY IN EIGHTEENTH-CENTURY AMERICAN MEDICAL TEACHING

Psychotic patients had not generally been considered to be a medical problem in the colonies until the eighteenth century. Despite humanitarian concepts of the treatment of the mentally ill advanced in the writings of Juan Luis Vives (1492–1540) and Johann Weyer (1515–1588), popular belief in demoniacal possession had continued in seventeenth-century Europe and America. It led in 1692 to the witchcraft hysteria at Salem, and the deaths of twenty-two persons, many clearly of unsound mind by contemporary criteria.[2] Persons with mild mental disorders were kept at home. Where public care for the insane was provided in the American colonies in the early eighteenth century, it was in almshouses, workhouses or jails. By 1756, when the first general hospital in North America—the Pennsylvania Hospital—was established, provision for insane persons was included, although in the cellar. The first hospital exclusively for the insane in North America was opened in 1773 in Williamsburg, Virginia.

Throughout the eighteenth century, existing knowledge of psychiatry and the nervous structure was acquired informally in general medical education. Young American physicians learned their professions as apprentices to established practitioners, absorbing instruction in "physic, surgery and pharmacy" for periods ranging from three to five years. In a few of the larger Eastern cities, public lectures supplemented apprentice training. Although the first medical school in the American colonies was founded in Philadelphia in 1765 at the College of Physicians, and a second

2. See, for example, *Narratives of the Witchcraft Cases, 1648–1706* (New York, 1914), pp. 374–76, as cited in Albert Deutsch, *The Mentally Ill in America: A History of Their Care and Treatment from Colonial Times*, 2nd ed. (New York: Columbia University Press, 1949), pp. 31–38; also Gregory Zilboorg (in collaboration with George W. Henry), *A History of Medical Psychology* (New York: W. W. Norton, 1941), pp. 180–95, 206–35.

two years later at New York's King's College, the apprenticeship system continued into the nineteenth century, supplemented by growing numbers of proprietary schools. After 1760, small but increasing numbers of young American physicians took advanced training abroad—in Edinburgh, in Paris by the 1830s, and (after the Civil War) in German medical centers.[3]

It was not until 1791 that the versatile Dr. Benjamin Rush (1745–1813) gave a series of lectures on mental disorder at the University of Pennsylvania's Institutes of Medicine and Clinical Practice. Probably the first lectures on insanity in the United States, they were accompanied by clinical instruction and were published in 1812 as *Medical Inquiries and Observations upon the Diseases of Man.*

Rush has been termed the Father of American Psychiatry; his lectures constituted the first textbook of psychiatry in North America, and became the standard work on the subject for many years.[4] Rush viewed insanity as a pathologist, seeing it as a disease of the brain. He believed that madness resulted when the blood vessels of the brain were overstimulated or overcharged with blood, causing morbid excitement or inflammation of the brain. Rush, however, classified the causes of mental disorders in two groups—those acting directly on the body or brain and those which affected the body or brain through the medium of the mind. While insanity was organic in nature to Rush, as George Mora points out, he recognized a psychogenic origin in many mental disorders.[5] His treatment included

3. On the general development of early American medical education see William Frederick Norwood, *Medical Education in the United States Before the Civil War* (Philadelphia: University of Pennsylvania Press, 1944); William Frederick Norwood, "The Mainstream of American Education, 1765–1965," *Ann. N.Y. Acad. Sci.* 128 (1965): 464–71; Wyndham B. Blanton, *Medicine in Virginia in the Eighteenth Century* (Richmond: Garrett and Massie, 1931); William Moll, "History of American Medical Education," *Brit. J. Med. Educ.* 2 (1968): 173–81; Byron Stookey, "America's Two Colonial Medical Schools," *Bull. N.Y. Acad. Med.* 40 (1964): 269–84; Richard H. Shryock, *Medical Licensing in America (1650–1965)* (Baltimore, Md.: Johns Hopkins University Press, 1967). An excellent review of the period from 1910 to 1956 is also available in Saul Jarcho's "Medical Education in the United States, 1910–1956," *J. Mt. Sinai Hosp.* 26 (1959): 339–85.

4. Henry Alden Bunker, "American Psychiatry as a Specialty," in *One Hundred Years of American Psychiatry* (New York: Columbia University Press for the American Psychiatric Association, 1944), p. 481.

5. Benjamin Rush, *Medical Inquiries and Observations upon the Diseases of the Mind* (Philadelphia: Kimber and Richardson, 1812). See also Russell de Jong, "The First American Textbook on Psychiatry: A Review and Discussion of Benjamin Rush's 'Medical Inquiries and Observations upon the Diseases of the Mind,' " *Ann. Med. Hist.*, 3rd ser., 2 (1940): 195–202; Eric T. Carlson and Meribeth M. Simpson, "Benjamin Rush's Medical Use of the Moral Faculty," *Bull. Hist. Med.* 39 (1965): 22–33; E. T. Carlson and M. M. Simpson, "The Definition of Mental Illness: Benjamin Rush (1745–1813)," *Am. J. Psychiatry* 121 (1964): 209–14; and George Mora, "Historical and Theoretical Trends in Psychiatry," in Alfred M. Freedman, Harold I. Kaplan, and Benjamin J. Sadock, eds.,

extensive bloodletting, emetics, and purgatives, standard therapeutic approaches in medical conditions at that time. Drugs such as nitre, Peruvian bark, opium, digitalis, and camphor were also recommended. Rush, nevertheless, accepted a need for cold baths and mechanical restraint, even devising a "tranquilizing chair" and circulating swing ("gyrator") as remedies in insanity. Rush insisted on a courteous and kind attitude towards patients, provision for occupational therapy, and the exclusion of visitors disturbing to patients.

NINETEENTH-CENTURY PSYCHIATRY

Despite the publication of Rush's lectures (which went through four editions), medical schools in Europe and the United States did not include instruction in psychiatry as a standard part of the medical school curriculum. A course of lectures on insanity was given about 1840 at the College of Physicians and Surgeons of New York City. In 1847 a Dr. Samuel Smith was appointed professor of medical jurisprudence and insanity at Willoughby University in Columbus, Ohio, and in 1853 Dr. Pliny Earle delivered a course of lectures on insanity at the College of Physicians. Earle was also appointed professor of psychological medicine in the Berkshire Medical Institute in 1863 and four years later the neurologist, Dr. William A. Hammond, surgeon general of the United States Army from 1862 to 1864, linked the two fields in his appointment to the new chair of diseases of the mind and nervous system at the Bellevue Hospital Medical College in New York City.

Franklin Ebaugh, in reviewing psychiatric education in 1944, noted that between Rush's death in 1813 and Hammond's appointment in 1867 it appeared no systematic course on mental diseases was given anywhere in America.[6] If psychiatry only began to appear in medical school training after the mid-nineteenth century, however, it was a recognized field within medicine for the care and hospitalization of psychotic patients well before. When the Association of Medical Superintendents for American Institutions for the Insane (AMSAII) was established in Philadelphia in 1844, there already existed twenty-two public and corporate American institutions for the mentally ill and three private institutions.[7] The popu-

---

Comprehensive Textbook of Psychiatry—II, 2nd ed., 2 vols. (Baltimore: Williams and Wilkins, 1975), 1:46–47.

6. Bunker, "American Psychiatry as a Specialty," p. 483; Franklin Ebaugh, "History of Psychiatric Education from 1844 to 1944," *Am. J. Psychiatry* 100 (1944): 151.

7. Samuel W. Hamilton, "American Mental Hospitals," in *One Hundred Years of American Psychiatry*, p. 76. The AMSAII became the American Medico-Psychological Association in 1893 and in 1921 was renamed the American Psychiatric Association.

lation of the United States in 1844 was estimated at 17,069,453 persons; the number of mentally ill at 17,457. Of these, however, only 2,561 persons were then hospitalized. Of the thirteen founders of the AMSAII, six headed state institutions for the insane, five were in charge of endowed incorporated institutions, and two owned private hospitals.[8] They had come to their positions with little or no formal training in psychiatry.

Consequently, nineteenth-century psychiatry was steeped in the hospital tradition, and developed in separation from the community and from general medicine. Psychiatry in the first half of the nineteenth century also reflected European reforms, with "moral treatment" propagated by Philippe Pinel and Jean Esquirol in France and William Tuke and John Conolly in England. Moral treatment was an early method of reeducating the patient in a humanistic environment (therapeutic milieu), with the attending physician serving as a kind, but firm, parental surrogate. Moral treatment was carried out by physician-superintendents in private mental hospitals. It was not, however, taught as a system and declined after 1860.

An increasing need for training programs in psychiatry in American medical schools began to be recognized in the last third of the nineteenth century, with growing numbers of admissions to state mental hospital facilities. In 1871 the AMSAII urged that every school conferring medical degrees in the United States should include a complete course of lectures on insanity, combined with clinical instruction. By 1882 the Association for the Protection of the Insane and Prevention of Insanity circularized every existing American medical school urging the introduction of a thorough system of instruction on mental disease. But until the 1890s psychiatry and psychiatric teaching were, for the most part, confined to mental institutions and isolated from medical schools.[9]

NINETEENTH-CENTURY NEUROLOGY

By the late 1860s a substantial body of knowledge on the structure and function of the nervous system had been delineated, and clinical neurology was evolving into a specialty. Moritz von Romberg's classic, *Lehrbuch der Nervenkrankheiten des Menschen*, published in 1846, was translated into English in 1853; it had a wide influence in the United States as well as in England.[10] G. B. A. Duchenne's clinical works on

8. Winfred Overholser, "Founding the Association," in *One Hundred Years of American Psychiatry*, pp. 45–46. Mora, "Historical and Theoretical Trends in Psychiatry," pp. 47–50.

9. Ebaugh, "History of Psychiatric Education from 1844 to 1944," pp. 151–52.

10. Henry R. Viets, "The History of Neurology in the Last One Hundred Years," *Bull. N.Y. Acad. Med.*, 2nd ser., 24 (1948): 773.

electrical stimulation of muscle, and his descriptions of progressive muscular atrophy, poliomyelitis, tabes dorsalis (which he termed progressive locomotor ataxia), and other conditions, were not published in English until 1883. But Duchenne had described clinically a number of significant neurological diseases for the first time.

Meanwhile, at Jean-Martin Charcot's pathological laboratory, established at the Salpêtrière in Paris in 1862, major contributions in the knowledge of structural disease of the nervous system were being formulated. In England John Hughlings Jackson (1835–1911) at the "Queen Square" Hospital and the Moorfields Eye Hospital was studying epilepsy and focal seizures and evolving theories of aphasia and of levels of function of the nervous system. At Heidelberg, Wilhelm Heinrich Erb (1840–1921) was developing instruction in neurology as "an integral part of the medical curriculum."[11]

In the United States, medical specialties began to coalesce after the Civil War. Prior to that time such neurology as was practiced was either a part of general medicine or ancillary to psychiatry. A number of physicians, in treating neurological disturbances resulting from war injuries or infections, became interested in the developing field. With few exceptions, like William Hammond, J. J. Putnam, and Edward Seguin, American physicians who became interested in clinical neurology started as general internists.[12] Several had held earlier university appointments in anatomy and physiology.

William Alexander Hammond (1828–1900) had been appointed Surgeon General of the United States Army Medical Corps in 1862 at the age of thirty-four. By May 1863 he had established the first separate Army hospital for the treatment of nervous diseases and nerve injuries. Hammond's far-seeing innovations in Army medicine brought about a confrontation with the domineering Secretary of War, Edwin Stanton, who dismissed him after a trial. Hammond was subsequently vindicated (1878) and his Army rank of brigadier general restored.[13] Meanwhile, he set up a private practice of neurology in New York City. A tall man with a power-

11. Ibid., p. 782. See, for example, Moritz H. Romberg, *A Manual of the Nervous Diseases of Man*, trans. and ed. by Edward H. Sieveking, 2 vols. (London: New Sydenham Society, 1853); Guillaume-Benjamin Duchenne, *Selections from the Clinical Works of Dr. Duchenne (de Boulogne)*, trans. and ed. George V. Poore (London: New Sydenham Society, 1883); and the discussion on clinical neurology in McHenry, *Garrison's History of Neurology*, pp. 269–341.

12. Morton Prince, "American Neurology of the Past: Neurology of the Future," *J. Nerv. Ment. Dis.* 42 (1915): 446.

13. Webb Haymaker in *The Founders of Neurology: One Hundred and Thirty-Three Biographical Sketches* (Springfield, Ill.: Charles C. Thomas, 1953), pp. 295–97.

ful voice, Hammond made a very effective lecturer as professor of mental and nervous diseases at Bellevue Hospital Medical College, to which he was appointed in 1867.

At the time, clinical neurology was still taught "from the rear section of classical textbooks of internal medicine."[14] Among these were Robley Dunglison's *Practice of Medicine*, third edition, 1848; Thomas Watson's *Principles and Practice of Physic*, third American edition, 1866; and George Wood's *Practice of Medicine*, fourth edition, 1855. In his second volume Wood devoted 228 pages to diseases of the brain, spinal marrow, nerves and nervous system in general. In his "Fifty Years of American Neurology," Smith Ely Jelliffe notes that when Hammond published his *Treatise on Diseases of the Nervous System* (New York: Appleton, 1871), it was the only text on neurology by an American author.[15.]

By 1874 the growing community of neurologists in New York had established a working professional organization—the New York Neurological Society—with William Hammond as president and Max Herzog as corresponding secretary. This was the first neurological society in America.[16] The following year, largely at the initiative of the New York group, the American Neurological Association (ANA) was founded. The first meeting was held in a lecture room of the Young Men's Christian Association Hall at New York's Fourth Avenue and Twenty-Third Street. Hammond and two New York colleagues, Dr. Meredith Clymer and Dr. E. C. Seguin, drew up a draft constitution and bylaws for the new association. Dr. Silas Weir Mitchell (1829–1914), the eminent Philadelphia physician, was elected president, but subsequently declined. Thus, the elected first vice-president, Dr. J. S. Jewell (1837–1887), professor of nervous and mental diseases at the Chicago Medical College (subsequently Northwestern University's Medical School) became the first president.[17]

Although many of the thirty-five members of the new national association still practiced general medicine, or neuropsychiatry, the group in-

14. Louis Casamajor, "Notes for an Intimate History of Neurology and Psychiatry in America," *J. Nerv. Ment. Dis.* 98 (1943): 605.
15. Smith Ely Jelliffe, "Fifty Years of American Neurology," in *Semi-Centennial Anniversary Volume of the American Neurological Association, 1875–1924* (Albany, N.Y.: American Neurological Association, 1924), pp. 406–7.
16. Byron Stookey, "Historical Background of the Neurological Institute and the Neurological Societies," *Bull. N.Y. Acad. Med.*, 2nd ser., 35 (1959): 708–9. The Neurological Society of New York actually dates from 1872, but did not become a working organization until 1874.
17. J. Ramsay Hunt, "The Foundation and Early History of the American Neurological Association," in *Semi-Centennial Anniversary Volume of the American Neurological Association, 1875–1924*, pp. 2–5; see also Haymaker, *The Founders of Neurology*, p. 332, on Mitchell.

cluded among its leaders physicians who were increasingly interested in clinical neurology. Even in the early decades of the twentieth century it was observed in medical circles that the so-called neuropsychiatrist found his pleasure in the study and treatment of patients with organic diseases of the nervous system, but earned his living treating psychiatric patients.[18] Far more than the state mental hospital psychiatrist, the practicing neurologist treated ambulatory neurotic patients and those suffering from functional disorders.

The founding of the ANA marked a significant event in the professionalization and the training of members of a now identifiable specialty. The early leaders of the ANA in the fifty-year period after 1875 numbered most of those who provided neurological instruction in medical schools in the United States for the next generation of American neurologists. Dr. James Stewart Jewell, the brilliant first president, founded and edited the *Journal of Nervous and Mental Diseases,* in addition to his regular lectures in neurology and psychiatry at Northwestern. James Jackson Putnam (1846–1918), clinical instructor and lecturer on diseases of the nervous system at Harvard Medical School when the ANA was founded, became professor of that subject in 1893. Charles Loomis Dana (1852–1935), an inspiring teacher and clinical investigator, who served first as professor of diseases of the mind and nervous system from 1884 to 1895 at the Postgraduate Hospital in New York and subsequently as professor of diseases of the nervous system at Cornell University Medical College, published a *Textbook of Nervous Diseases and Psychiatry for the Use of Students and Practitioners of Medicine* (1892), which went through ten editions by 1925.[19]

Writing in 1915, Dr. Morton Prince, then professor of nervous diseases at Tufts College Medical School, observed that the early American neurologists were "mostly clinicians, but the problems they solved were more than clinical; they were pathological, physiological, anatomical, etiological, and surgical, and, to an extent, psychological."[20]

By 1900 fourteen academically affiliated medical training centers had established divisions or other organizational units for the teaching of medical neurology.[21]

18. H. Houston Merritt, "The Development of Neurology in the Past Fifity Years," *Centennial Anniversary Volume, American Neurological Association, 1875–1975* (New York: Springer, 1975), p. 4.

19. *Centennial Anniversary Volume, American Neurological Association,* pp. 64–68, 86–91, 96–101.

20. Prince, "American Neurology of the Past," p. 447.

21. See the listing of academic training centers for medical neurology in the *Centennial Anniversary Volume, American Neurological Association,* pp. 553–64.

While the majority of the early neurologists grew increasingly concerned with problems of organic neurology, many continued serious interests in psychiatric problems. Among the most notable were Dr. George M. Beard, who in 1869 had described "neurasthenia"; Edward C. Spitzka, professor of nervous diseases at the New York Postgraduate Medical College; James Jackson Putnam, who later became the first president of the American Psychoanalytic Society; and Dr. S. Weir Mitchell, who developed the celebrated "rest cure" for neurotic conditions.

YEARS OF CHANGE AND GROWTH: PSYCHIATRY, 1900–1941

The distinguished neurologist Silas Weir Mitchell, in his widely quoted address of 1894 to the fiftieth annual meeting of the American Medico-Psychological Association, rebuked the country's psychiatrists for their isolation from developments in American medicine, their poor teaching programs, and the absence of programs of scientific investigation into the nature of mental illness.[22] Some of Mitchell's charges were refuted in the presidential address given the following year by Dr. Edward Cowles. But it could not be denied that the alienists (as psychiatrists were then called in England and the United States) had failed to keep pace with the brilliant scientific advances of the great nineteenth-century neurologists.[23]

Franklin Ebaugh and Charles Rymer, in their 1942 survey, have described American psychiatry before 1914 as isolated, and the teaching focussed on a didactic, descriptive presentation of the frank insanities. Teaching personnel were inadequate, medical students were uninterested in the field, and teaching was limited to the clinical years. Further, the organic point of view was dominant, the practice of psychiatry marked by therapeutic nihilism, and mental disease isolated from medicine and mental hospitals from universities.[24]

By using 1914 as a convenient watershed year, this survey postponed recognition of profound changes in the practice, theory, and teaching of

22. Edward Cowles, "Progress in the Care and Treatment of the Insane During the Half Century," *Am. J. Insan.* 51 (1894): 10–22; S. Weir Mitchell, "Address Before the Fiftieth Annual Meeting of the American Medico-Psychological Association Held in Philadelphia, May 16, 1894," *J. Nerv. Ment. Dis.* 21 (1894): 413–38. See the discussion on Mitchell's address by John C. Whitehorn, "A Century of Psychiatric Research in America," in *One Hundred Years of American Psychiatry*, pp. 167–69.
23. Zigmond M. Lebensohn, "Neurology and Psychiatry: Separable or Inseparable," *Med. Ann. of D.C.* 34 (1965): 516.
24. Franklin G. Ebaugh and Charles A. Rymer, *Psychiatry in Medical Education* (New York: Commonwealth Fund, 1942), p. 19.

psychiatry underway in the first decade of the twentieth century. Starting in 1902 psychiatric wards (then termed psychopathic pavilions) began to provide treatment facilities within general hospitals for mental patients. Further steps in breaking down the isolation of state hospital treatment were the development (1906) of social work programs, the initiation of outpatient and aftercare programs, and the start in 1909 of the mental hygiene movement.[25] The establishment in populous American cities of new "psychopathic" hospitals for the examination and initial care of mental patients also provided further educational facilities for medical students.[26]

By the fall of 1909, when Sigmund Freud was invited by Stanley Hall to lecture at Clark University, psychodynamic concepts had already bridged the Atlantic through the literature in the field. The young Abraham Brill (1874–1948) had completed a year of psychoanalytic study with Freud in Vienna and Eugen Bleuler in Zurich and returned to the United States by 1908. Freud's controversial doctrines, which were to affect the theory, teaching, and practice of psychiatry so deeply, were already championed by three distinguished neurologists—James Jackson Putnam, Smith Ely Jelliffe, and Ernest Jones (then practicing in Toronto). By 1910 the American Psychopathological Association had been founded in Washington, D.C., by Dr. Morton Prince, in association with Putnam, Jones, August Hoch of New York, George Waterman of Boston, Adolf Meyer, and others. The spring of 1911 saw the birth of the American Psychoanalytic Society with Putnam as president and Jones as secretary.

The Swiss-born Adolf Meyer (1866–1950) has been described by William Alanson White and others as the outstanding influence in the development of American psychiatry for some forty years.[27] Through his teaching—first in clinical neurology at the Eastern State Hospital in Kankakee, Illinois, later at Clark University; as director of the Pathological Institute of the New York State Hospital and as professor of psychiatry at Cornell; and from 1910 to 1941 as the professor of psychiatry and director of the new Henry Phipps Psychiatric Clinic at the Johns Hopkins Medical School and Hospital—Meyer left an indelible imprint on several generations of young psychiatrists. In his years at Johns Hopkins, Meyer

25. Jeanne L. Brand, "The United States: An Historical Perspective," in Richard H. Williams and Luey D. Ozarin, eds., *Community Mental Health: An International Perspective* (San Francisco: Jossey-Boss, 1968), pp. 21–23.

26. Franklin G. Ebaugh, "History of Psychiatric Education in the United States from 1844 to 1944," *Am. J. Psychiatry* 100 (1944): 153.

27. W. A. White in *Forty Years of Psychiatry* (New York and Washington, D.C.: Nervous and Mental Disease Publishing Co., 1933), as cited in Brand, "The United States: An Historical Perspective," p. 22.

established a model university training center for young psychiatrists and was able to introduce both dynamic psychiatry and his concepts of psychobiology into the medical school curriculum.

Meyer was also a major figure in the development of psychiatric research, social psychiatry, and the mental hygiene movement. A careful clinical observer, Meyer insisted on the importance of the psychiatrist's taking a holistic, body-mind approach to mental illness, developing detailed scientific case histories, including the patient's life, his family, his social setting, mental and physical condition. He favored early intervention in the development of psychiatric illness by a patient's school, family and community, and the organization of aftercare programs. Although Meyer accepted psychoanalysis with some reservations and was critical of its lack of methodology, he is credited with being the most important early disseminator of psychoanalysis to young psychiatrists.[28]

Psychoanalysis contributed both a new model for the etiology of mental illness and a new method of treatment for a number of nervous and mental disorders. At least three influential medical texts written from 1907 to 1915 included psychoanalytic concepts—W. A. White's *Outlines of Psychiatry;* the voluminous compendium, *The Modern Treatment of Nervous and Mental Disease,* edited by White and Jelliffe; and the shorter treatise written by White and Jelliffe, *Diseases of the Nervous System, a Textbook of Neurology and Psychiatry.*[29]

With the catalytic impact of the Flexner Report after 1910, medical education in the United States began to move toward a uniformity of standards. But despite the challenging new concepts and developments within psychiatry generated by Adolf Meyer, E. E. Southard, W. A. White and other brilliant leaders of American neuropsychiatry at the time, a report in 1914 on the status of psychiatric education throughout the country's medical schools pointed to the lack of time allotted to both neurology and psychiatry. Writing in the *Journal of the American Medical Association,* Dr. William Graves deplored "the almost universal feeling of incompetence in the recognition of nervous and mental diseases by

28. No full-length biography of Meyer has yet been published. But see Nathan G. Hale, Jr., *Freud and the Americans: The Beginnings of Psychoanalysis in the United States, 1876–1917* (New York: Oxford University Press, 1971), p. 157. See also the assessment of Meyer by Henry Alden Bunker in *One Hundred Years of American Psychiatry,* pp. 490–96; John Burnham, *Psychoanalysis and American Medicine, 1894–1918* (New York: International Universities Press, 1967); David M. Rioch's sketch of Meyer in *Centennial Anniversary Volume, American Neurological Association,* pp. 153–59; the excellent article by Theodore Lidz, "Adolf Meyer and the Development of American Psychiatry," *Am. J. Psychiatry* 123 (1966): 320–32; and the recent, thoughtful assessment of Meyer by George Mora in "Historical and Theoretical Trends in Psychiatry," pp. 626–32.

29. Hale, *Freud and the Americans,* pp. 437–38.

recent graduates."[30] Five of the eighty-five American medical schools whose catalogues Graves reviewed had no instruction in either neurology or psychiatry; in many schools where the subject was given, neurology received more time and attention than psychiatry, and the teaching of both was limited to the clinical years.

By 1932, with a survey of sixty-eight American medical schools sponsored by the Division of Psychiatric Education of the National Committee for Mental Hygiene (NCMH), the situation had improved. Twenty-nine schools offered some preclinical instruction in psychiatry and thirty-five taught psychiatry in the clinical years only. Psychiatry received an average of 77 hours of instruction per school, neurology 74. The actual hours of psychiatric instruction, however, varied from zero to 207, and of neurological training, from zero to 236.[31] Some of the improvement was related to a wider public interest in the importance of psychiatric understandings, fostered by neuropsychiatric casualties in World War I and the developing mental hygiene movement.

Within psychiatry and neurology, there was yet no formal professional yardstick to establish national training standards or to measure minimal professional competence. With the rapid growth of medical specialism in the first quarter of the twentieth century, several medical groups had already established certifying boards: opthalmology in 1916, otolaryngology in 1924, obstetrics and gynecology in 1930, and dermatology and syphilology in 1932. In his 1928 presidential address to the American Psychiatric Association, Adolf Meyer had pointed to the need for a certificate to confirm professional competence in the practice of psychiatry and neurology.

The subsequent steps leading to the final establishment of the American Board of Psychiatry and Neurology in 1934 have been detailed by Doctors Walter Freeman, Franklin Ebaugh, and David A. Boyd, Jr.[32] The first of a series of conferences on psychiatric education, sponsored by the NCMH, convened in the spring of 1933 and called for the establishment of an examining board by the American Psychiatric Association with

30. William W. Graves, "Some Factors Tending Toward Adequate Instruction in Nervous and Mental Diseases," *J. AMA* 63 (1914): 1707 (cited by Ebaugh and Rymer, *Psychiatry in Medical Education*, p. 9, and by Bunker, "American Psychiatry as a Specialty," pp. 486–87).

31. Franklin Ebaugh, "The History of Psychiatric Education in the United States from 1844 to 1944," p. 155; and "The Evolution of Psychiatric Education," *Am. J. Psychiatry* 126 (1969): 97–100; Franklin Ebaugh and Charles Rymer, *Psychiatry in Medical Education*, pp. 13–18.

32. Walter Freeman, Franklin Ebaugh, and David A. Boyd, "The Founding of the American Board of Psychiatry and Neurology, Inc.," *Am. J. Psychiatry* 115 (1959): 769–78.

specific training requirements for candidates seeking a diploma in psychiatry. Further stimulus for certification came in June 1933 from the Section on Nervous and Mental Diseases of the American Medical Association. Meanwhile the American Neurological Association had expressed interest in certification for neurologists.

By December 1933 representatives of the three groups gathered in New York, and at the outset were widely split on the question of whether psychiatry and neurology belonged together. It was not surprising, in view of their diverse backgrounds and their respective orientations in dynamic psychiatry and organic neurology, that the representatives "got along like a couple of strange bulldogs" at the organizing meetings in 1933 and 1934. Common standards were worked out, however, and separate qualifying requirements and examinations were agreed upon. Certification as both a neurologist and psychiatrist required an applicant to pass both examinations. Training requirements for psychiatrists required a medical degree from an approved medical school; a license to practice medicine; three years of study in psychiatry following the general internship in approved hospitals, clinics and laboratories; and two years of hospital or other practice limited to psychiatry. A "grandfather clause" permitted blanket certification of applicants who had graduated from medical school in 1919 or earlier and who had carried out a specialized practice for fifteen years.[33]

In the years after 1934 the requirements established by the American Board of Psychiatry and Neurology at minimum set the skeletal outlines for the development of training programs in both specialties. Within the broad framework established, there continued to be wide variations in the content and the type of residency training provided for each field. John Romano, who subsequently developed one of the country's leading psychiatric training programs at the University of Rochester School of Medicine, described one of the best of the psychiatric residency programs in operation by the mid-thirties at the University of Colorado Medical Center. Colorado then provided an opportunity for graduate study in clinical psychiatry "within a major university hospital, housed in a psychopathic hospital, woven into the fabric of a medical school, with the rare support of fellowship stipends" (one hundred dollars per month!). Little or no formal instruction, through tutorials, seminars, conferences or lecture series, was provided. Romano notes the "endless number" of acutely disturbed patients with emergency needs to which the young residents, together with their nurses and attendants, would respond

33. Ibid.

"with the prompt devotion and gusto of seasoned firehorses." Psychology and social work he recalled as being "represented by only a few valiant souls, who served principally as handmaidens."[34]

At St. Elizabeths Hospital in Washington under William Alanson White in 1935, Dr. Zigmond Lebensohn, now clinical professor of psychiatry at Georgetown University, recalled the "on-the-job training." Dr. White would give an occasional lecture and visiting lecturers would address the residents from time to time. But both at Colorado and at St. Elizabeths relatively little formal training or evaluation of the resident was undertaken, and residents at that time often worked out their patients' problems themselves or in discussion with their fellow residents. The learning experience, if crude, was one of the most challenging possible, Dr. Lebensohn notes today.[35]

By the late 1930s treatment modalities for neurotic and psychotic patients had expanded. Both Adolf Meyer and William Alanson White had emphasized the need for preventive psychiatry and the treatment of children and adolescents. By 1932 twenty-seven of the largest American cities had a full-time child guidance clinic service, with some 232 whole or part-time clinics operating throughout the country.[36] For the hospitalized psychotic patient new shock therapies were being tried—Manfred Sakel's insulin therapy (first reported in 1933 from Berlin), Metrazol convulsive shock (Ladislaus von Meduna at Budapest) in the same year, and electric convulsive shock (Ugo Cerletti and Lucio Bini in Rome, 1938), which largely replaced the first two by the 1940s. Although the shock therapies were empirical and the physiological effects not understood, some psychiatrists believed they facilitated the use of psychotherapy. Shock treatment had a share in changing the pessimistic view of recovery from schizophrenia and subsequently the endogenous depressions.[37]

Still a further area of growth within psychiatry in the thirties lay in the extension of Adolf Meyer's psychobiological approach to medical problems and the development of psychosomatic medicine, exploring the relationships between normal and pathological bodily processes and a pa-

34. John Romano, "The Teaching of Psychiatry to Medical Students: Past, Present, and Future," *Am. J. Psychiatry* 126 (1970): 1115–16. See also John Romano's "Twenty-Five Years of University Department Chairmanship," *Am. J. Psychiatry* 122 (1966): suppl. pp. 7–27.

35. Personal communication with Zigmond M. Lebensohn, M.D., 15 July, 1975.

36. Bunker, "American Psychiatry as a Specialty," p. 498. The first American textbook on child psychiatry, written by the Johns Hopkins psychiatrist Leo Kanner, was *Child Psychiatry* (Springfield, Ill.: Charles C. Thomas, 1935).

37. William Malamud, "Psychiatric Therapies," in *One Hundred Years of American Psychiatry*, pp. 319–22; Garfield Tourney, "History of Biological Psychiatry in America," *Am. J. Psychiatry* 126 (1969): 29–42.

tient's personality and life stresses. Clinical instruction and contemporary medical textbooks in the first quarter of the twentieth century had paid little attention to mind-body problems in either the etiology or treatment of medical disorders.[38] Then, drawing on the basic studies in neurophysiology of Walter B. Cannon, psychiatrists of the thirties, led by Franz Alexander and Harold Wolff, began to reexamine physiological disorder in relation to psychological stress. It was an orientation which created new links between psychiatry, neurophysiology, and medicine.

ADVANCES IN NEUROLOGY: 1900–1941

During the first quarter of the nineteenth century, when Freud's concepts were changing the theoretical basis of psychiatric practice, a number of neuropsychiatrists began to confine their interests more to clinical and organic neurology. Indeed, as Dr. Charles Mills pointed out in reviewing the published papers from the first fifty years (1875–1925) of meetings of the American Neurological Association, 78 percent of all the publications could be classified as organic neurology, another 11 percent dealt with functional nervous diseases, and the rest (11 percent) with psychiatry and psychology.[39]

The conditions for both training in and the practice of clinical neurology, however, still lagged behind some of the other rapidly developing medical specialties at the start of the twentieth century. Speaking before the AMA's Section on Nervous and Mental Diseases at the annual meeting of 1910, Doctors Joseph Collins and Pearce Bailey, two of the three founders of the newly opened Neurological Institute of New York—the only hospital at that time in the United States devoted to neurological diseases—made an impassioned plea for greater attention to clinical neurology:

> In all America there is scarcely a general hospital with neurologic wards worthy of the name, with the exception of a few hospitals and inaccessible city almshouses in which cripples and dotards are crowded together under the care of untrained housestaffs without laboratory facilities. Magnificent endowments almost yearly furthur the advances in surgery, medicine, and psychiatry, but neurology is left to take care of itself. Few nurses receive special training in nervous diseases; the objective teaching of students is limited

38. L. L. Langley and Jeanne L. Brand, "The Mind-Body Issue in Early Twentieth-Century American Medicine," *Bull. Hist. Med.* 46 (1972): 178–79.
39. *Semi-Centennial Anniversary Volume of the American Neurological Association, 1875–1924*, p. 37.

chiefly to ambulatory cases. The profession who teach them, having no hospital patients of their own, can demonstrate only such patients as are able to walk to the clinic. In the recognition of brain abscess, meningitis, acute intoxications and injuries of the nervous system, the student either goes uninstructed, or else gets his instruction from men neither particularly interested nor particularly versed in these subjects. Hospital section-teaching, the most valuable of all modern teaching methods, is practically unknown in nervous diseases. The clinical facilities of the professors of neurology are not much better than those of the students. Without wards, without laboratories, without means for the continuous daily observations of patients, the holders of these chairs cannot obtain the intimate knowledge of disease, and the stimulus to investigate it, which is necessary to keep them abreast of modern progress.[40]

It was not until the publication of Judson Herrick's *Introduction to Neurology* in 1915 and S. W. Ranson's textbook, *The Anatomy of the Nervous System from the Standpoint of Development and Functions*, five years later that adequate textbooks were available for the few medical students entering neurology at the time.[41]

To the eyes of the present-day neurologist, training in clinical neurology—even by 1925—lagged far behind the advances being made in basic knowledge of the anatomy, physiology and pathology of the nervous system. Only a few residencies in neurology were available to young physicians, and the existing training programs lasted only about a year. Even two years after the establishment of the American Board of Psychiatry and Neurology in 1934, only sixteen hospitals in the United States had approved neurological residency training.

In most medical schools, with the exceptions of Harvard, Columbia University, and the University of Pennsylvania, neurology in the 1920s was still an integral part of internal medicine or psychiatry.[42] Beginning in 1928, with the assistance of funding from the Rockefeller Foundation, full-time teaching and research units in medical neurology began to be developed. But not until after World War II did full-time departments of neurological medicine become a pattern in American medical schools.

The advances taking place in the basic sciences during the first half of the twentieth century—major developments within neurochemistry, neurophysiology, neuropathology, electrophysiology, and genetics—

40. Joseph Collins and Pearce Bailey, "The Dependence of Neurology on Internal Medicine," *J. AMA* 55 (1910): 393.
41. Aura E. Severinghaus, *Neurology: A Medical Discipline Takes Stock*, DHEW Publication, NIH 72–175 (Bethesda, Md.: National Institutes of Health, 1971).
42. Merritt, "The Development of Neurology in the Past Fifty Years," p. 4.

meanwhile extended the baselines for later advances in clinical neurology. Changes in other medical fields also profoundly affected neurological practice. As the late historian of neurology Dr. Henry Viets pointed out in 1951, syphilis and tuberculosis were two of the primary causes of diseases of the nervous system in 1900, but neither was significant in neurological practice by mid-century. Antibiotics virtually eliminated tabes dorsalis and neurological sequelae of typhoid fever, pneumonia, smallpox, and many other diseases. New drugs had already become available to alleviate some neurological disorders—neostigmine in myasthenia gravis, dilantin in epilepsy. Viets concluded that the outstanding features of the previous half century of neurology were the integration of laboratory research with clinical practice, the spectacular growth of neurosurgery, and the development of such diagnostic aids as myelography, electroencephalography, and pneumoencephalography.[43]

POSTWAR TRAINING DEVELOPMENTS IN NEUROLOGY AND PSYCHIATRY: THE FEDERAL PROGRAM

The Establishment of NIMH-NINDB

The American people emerged from World War II not only with a sense of deep gratitude for the end of hostilities, but with a feeling of strong identification with a successful national achievement. Scientific research had a new value, and the federal government had assumed new responsibilities for science and the national welfare. This climate facilitated the remarkable postwar growth of federal support for health research and the programs of the National Institutes of Health.[44]

The new federal programs in support of mental health and neurology were built upon administrative roots within the Public Health Service—the Division of Mental Hygiene. Even before the entry of the United States into World War II, the director of the Division of Mental Hygiene, Dr. Lawrence Kolb, had drafted plans for a neuropsychiatric institute to expand support for nervous and mental diseases, as well as plans for a coordinating research center within the PHS. Dr. Kolb was fully supported in this by the surgeon general, Dr. Thomas Parran. By 1940 endorsements for the new institute had been obtained from the National

43. Henry R. Viets, "Medicine as a Science: Neurology," *N. Eng. J. Med.* 244 (1951): 400–407. See also Erik Lindgrens's chapter, "A History of Neuroradiology," in Thomas H. Newton and D. Gordon Potts, eds., *Radiology of the Skull and Brain*, 3 vols. (St. Louis: C. V. Mosby, 1971–1977), 1–25.

44. Jeanne L. Brand, "The National Mental Health Act of 1946: A Retrospect," *Bull. Hist. Med.* 39 (1965): 231–45.

Committee for Mental Hygiene, the American Neurological Association, the American Psychiatric Association, and the Section on Nervous and Mental Disease of the American Medical Association. But when the idea was, in turn, broached to the House of Delegates of the American Medical Association, the spectre of state medicine breathed down the assembled medical necks, and the endorsement was flatly disapproved. Nevertheless, Dr. Kolb proceeded to draw up a bill. With the outbreak of the war shortly thereafter, however, it was never introduced into Congress.[45]

Mental and neurological disorders formed the largest group of causes for medical rejection of draftees in World War II, however, and by 1946, 60 percent of all hospitalization under the Veterans Administration was caused by psychiatric disorders at a cost of forty thousand dollars or more per case.[46]

The draft bill for a National Neuropsychiatric Institute was introduced into the Congress on March 10, 1945, and signed into law on July 3, 1946, as the National Mental Health Act. During the bill's passage through the Congress the name of the institute was changed to the National Institute of Mental Health. It was established in April 1949.

Neurology was at first supported as a part of NIMH program interests. In 1949 the young National Multiple Sclerosis Society petitioned the Congress for a new institute, specifically devoted to multiple sclerosis.[47] Fifty multiple sclerosis patients attended the Senate Committee on Labor and Public Welfare hearings. Senator Charles Tobey of New Hampshire, whose daughter had been stricken with the disease, led the movement for a new institute. The Congressional response was the passage of Public Law 692, signed on August 15, 1950, authorizing establishment of a National Institute of Neurological Diseases and Blindness, the seventh of the National Institutes of Health in Bethesda. In 1968 legislation established a National Eye Institute, and the name of NINDB was changed to National Institute of Neurological Diseases and Stroke, and subsequently to the

45. Lawrence Kolb, "The Need for a Neuropsychiatric Institute in the U.S. Public Health Service for the Study of Nervous and Mental Diseases," c. December 1939 (Records of the Division of Mental Hygiene, Files of the National Institute of Mental Health, Rockville, Md.); Letter, Lawrence Kolb, M.D., to Jeanne L. Brand, Ph.D., 7 April 1964; "Resolution from the Section on Nervous and Mental Diseases Endorsing the Formation of a Central Neuropsychiatric Institute in the United States Public Health Service," Minutes of the Ninety-First Annual Session of the American Medical Association, House of Delegates, Held in New York, June 10–14, 1940, *J. AMA* 114 (1940): 2570.

46. *Senate Report on the National Mental Health Act*, 79th Congress, 2nd Session, Report No. 135 (Washington, D.C.: U.S. Government Printing Office, 1946), pp. 2–3.

47. Merritt, "The Development of Neurology in the Past Fifty Years," p. 6.

National Institute of Neurological and Communicative Disorders and Stroke in 1975.

The overall significance for the development of both psychiatry and neurology of the postwar establishment of these two new categorical disease institutes cannot be minimized. For the first time large-scale funding, knowledgeable leadership within the Public Health Service, and the expert professional consultation available through the NIH advisory councils, training committees, and research study sections were focussed on solving the scientific and neurologic problems of mental and neurological disorder.

Postwar Training in Neurology

In 1952, before the start of the NINDB training grant support, there were only 250 qualified neurologists in the United States. Six states had no board-certified neurologist, and in some regions of the American South only a single neurologist was available to serve almost one million persons. Existing medical school training programs were concentrated in the East and Midwest. Only fifteen of the existing medical schools offered training programs in neurology. Only about 50 percent of all American medical students graduated each year had instruction in an organized course in neurology given by a trained neurologist.[48]

The first director of NINDB, Dr. Pearce Bailey, Jr., had served as chief of neurology for the Veterans Administration. With his colleagues and consultants, Dr. Bailey made the training of more clinical neurologists one of the principal NINDB goals. Teachers were also in short supply, and as the institute's programs moved ahead funds were channelled into the training of capable teacher-investigators in clinics and laboratories. In succeeding years training grant support was extended for research training in related sensory fields—opthalmology, otolaryngology, and medical audiology and speech. In recognition of the need for neurologists to become more familiar with the basic neurological sciences, graduate training funds were awarded to expand training capabilities in neuropathology, neurochemistry, neuroanatomy and neuropharmacology at a small number of basic science centers. By 1957 fellowship, traineeship, and training grant support was extended to graduate training in pediatric neurology, and later to neurosurgery and neuroradiology.[49]

The growth in numbers of neurologists was dramatic. By 1960 a total of 1,396 physicians had registered with the American Medical Association as

48. Elizabeth Hartman, "Impact of NINDB on Neurology," in *Neurology: A Medical Discipline Takes Stock*, pp. 30–33.
49. Ibid.

primary neurologists; by 1970 the number had increased to 2,727.[50] From the start of the NINDB training programs through fiscal year 1974, a total of eighty-six million dollars was funneled into training in medical and child neurology.[51] Reviewing the NINDB training programs in 1975, Dr. Pearce Bailey, Jr., pointed out that the vast majority of NINDB trainees had continued to pursue academic careers, and that many held chairs in leading American medical schools and hospitals.[52]

Postwar Training in Psychiatry

The large-scale training programs mounted by NIMH since its establishment in 1949 have had a quantitative and qualitative impact on the development of the four core mental health professions—psychiatry, psychology, psychiatric nursing, and psychiatric social work.[53] In his substantive review of the national mental health program in 1972, Dr. Richard Hays Williams points out that four qualitative issues have characterized the NIMH training programs. First has been the uneven geographical distribution of specialists in the field; next, a system whereby only a small proportion of the population has access to and purchasing power for the services of highly qualified trained personnel; third, a need to broaden the base of manpower, including consideration of the changing roles of health professionals to increase their utility in health care; and fourth, social demands for special training programs in child and family mental health and for minority groups and such social problems as suicide, crime, delinquency, alcoholism and the abuse of drugs.[54]

The immediate concern in the development of federally supported psychiatric training programs after World War II was the small number of qualified American psychiatrists—3,600. The largest share of NIMH training grant support, consequently, flowed into basic psychiatric residency programs, without regard to geographic distribution or equity of access.[55] Large-scale psychiatric training programs were also mounted by the Veterans Administration.

50. Severinghaus, *Neurology*, p. 35.

51. Personal communication with Dr. Murray Goldstein, Associate Director for Extramural Programs, NINCDS, August 1975.

52. Pearce Bailey, Jr., in *Centennial Anniversary Volume, American Neurological Association*, p. 524.

53. NIMH was transferred administratively within the Public Health Service in 1967 from the National Institutes of Health to the Health Services Mental Health Administration and is today a part of the Alcohol, Drug Abuse, and Mental Health Administration.

54. Richard H. Williams, *Perspectives in the Field of Mental Health: A View of the National Program* (Rockville, Md.: NIMH, 1972), p. 119.

55. James S. Eaton, Jr., M.D., and R. A. Daniels, M.D., "Psychiatric Education in the United States," paper presented at the First Pacific Congress of Psychiatry, Melbourne, Australia, 15 May 1975, p. 3.

The quantitative results were even more dramatic than those that had taken place in neurology. By 1975 the number of American psychiatrists had risen to 27,000, and psychiatry had become the third largest medical specialty.[56] As early as 1951, when the first NIMH-funded Conference on Psychiatric Education met in Ithaca, separate departments of psychiatry had been established at almost all American medical schools, and psychiatric and behavioral science was being taught in at least two of the four years of medical school. The second working conference held in Ithaca the following year, in reviewing the training of career psychiatrists, took note of the recommended three-year program formulated in 1946 by the American Board of Psychiatry and Neurology:

> This training for psychiatrists should include clinical work with psychoneurotic and psychotic patients, combined with the study of basic psychiatric sciences, medical and social psychology, psychopathology, psychotherapy, and the physiological therapies, including a basic knowledge of the form, function, and pertinent pathology of the nervous system. This training should be supervised and guided by teachers competent to develop skill and understanding in the utilization of such basic knowledge in dealing with patients. Mere factual knowledge is not sufficient. This training period should include instruction in the psychiatric aspects of general medical and surgical conditions and the behavior disorders of children and adolescents sufficient to develop practical ability to direct the treatment of such conditions. It should also include collaborative work with social workers, clinical psychologists, courts and other social agencies. The training program of the candidate for certification in psychiatry should include sufficient training in neurology to enable him to recognize and to evaluate the evidences of organic neurological disease.[57]

The range of psychiatric training centers by 1953 spread far beyond the university teaching hospital, and included Army and Navy general hospitals; United States Public Health Service and other federal mental hospitals; Veterans Administration hospitals; state mental hospitals; municipal, county and private hospitals (both general and mental); and other specialized institutions, such as child guidance clinics, prisons, rehabilitation centers.[58]

56. George Mora, "Recent Psychiatric Developments (Since 1939)," *American Handbook of Psychiatry*, 3 vols. (New York: Basic Books, 1974), 1:78.
57. American Psychiatric Association, *The Psychiatrist, His Training and Development: Report of the 1952 Conference on Psychiatric Education Held at Cornell University, Ithaca, New York, June 19–25, 1952* (Washington, D.C.: American Psychiatric Association, 1953), p. 3.
58. Ibid., p. 73–74.

The 1952 conference also pointed out that "it is now almost universally agreed that a necessary part of the preparation of a competent psychiatrist was the development of an understanding of the principles of psychodynamics," stating that "by far the greatest contributions in data, methods, and operational principles are those of Freud and psychoanalysis."[59] There was virtually unanimous agreement at the conference, however, that while it was not necessary to be psychoanalyzed in order to develop competence as a psychiatrist, it was highly desirable.

Psychoanalytic understanding, however, was only a part of the educational armamentarium which the young psychiatrist was expected to absorb. By 1962, an APA-sponsored conference in graduate psychiatric education pointed to the new emphases on sociologic, psychologic and ecologic aspects of human behavior which, together with the expansion of knowledge in the biological sciences, had "significantly widened the base of psychiatric education."[60] By the early sixties reserpine, chlorpromazine and other psychopharmacologic agents were in wide use. Tranquilizers became a significant factor in the extension of community care for psychotic patients. Drawing on English, Dutch and other foreign examples for open hospitals, day hospitals, and milieu therapy, American psychiatrists began to use new treatment methods which also entered into psychiatric training.

Spurred by the final report in 1961 of the Joint Commission on Mental Illness and Health, and the tragic assassination of President Kennedy in 1963, the Congress passed the Community Mental Health Centers Act of 1963 to finance construction of community mental health centers. Two years later Public Law 89–105 authorized funds to assist in staffing the centers. New population groups were now receiving psychiatric care, and residents in psychiatry were drawn closer to minority and urban problems through participation in the inner city, rural clinics, and the expansion of the community mental health center program. Mora has noted that in recent years many young psychiatrists have become interested in humanistic medicine, in the "comprehensive approach to patients of any social class and their families and communities."[61]

59. Ibid., p. 91. Karl Menninger, reviewing the contribution of psychoanalysis to American psychiatry in 1954, pointed to negative effects. He believed psychoanalysis impaired clinical observation and fostered "an attitude of patronizing indifference toward the acquisition of systematic historical material" (*Bull. Menninger Clinic* 18 [1954]: 89–90).

60. American Psychiatric Association, *Training the Psychiatrist to Meet Changing Needs* (Washington, D.C.: American Psychiatric Association, 1963), p. viii.

61. Mora, "Recent Psychiatric Developments (Since 1939)," p. 78. See also George Mora, "The Development of Psychiatry in New York City," *Bull. N.Y. Acad. Med.* 47 (1971): 550–66.

In the spring of 1975 the American Psychiatric Association's Division of Manpower, Research and Development published results of a survey of academic resources in psychiatric residency training.[62] Directors of 288 programs responded, reporting on a total of 4,750 residents. Only ninety-seven residency programs were in medical school settings; the majority were in psychiatric hospitals not part of a medical school. Ten states were found to be training 70.4 percent of all American psychiatric residents, with New York and California leading. One of the most noteworthy findings documented in the survey was the large number of psychologists and social scientists with full-time appointments to teach residents in psychiatry. Nevertheless, little systematic preparation was given for residents "to work collaboratively with either the more traditional multidisciplinary mental health team or the newer paraprofessional."[63]

Treatment methods that the survey found "almost universally" taught to residents included individual and group psychotherapy, the use of psychotropic drugs, crisis intervention, and, to a lesser extent, electroconvulsive shock treatment. Therapies which were characterized as "used very infrequently" included insulin coma and subcoma therapy, psychoanalysis (as such), sensitivity training and psychodrama.

Fifty-nine of the 288 programs responding reported they made an explicit effort to provide training in the understanding of minority subcultures. Forty-six programs reported extensive involvement in community psychiatry. Instruction in the medical management of alcoholism and drug dependency was quite standard in residency programs, but very few programs included didactic or clinical training in other social problems such as aging, unemployment, suicide, and abortion.

Not infrequently the psychiatrist's role today is described as "in flux" or "undergoing an identity crisis." With the heavy influence of the behavioral sciences on psychiatry in the 1950s and the increasing humanistic and ecological concerns of Americans in the sixties and seventies, the potential responsibilities of the psychiatrist have been stretched far from the medical model. Medical school residency training in psychiatry, however, has remained more traditional in its orientation, although paying tribute to a broader social commitment by participating in community-

62. Lee Gurel, "Some Characteristics of Psychiatric Residency Training Programs," *Am. J. Psychiatry* 132 (1975): 363–72. After New York and California, the ten states which had the largest number of psychiatric residents were (in descending order) Massachusetts, Pennsylvania, Ohio, Michigan, Illinois, Maryland, Connecticut and Missouri.

63. Ibid., p. 369. It should be noted that the Gurel survey covered both general psychiatric residency programs and specialized residency programs, as in child psychiatry.

based programs, sponsoring some attempts at training in subculture value systems, and reducing emphasis on psychoanalysis per se.

Psychiatry and behavioral science have also been significantly expanded in the teaching of medical students since World War II. Where prewar psychiatric instruction was often limited to "museum teaching of flagrant and bizarre psychotic states," medical students now studied the psychoneuroses, psychophysiological states and the effects of emotion on illness.[64]

John Romano has pointed out the value to the medical student which psychiatry has demonstrated—in broadening his understanding of personality and improving methods of observation, both central to the physician-patient relationship. At the same time Romano regrets the frequent failure of many American medical schools to include within their teaching programs current contributions from the biological sciences, particularly functional neuroanatomy, behavioral genetics, neurohumoral and hormonal chemistry, and behavioral neurophysiology.[65] In a number of American medical schools, however, psychiatry has been used to broaden the students' perspectives on the healing role—utilizing a comprehensive approach to medicine and focussing on the patient rather than on the illness.

Federal funds had both a qualitative and quantitative impact on the development of neurological and psychiatric training. By the early 1970s, however, public support for advanced medical specialty training, including neurology and psychiatry, had come under fire. No consensus had been reached on the optimum number of psychiatrists and neurologists for the country's needs. More broadly, it was not unreasonable to question whether, amongst competing national needs, federal funds should continue to underwrite advanced medical specialty training for physicians, who could then anticipate an annual income far above that of the average taxpayer. Despite some congressional resistance, efforts of the administration from 1970 onward to curtail support for specialty training in medical fields have substantially slowed the growth both in the numbers of specialists trained and in the amount of funding available for their education.

64. American Psychiatric Association Committee on Medical Education, "An Outline for a Curriculum for Teaching Psychiatry in Medical Schools," *J. Med. Educ.* 31 (1956): 117; Ebaugh, "The Evolution of Psychiatric Education," p. 98.

65. Romano, "The Teaching of Psychiatry to Medical Students," pp. 1122–23. See also Sidney L. Werkman, *The Role of Psychiatry in Medical Education: An Appraisal and a Forecast* (Cambridge, Mass.: Harvard University Press, 1966), pp. 54–57.

Public Health and Preventive Medicine

JUDITH WALZER LEAVITT

PUBLIC health and preventive medicine have never been key elements in the curricula of American medical schools. Nor have they been totally ignored. Alternately referred to as *medical police, personal* or *public hygiene, sanitation, sanitary science, social medicine, preventive medicine* or *public health*—terms used interchangeably to describe similar course contents—public health material frequently found its way into the lecture schedules of nineteenth-century medical students and almost always has been part of the twentieth-century curriculum. However, its status in the medical curriculum has been low and its impact negligible. This essay examines the extent to which instruction in public health and preventive medicine has been included in American medical schools, as well as its contribution to the education of physicians.

The typical mid-nineteenth-century medical curriculum did not include public health as a separate course. In a survey conducted by the American Medical Association (AMA) in 1849, only two of thirty-eight

I would like to thank Doctors John Duffy and Chester Burns for their helpful suggestions. Linda Jameson and Larry Lynch provided useful research assistance.

medical colleges mentioned hygiene as a subject taught.[1] This figure is misleading, since hygiene was often included in more comprehensive courses. For example, Western Reserve University School of Medicine taught hygiene as part of its medicine course.[2] Few schools saw the need for a chair in hygiene in this period, but most established professorships of anatomy, surgery, physiology, pathology, medicine, obstetrics or materia medica.[3] The exceptions to this pattern were the women's medical colleges, which showed a deep concern for personal and public hygiene in their early curricula. The Woman's Medical College of Pennsylvania, for example, was particularly dedicated to the teaching of preventive medicine and personal and public hygiene from its establishment.[4] But careful observers of mid-century medical colleges despaired at the general neglect of public hygiene courses. Noting the subject's "intimate relation to the preservation of human life," one AMA writer described it as "not only one of the most interesting but useful of the sciences."[5]

Despite strong AMA interest in the subject, it was the Civil War that turned the attention of medical colleges to public health. The Union army required its medical staff to attend lectures in hygiene, and medical schools responded by establishing such courses and hiring professors to teach them.[6] One of the earliest schools to do so was the University of Michigan, which required hygiene and military surgery in 1863.[7]

1. "Rules, Requirements, etc., etc., etc., of the Several Medical Colleges of the United States," *Trans. AMA* 2 (1849): 284–99. The two schools that offered instruction in hygiene were the Medical Department of the University of Maryland, Baltimore, and the Medical Department of Washington University, Baltimore.

2. Frederick C. Waite, *Western Reserve University Centennial History of the School of Medicine* (Cleveland: Western Reserve University Press, 1946), p. 112. See also John A. Wyeth, "A Medical Student in 1867," *Proc. AAMC* 19 (1909): 23–24.

3. See, for example, the recommended professorships in James R. Wood, "Report of the Special Committee on Medical Education," *Trans. AMA* 11 (1858): 258.

4. Gulielma Fell Alsop, *History of the Woman's Medical College of Philadelphia, Pennsylvania, 1850–1950* (Philadelphia: J. B. Lippincott, 1950), p. 207. The New York Infirmary Women's Medical College established a chair in hygiene in 1868, possibly the first single chair in the subject in this country (Elizabeth Blackwell, *Pioneer Work in Opening the Medical Profession to Women* [New York: Longmans, Green, 1895], p. 239). I am grateful to Regina Markell Morantz for calling my attention to this. See also Nancy Sahli, "Elizabeth Blackwell, M.D., 1821–1910: A Biography" (Ph.D. diss., University of Pennsylvania, 1974), p. 164. The University of Vermont may have had a chair earlier than Women's (see "Synopsis of Education in American Medical Schools, 1865," *Trans. AMA* 16 [1865]: 605).

5. Christopher C. Cox, "Report of the Committee on Medical Education," *Trans. AMA* 14 (1863): 90–91. See also D. Meredith Reese, "Report of the Standing Committee on Medical Education," ibid. 13 (1860): 741–42.

6. Cox, "Report of the Committee on Medical Education," p. 91.

7. Wilfred B. Shaw, ed., *The University of Michigan: An Encyclopedic Survey in Nine Parts*, part 5, *The Medical School, the University Hospital, the Law School, 1850–1940* (Ann Arbor: University of Michigan Press, 1951), p. 803. The course was discontinued after the

The effects of hygiene's new status were evident by the end of the war. In 1865 one-third of America's medical colleges offered courses in the field.[8] The AMA recommended that every medical college "embrace" public hygiene in its curriculum, even if it meant adding an extra summer course.[9] In its proposed four-year sequential curriculum of 1871 the AMA included hygiene and medical police as part of the regular studies.[10] By 1876 over half of American medical colleges indicated that they at least "paid attention" to hygiene, while five of them had a special professorship of hygiene and offered a full course in the field. Henry I. Bowditch, in his survey of public hygiene in America, attributed the steadily rising interest in the subject to "the influence of the war upon the private practitioner, by convincing him of the great value of preventive medicine."[11]

Despite this optimistic trend, sanitarians were not satisfied with the place of hygiene in the medical curriculum. In the 1870s the American Public Health Association (APHA) called for reforms in medical education that included a major role for sanitary science.[12] The AMA also continued to urge that sanitation be made a "distinct branch, not merely to appear in the general fabric as some sprig or vine is stamped upon a carpet, but interwoven as part of the web and the woof—a foundation study, a base upon which is to be elaborated a glorious superstructure."[13] During the

---

Civil War, and Michigan did not again offer a course in hygiene until 1884, when Victor Vaughan became professor of hygiene.

8. "Synopsis of Education in American Medical Schools, 1865," p. 605. Of twenty-two colleges surveyed, the seven offering courses were Buffalo Medical College, Berkshire Medical College, Georgetown College Medical Department, Long Island College Hospital, University of Michigan Medical Department, University of Vermont Medical Department, and the University of New York.

9. See, for example, S. D. Gross, "Report of the Committee on Medical Education," *Trans. AMA* 18 (1867): 371–72, 365, 380.

10. "Report of the Committee on Medical Education," *Trans. AMA* 22 (1871): 140–41.

11. Henry I. Bowditch, *Public Hygiene in America: Being the Centennial Discourse Delivered Before the International Medical Congress, Philadelphia, September, 1876* (Boston: Little, Brown, 1877), p. 298n. His survey is discussed and tables presented on pp. 281–98. The colleges with chairs in hygiene were Medical College of Alabama (chair established 1871), Buffalo Medical College, Harvard University (chair, 1871), Miami Medical College, and Medical Department of the University of Pennsylvania. Bowditch did not include Woman's Medical College of Pennsylvania in his survey. See also Harvard University, *The Harvard Medical School 1782–1906* (Boston, 1906), pp. 109–11. It should be noted that hygiene often was taught at the premedical level; for example, at the University of Minnesota beginning in 1873 (Philip D. Jordan, *The People's Health: A History of Public Health in Minnesota to 1948* [St. Paul: Minnesota Historical Society, 1953], p. 61).

12. See, for example, Stephen Smith, "On the Limitations and Modifying Conditions of Human Longevity: The Basis of Sanitary Work," *Public Health: Reports and Papers APHA* 1 (1873): 1–17, and Andrew D. White, "Sanitary Science in Its Relations to Public Instruction," ibid., pp. 139–46.

13. E. M. Hunt, "The Deeds and the Needs of Sanitation," *Trans. AMA* 28 (1877): 405.

1880s, additional chairs of hygiene appeared in medical schools throughout the country.[14] At the end of the decade John H. Rauch's report on medical education showed that of 118 medical schools, 117 taught hygiene in some form.[15] Not only were courses offered almost everywhere, but some of them were utilizing bacteriological laboratories in addition to the usual didactic lectures.

The popularity of public health in the medical school curriculum of the 1880s was an indication of the extent to which the field reflected established medical priorities: it was practical and scientific. The Civil War had demonstrated the practical importance of public hygiene, and the lesson was easily applied to urban areas after the war. In addition, laboratory advances in Europe established its scientific value. Almost every medical school in America considered bacteriology a "subject worthy of most careful consideration," and a majority of them were teaching the subject by 1888.[16] The acceptance of the germ theory in this period was an important factor in the increased status of its complement, public hygiene.[17] One optimistic writer in *The Journal of the American Medical Association*, convinced that the importance of preventive medicine was established, proclaimed "the day is at hand when the sanitary counsellor shall be a potentate in the community."[18]

There was reason to believe in the last decade of the nineteenth century that the progressive trend in medical education toward prevention would continue. Increasing numbers of jobs were becoming available for physicians on local and state boards of health, and this put pressure on the medical colleges to train people for the positions.[19] Instruction, however,

14. See, for example, *J. AMA* 1 (1883): 32; James Cassedy, *Charles V. Chapin and the Public Health Movement* (Cambridge: Harvard University Press, 1962), p. 37; *J. AMA* 2 (1884): 488–89; *J. AMA* 13 (1889): 782; Carleton B. Chapman, *Dartmouth Medical School: The First 175 Years* (Hanover, N.H.: University Press of New England, 1973), p. 71; Waite, *Western Reserve*, p. 184; John Eaton, "Sanitation and Education," *Public Health: Papers and Reports of the APHA* 6 (1880): 259–60.

15. John H. Rauch, *Report on Medical Education, Medical Colleges and the Regulation of the Practice of Medicine in the U.S. and Canada, 1765–1890* (Springfield, Illinois: H. W. Rokker for the Illinois State Board of Health, 1890), p. iv. See also "The Illinois Report on Medical Education," *J. AMA* 12 (1889): 308.

16. H. W. Conn, "Bacteriology in Our Medical Schools," *Science* 11 (1888): 125.

17. A strong advocate of public hygiene measures after the Civil War was C. N. Hewitt, secretary of the Minnesota State Board of Health, who tried to add hygiene to the University of Minnesota medical courses. He taught university undergraduates personal and public hygiene but was not successful in his attempt to make preventive medicine the core of the medical student's training. See Jordan, *The People's Health*, pp. 63–64.

18. Albert L. Gihon, "The Hospital: An Element and Exponent of Medical Education," *J. AMA* 18 (1892): 380.

19. "The Necessity for Trained and Educated Health Officials," *J. AMA* 20 (1893): 189; "A New Field for the College," ibid. 23 (1894): 730.

continued to vary from school to school. "In one college the student would be offered a thorough course of instruction in hygiene; in another no instruction whatever."[20] Frequently the subject was available only as an elective. Sometimes medical schools offered it early in the students' training, before they understood its importance. Occasionally they gave it only in combination with another course, devoting only a few lectures to hygiene.[21] With such haphazard instructional patterns, individual physicians often lacked familiarity with the field upon graduation. Those who felt hygiene was important in the daily practice of medicine concluded that "hygiene does not yet hold the place it merits in medical studies."[22]

An examination of the hygiene course at the University of Michigan Medical Department illustrates the content and methodology of one of the most comprehensive courses offered at the end of the nineteenth century. Victor C. Vaughan developed the Michigan course in 1884, adding a hygienic laboratory to it in 1889 and refining his instruction throughout the 1890s. Vaughan believed hygiene was "boundless" and as important as curative medicine to the practicing physician.[23] The lecture schedule of approximately eighty hours, divided into twelve parts, reflected his broad conception of the field. First came personal hygiene, including foods, clothing, baths and exercise. These subjects were extremely important to Vaughan, and he devoted thirty-eight lectures to them. Next he covered hygiene of the home, including heating, ventilation and disposal of excreta and garbage (four lectures); school hygiene, with emphasis on diseases attributable to dust, poisons and certain hazardous occupations (six lectures); municipal hygiene, including water supplies, sewage and garbage disposal, tenement houses, hospitals, laboratories and boards of health (nine lectures); rural hygiene (two lectures); state hygiene, including state boards of health, laboratories and quarantines (four lectures); national hygiene, addressing the questions of national health services and the inspection of immigrants (two lectures); hygiene of transportation (one lecture); the influence of climate on health,

20. "The Present Status of Medical Education in the United States," *J. AMA* 23 (1894): 203.

21. C. O. Probst, "Instruction in Hygiene in Schools and Colleges," *Public Health: Reports and Papers APHA* 20 (1895): 255. At Harvard, hygiene was offered only as an elective (John H. Rauch, *Report on Medical Education, Medical Colleges and the Regulation of the Practice of Medicine in the U.S. and Canada 1765–1893* [Springfield, Illinois: H. W. Rokker for the Illinois State Board of Health, 1893], p. 51).

22. J. I. Desroches, "Hygiene in Medical Education," *Public Health: Reports and Papers APHA* 20 (1894): 298.

23. Victor C. Vaughan, "Methods of Teaching Hygiene," *Phila. Med. J.* 6 (1900): 403. See also Shaw, *Michigan*, pp. 822–26, and Victor C. Vaughan, "Syllabus of Lectures on Hygiene," *J. AMA* 25 (1895): 22.

covering the geographical distribution of certain infectious diseases (four lectures); and the public health duties of the physician (three lectures). The course ended with a lecture on military hygiene, perhaps reflecting the influence of the Civil War on public health education. In addition to attending these lectures, Vaughan's students worked in the hygiene laboratory doing food and water analyses.[24]

Although he offered an extremely comprehensive course, Vaughan did not attempt to make sanitarians out of his medical students. He felt that individual physicians needed to be aware of all the above topics to practice successfully, and he was not alone in this opinion. With the expansion of many medical schools to four-year terms, time became available for nontraditional courses like hygiene, and the status of preventive medicine advanced accordingly. Medical schools, including the Woman's Medical College of Pennsylvania, the College of Physicians and Surgeons in New York, the Johns Hopkins University, and the universities of Illinois and North Carolina, joined Michigan in adding to or improving their courses in public health and preventive medicine.[25] Medical societies in Ohio, Illinois, and North Carolina, convinced of the subject's importance, requested medical colleges in their respective states to offer courses in hygiene. They also asked that state boards of health require health officers to enroll in such courses.[26] Such surprising progress moved one physician to predict "that the day is not far distant when . . . a chair [in preventive medicine] will become the most important in medical colleges."[27]

In spite of the optimistic trend of the late nineteenth century, public health and preventive medicine did not thrive in the medical schools of the early twentieth century. Many educators acknowledged its importance, and curriculum proposals continued to include hygiene among the increasing number of courses offered. But the actual practice within medical schools belied the rhetoric. Dr. A. C. Abbott, who taught hygiene and bacteriology at both the University of Pennsylvania and the Johns

24. The lectures and topics are listed in Vaughan, "Syllabus," pp. 22–24, and Vaughan, "Methods," p. 403.

25. See, for example, J. M. G. Carter, "Teaching in Medical Colleges," *J. AMA* 23 (1894): 922; "Woman's Medical College of Pennsylvania," ibid. 27 (1896): 639; Alan M. Chesney, *The Johns Hopkins Hospital and the Johns Hopkins University School of Medicine: A Chronicle*, 4 vols. (Baltimore: Johns Hopkins Press, 1943–1974), 2:133, 139; John Shrady, ed., *The College of Physicians and Surgeons, New York, and Its Founders, Officers, Instructors, Benefactors and Alumni: A History* (New York: Lewis, n.d.), p. 297.

26. "Hygiene in Medical Education," *J. AMA* 23 (1893): 88; "State School of Health," ibid. 32 (1899): 1067.

27. L. Webster Fox, "An Introductory Address to the Students of the Medico-Chirurgical College [Philadelphia]," *J. AMA* 23 (1894): 722. See also C. A. Lindsley, "Sanitary Administration," *J. AMA* 21 (1893): 593; "Hygienic Measures in Relation to Infectious Disease," ibid. 20 (1893): 514; and Chesney, *Hopkins*, 2:334.

Hopkins University, noted with dismay in 1901 that only three medical schools required laboratory work with their hygiene courses. Thirteen schools required the subject without laboratory work, and fifteen offered courses but required no examination in the field. He sadly concluded that "in this country there is little or no consensus of opinion upon the importance of this subject to medical education."[28] The lack of consistency in American schools was particularly dismaying when compared with Great Britain and Germany, where the subject was required.

Abbott feared that the neglect of hygiene in America was an indication of the lack of demand for trained people in the field. William T. Sedgwick of Boston similarly observed that "hygiene is allowed only a modicum of time in our medical schools."[29] Sedgwick agreed that as long as jobs in the field of public health were unattractive, the subject would remain unpopular in medical schools. He thought the major problem was that sanitation had become too large a part of hygiene. It was "absurd," he asserted, to expect medical students to become experts in matters of sanitary engineering.[30] If a separation could be made between hygiene (the jurisdiction of physicians) and sanitation (the jurisdiction of engineers), then the former would reasonably fit into the medical curriculum. The focus would be on the individual and his or her diseases instead of on the technology of sanitation, which would be offered in technical schools.[31]

The Committee on the Teaching of Hygiene of the APHA, also sensitive to the perilous position of public health in the medical schools at the beginning of the twentieth century, hoped to solve the problem by dividing its study into three parts. The committee suggested, first, that practical training in the field be compulsory for all medical students: its object would be to enable doctors to cooperate intelligently with health boards and to carry out the hygienic work in their own practices. Second, a more

---

28. A. C. Abbott, "University Teaching in Hygiene," *Public Health: Papers and Reports APHA* 27 (1901): 94. Many others noted the general absence of the subject in most schools. See, for example, Milton G. Linthicum, "The Advancement of Medical Education," *Proc. AAMC* 20 (1910): 18; William H. Welch, "The Medical Curriculum," ibid., p. 64.

29. William T. Sedgwick, "The Readjustment of Education and Research in Hygiene and Sanitation," *Public Health: Reports and Papers* 31 (1905): 117.

30. Ibid., pp. 117–18. J. R. Jones agreed with Sedgwick's conclusions for different reasons. He thought sanitary science courses attempted to teach "everything," cramming the student with "conglomerate stuff" that in such diffuse proportions was "useless" (J. R. Jones, "Medical Education," *J. AMA* 37 [1901]: 743).

31. There were others who, along with Sedgwick, hoped to improve the medical curriculum by changing the content or methodology of the hygiene courses. For example, efforts were made to add dietetics to hygiene courses. See R. O. Beard, "The Teaching of Practical Dietetics in Medical Schools," *J. AMA* 38 (1902): 299–300.

advanced optional course should be available to medical students who wished further instruction. Third, a postgraduate course in public health should be specifically developed for those who wanted to be specialists in hygiene.[32] This committee, and others that were to follow it within the APHA, together with the AMA and the Association of American Medical Colleges (AAMC), supported advanced training for specialists in public health in addition to basic training in hygiene for all medical students.

Reforms sought in the teaching of hygiene during the first decade of the twentieth century were part of a larger movement to improve the entire medical curriculum. The AMA's Council on Medical Education studied existing curricula in 1905 and was "struck with the great variations not only in the arrangement of the [medical] course, but in the methods of instruction, as well as in the hours which are allotted to each."[33] In some schools anatomy received 20 lectures, in others 160. The Association of American Medical Colleges noted similar disparities.[34] To remedy the inequalities, both the AMA Council and the AAMC recommended standard curricula for four-year medical schools. In the AMA's 1909 recommendations, hygiene and public health received approximately sixty hours.[35] The AAMC allotted less time to hygiene but noted that the bacteriology laboratory also had a "trend toward hygiene."[36]

32. "Report of Committee on Teaching of Hygiene and Granting of Diploma of Doctor of Public Health," *Public Health: Papers and Reports APHA* 27 (1901): 87. See also Leander P. Jones, "A Scheme for Preventive Medicine," ibid. 26 (1900): 133, who suggested establishment of an institute in which health officers could be educated, which he hoped could be funded through private charity. In 1905 the APHA committee reiterated its opinion that hygiene teaching need not be comprehensive in the medical schools, which should not "turn out specialists" (Benjamin Lee, "Report of the Committee on the Teaching of Hygiene and the Conferring of a Degree in Public Health," *Public Health: Reports and Papers APHA* 29 [1903]: 127). See also Wyatt Johnston, "On the Practical Clinical Teaching of State Medicine," *Phila. Med. J.* 6 (1900): 407–9, who advocated a one-year postgraduate course in practical sanitary and laboratory work leading to a diploma in public health.

33. "Council on Medical Education of the AMA," *J. AMA* 44 (1905): 1472. For earlier critiques, see "Report of the Committee on Syllabus," *Proc. AAMC* 6 (1896): 7–9; "AAMC Report of the Committee on Syllabus," *J. AMA* 26 (1896): 771; Henry M. Lyman, "Medical Education," *J. AMA* 21 (1893): 959; George M. Kober, "A Plea for a Standard Medical Curriculum," *J. AMA* 43 (1904): 457–60.

34. George M. Kober, "A Plea for a Standard Medical Curriculum," *Proc. AAMC* 14 (1904): 7–9, 41–45.

35. "Council on Medical Education of the American Medical Association: Report on Medical Curriculum," *J. AMA* 52 (1909): 1521–22. See also "Report of the Committee on Syllabus," *Proc. AAMC* 6 (1896): 7–9, rpt. in *J. AMA* 26 (1896): 771. An earlier curriculum proposal is Henry M. Lyman, "Medical Education," *J. AMA* 21 (1893): 959. See also "AAMC," *J. AMA* 22 (1894): 484; "Report of the Committee on Curriculum," *J. AMA* 54 (1910): 1227–28.

36. *Proc. AAMC* 10 (1900): 95. If dietetics were included, the AAMC recommendations for hygiene would be closer to those of the AMA.

One of the biggest obstacles to the inclusion of public health in the medical school curriculum was cost.[37] Many educators admitted the value of the subject for the general practitioner. Yet budgets and facilities limited their options. If extra money became available, complained one public health official, it was more likely to be spent on preparing the student to cope with an individual patient than for the "betterment of the public at large."[38] By the end of the first decade of the twentieth century, the alleged crowding of the medical curriculum was further complicating the situation.[39] The commitment to teaching all physicians the principles of sanitary science remained, but it received low priority in a medical school curriculum that was increasingly emphasizing the laboratory sciences.[40]

Actual hourly allotments for public health closely reflected the AMA and AAMC recommendations for the distribution of curriculum time. Statistics from fifty medical schools in 1910 indicated that an average of fifty-eight hours were devoted to hygiene.[41] Georgetown University School of Medicine offered ninety hours: sixty in hygiene and dietetics with George M. Kober and thirty in state medicine (including jurisprudence) with William C. Woodward.[42] A comparison of Vaughan's University of Michigan course in the 1890s with Kober's and Woodward's in 1910 indicates that hygiene for medical students did not change greatly in these years—the very years when the medical curriculum was moving in a laboratory direction. Hygiene continued to be seen as a practical science, covering by 1910 such topics as river pollution, meat preservation, care of the skin, exercise and house sanitation. Sedgwick's advice to separate hygiene from sanitation had not been heeded.

Perhaps because of its broad and sometimes nebulous scope, and despite AAMC and AMA recommendations to include it in the curriculum, hygiene occupied only a small place in the otherwise expanding medical

37. "Teaching Preventive Medicine in Universities and Normal Schools," *J. AMA* 57 (1911): 311–12.
38. Herbert D. Pease, "Sanitary Conferences," *Public Health: Reports and Papers APHA* 31 (1905): 146.
39. See, for example, *J. AMA* editorial "The Crowded Medical Curriculum," 53 (1909): 560–61.
40. Walter Wyman, "Relation of the Physician in Private Practice to the Public Health," *J. AMA* 52 (1909): 1899–1904.
41. Horace D. Arnold, "Report of the Subcommittee for the Clinical Years," *Proc. AAMC* 20 (1910): 134–35. The AMA had recommended 120 hours for hygiene and public health combined with medical jurisprudence and ethics. The actual breakdown between these subjects in the various medical schools is unclear, making comparisons between the recommendations and actual practice difficult. The situation is further complicated by dietetics, which was sometimes included as personal hygiene and alternately counted as part of the medicine course. See ibid., p. 142.
42. George M. Kober, "Hygiene and Dietetics," *Proc. AAMC* 20 (1910): 145–52.

school timetable after 1910. Abraham Flexner did not emphasize public health in his prescription for curriculum changes, and medical colleges attempting to meet his standards did not rush to include or expand courses in preventive medicine. Educators in the various schools frequently bemoaned that it was not allotted enough time, or that it was still ignored in many places. M. J. Rosenau of Harvard noted in 1917 that only six medical schools treated public health as a major subject: Harvard, Pennsylvania, Yale, Michigan, Columbia and Chicago.[43] He pushed for a deeper commitment to preventive medicine, at the same time recognizing that "the purpose of teaching public health in medical schools is not to make health officers of medical students, but to broaden their training so as to fit them better for the practice of medicine."[44]

Many physicians, fully aware of what Abbott called the increasing "complexities of our medical curriculum," refused to alter their belief in the importance of public health for the general practitioner. Doctors performed many sanitary duties in their daily practices and could not meet their obligations without a knowledge of preventive medicine. In addition to its practical objectives, sanitarians felt hygiene would broaden the point of view of medical students and influence their thinking on all medical matters. They wanted each medical school to hire a full-time person to teach hygiene and to allot one hundred hours for this basic training.[45] Both Rosenau and Vaughan hoped that preventive medicine would also be taught in conjunction with other courses in the medical school. In this way hygiene would attain its rightfully important place in the curriculum.[46]

Aware of the sentiments to limit the teaching of hygiene in the regular curriculum, sanitarians also worked to introduce postgraduate courses to train specialists for careers in public health. The University of Pennsylvania offered the first such course in 1909. Harvard followed in 1910, the University of Michigan and the University of Wisconsin in 1911, Detroit College of Medicine and Surgery in 1913, the University of Minnesota in 1914, the University of California in 1915, and Bellevue Hospital in 1916.

43. M. J. Rosenau, "Public Health Instruction in Medical Schools," *J. AMA* 68 (1917): 1613.

44. Ibid. See Abraham Flexner, *Medical Education in the United States and Canada* (New York: Carnegie Foundation for the Advancement of Teaching, 1910), pp. 67–68.

45. A. W. Abbott and E. O. Jordan, commenting on Rosenau's paper, *J. AMA* 68 (1917): 872.

46. Other than the medicine department, one natural overlap of departments was pediatrics. Preventive hygiene was seen as extremely important for infant health. See Henry Koplik, "The Education of the Physician and Post Graduate Study in the Hygiene and Diseases of the Nursing Infant," *J. AMA* 58 (1912): 75–78.

The Johns Hopkins opened its School of Hygiene and Public Health in 1918.[47] Most of the professional courses required a medical degree for admission, although this policy was later modified. Public health increasingly assumed the role of a separate profession for which specialized training was necessary. Ordinary medical training could not qualify a person to be a municipal health officer. With increased and better training available, many sanitarians hoped that jobs in the field of public health could escape traditional urban political influences and begin to reflect the health officer's improved professional training. The result would be better health for America's cities.[48]

Shortly after the turn of the century another war intervened to aid the cause of public health. Convinced of the importance of preventive measures, military surgeons returning from the war helped to raise the status and the public image of hygiene in the 1920s.[49] Consequently the medical profession grew increasingly tolerant of public health studies in the postwar period.[50] In 1920 the president of the AAMC noted that "several graduates deplore the lack of training in most medical schools in personal and occupational hygiene, in public health in the broader sense, and in preventive medicine."[51] Medical journals in the 1920s contained more articles on the importance of public health to physicians than in any previous decade. They advised physicians not only to practice preventive medicine but to teach their patients hygienic practices and to contribute

47. George E. Vincent, "Public Health Training in Universities," *J. AMA* 68 (1917): 1013; "Graduate Courses in Public Health," *J. AMA* 73 (1919): 516. The dates vary slightly according to source. See also Eugene C. Howe, "Professional Instruction in Public Health in the United States and Canada," *Am. J. of Public Health* 8 (1918): 600–607; "Preventive Medicine at the University of California," *J. AMA* 64 (1915): 169; "Another School of Public Health," *J. AMA* 63 (1914): 682; *J. AMA* 57 (1911): 335, 653.

48. This argument is found often; see M. J. Rosenau, "Courses and Degrees in Public Health Work," *J. AMA* 64 (1915): 794–96; F. F. Wesbrook, "Instruction in Hygiene in Medical Colleges and the Training of Health Officers," *J. AMA* 60 (1913): 427–28; James Ewing, "Principles and Experiments in Medical Education," *J. AMA* 66 (1916): 635–39; W. S. Rankin, "The New Public Health," *J. AMA* 69 (1917): 1391–94.

49. C. St. Clair Drake, "The Influence of the War on Preventive Medicine and Public Health," *J. AMA* 73 (1919): 803–5; "The Universities and the Public Health," *J. AMA* 72 (1919): 1229. Samuel Haythorn maintained that "the greatest single factor in precipitating the present day activities in preventive medicine was probably that of the war" ("The Problem of Preventive Medicine in Practice and in Medical Education," *J. AMA* 80 [1923]: 886). See also J. R. Darnell, "Contributions of the World War to the Advancement of Medicine," *J. AMA* 115 (1940): 1448–49.

50. The other important factor stimulating interest in hygiene, according to one observer, was "organized womanhood" (Walter M. Dickie, "The Place of Medicine in Public Health," *J. AMA* 81 [1923]: 1247–50). This view needs further examination.

51. George Blumer, "The General Practitioner's View of the Defects of Medical Education," *Proc. AAMC* 30 (1920): 12.

to general knowledge in the public schools.[52] According to William T. Sedgwick, a medical school that graduated students untrained in public health and preventive medicine was "sending out its graduates unprepared for some of the most serious problems they will have to face in the immediate future."[53] "The physician of tomorrow," wrote another health officer, "must live and work as much for his community as he does for his individual patient."[54]

The Committee on Public Health and Preventive Medicine of the AAMC recommended in 1920 that curriculum time for preventive medicine be doubled—not to make expert epidemiologists out of the medical students but to provide "what the ordinary practitioner needs."[55] With additional hours allotted to public health, it would be possible to continue with didactic lectures and laboratory exercises while adding "demonstrative excursions to places of sanitary interest," and, on the Harvard model, a required sanitary survey of a town, village, or city.[56] The AAMC model curriculum of 1909 had included only 54 hours for preventive medicine and hygiene, but the 1921 recommendation was 170

52. Frederick Peterson, "The Future of the Physician," *J. AMA* 75 (1920): 359; W. C. Braisted, "The Obligations of Medicine in Regard to General Education," *J. AMA* 74 (1920): 1203–15; "Introduction of Public Health Information into the Undergraduate Curriculum," *J. AMA* 78 (1922): 814–16; John M. Dodson, "The Growing Importance of Preventive Medicine to the General Practitioner," *J. AMA* 81 (1923): 1427–29. See also Dodson's "Preventive Medicine and the General Practitioner," *J. AMA* 80 (1923): 1–6, in which he claims that "preventive medicine is the 'best goods' which the physician has to sell" (p. 3).

53. Quoted in Ira V. Hiscock, "Public Health Courses in Medical Schools," *J. AMA* 81 (1923): 1899, from an address given at the Medical College of the University of Cincinnati, November 1920. See also John Kolmer, "A Five or Six Year Course in Medicine," *J. AMA* 75 (1920): 360–61; George E. Vincent, "Ideals and Their Function in Medical Education," *J. AMA* 74 (1920): 1067; Frederick R. Green, "The Social Responsibilities of Modern Medicine," *J. AMA* 76 (1921): 1477–83.

54. Walter M. Dickie, "The Place of Medicine in Public Health," *J. AMA* 81 (1923): 1249. Also there loomed the specter of public health being lost to physicians if they ignored the subject. See "Report of Special Committee on Teaching Hygiene," *Proc. AAMC* 31 (1921): 86.

55. Victor C. Vaughan, "Report of Committee on Public Health and Preventive Medicine," *Proc. AAMC* 30 (1920): 119. The committee members were Vaughan, M. J. Rosenau, and C.-E. A. Winslow.

56. "Report of Special Committee on Teaching Hygiene," *Proc. AAMC* 31 (1921): 84. In addition to lecture and laboratory time, Harvard required students to make a sanitary survey of a city or town in the vicinity of the medical school and submit a written report interpreting their findings (Rosenau, "Public Health Instruction in Medical Schools," p. 1616). See also M. J. Rosenau, "The Value of a Sanitary Survey in the Teaching of Hygiene," *J. AMA* 64 (1915): 321. University of Buffalo students were required to do field work with the Buffalo Department of Health (Francis E. Fronczak, "Present-Day Public Health Activities," *J. AMA* 63 [1914]: 1716). University of Cincinnati also worked out a cooperative course in public health with the city health department (*J. AMA* 57 [1911]: 653).

hours, or 3 to 4 percent of total curriculum time.[57] A study of public health courses given to medical undergraduates in fifty-seven medical schools in 1922/23 indicated that most institutions fell far short of the AAMC standards. Twenty offered courses of less than 54 hours, eighteen provided 54 to 80 hours, and only nineteen of those surveyed gave public health courses of over 80 hours.[58] Field work including sanitary surveys was available in six: Arkansas, Buffalo, California, Creighton, Harvard and Syracuse.

It was clear that a "new ideal and vision" was needed to overcome the resistance to increasing and improving the teaching of public health and preventive medicine in the medical schools of this country.[59] Many physicians professed a commitment to such instruction, and curriculum experts agreed on its importance; yet the actual experience of the medical student was severely limited. Health officers and students found available courses dull and impractical.[60] In the 1920s, encouraged by support of both the profession and the public, various schools searched for new ways to approach the teaching of public health and preventive medicine.

Haven Emerson of Columbia's College of Physicians and Surgeons urged that the teaching of preventive medicine concentrate on developing an "attitude of mind" and "altered emphasis" rather than on the transmission of a body of facts. With this focus, every department in the medical school could teach prevention along with cure. Except for a brief introduction in medical school, public health training would take place at the postgraduate level.[61]

Emerson voiced the opinion of many when he observed that the medical curriculum was already overcrowded and could ill afford more time for preventive medicine. Educators agreed that a logical solution would be to integrate the teaching of prevention with curative medicine. Samuel Haythorn at the University of Pittsburgh School of Medicine developed a

57. Hugh Cabot, "Report of Committee on Curriculum of the AAMC," *Proc. AAMC* 32 (1922): 73–91. See particularly pp. 77–78. This report is also available in *J. AMA* 78 (1922): 738–40.

58. Ira V. Hiscock, "Public Health Courses in Medical Schools," *J. AMA* 81 (1923): 1897–99. Following a tradition noted earlier (see n. 4), the Woman's Medical College of Pennsylvania was the only medical school to offer instruction in hygiene and disease prevention during every year of a four-year course.

59. T. A. Storey, "Teaching of Hygiene in Normal Schools, Colleges and Universities," *Proc. AAMC* 33 (1923): 141–44 (Dr. W. S. Leathers's phrase, p. 143).

60. "What Definite Plan Should Be Put into Effect to Insure to Medical Students Knowledge of Public Health Work and an Opportunity to Gain Practical Field Experience?," *U.S. Public Health Bull.* 139 (1923): 143–55.

61. Haven Emerson, "Education in Preventive Medicine in the Regular Curriculum," *Proc. AAMC* 35 (1925): 36–49. See also Charles P. Emerson's "Environmental Medicine: Medical Sociology," ibid., pp. 11–23; and *J. AMA* 84 (1925): 1296–97.

practical means of implementing such a plan: a "key course" in preventive medicine. Fifty to seventy-five hours were devoted to preventive medicine during the third year of medical study. The purpose of this key course was to present the broad idea of preventive medicine, its aims and general possibilities. This core then served as the basis for all other teaching of prevention in the clinical years. Haythorn thought that bedside instruction made prevention more palatable to students and also aided them more in their future medical practices. When students saw a case of typhoid, they studied not only how to cure it but how the infection spread and how it could be prevented.[62]

Haythorn was not the first public health instructor to integrate clinical and preventive teaching, although the Pittsburgh plan was one of the best coordinated and thoroughly executed. Stanford University included public health concerns with ward teaching.[63] W. S. Leathers at Vanderbilt University, who also thought didactic courses were insufficient, brought students in his course into "intimate contact with the practical problems of public health."[64] In addition to their lectures and laboratory work, Vanderbilt students received practical training with health agencies, infectious disease clinics, and sanitary surveys in the community; and the clinical departments further exposed them to preventive medicine. Leathers imbued his students "with the ideal that the physician's responsibility is just as binding in the protection of the individual and community against the spread of disease as the diagnosis and scientific application of measures for the relief of the patient."[65] Charles P. Emerson, at the Indiana School of Medicine, made significant efforts to teach students the relationships between medical and social conditions, providing clinics in which medical students and social workers could interact.[66]

The medical student of the 1920s probably benefitted from the practical emphasis. This approach did not, however, increase curricular hours de-

62. Samuel R. Haythorn, "Cooperative Plan of Teaching Preventive Medicine," *Proc. AAMC* 35 (1925): 50–58; discussion, pp. 58–68. See also Haythorn's "The Pittsburgh Plan," *Bull. AAMC* 1 (1926): 5–11; "Teaching Preventive Medicine," *J. AMA* 87 (1926): 1509; Haythorn, "Cooperative Plan," is also in *J. AMA* 84 (1925): 1–2.

63. Ernest C. Dickson, "Teaching of Public Health and Preventive Medicine," *Bull. AAMC* 1 (1926): 1–2.

64. W. S. Leathers, "The Place of Preventive Medicine in the Medical School," *J. AMA* 88 (1927): 974. His article is reprinted, in part, in *Bull. AAMC* 2 (1927): 278–80.

65. W. S. Leathers, "The Place of Preventive Medicine" (*J. AMA*), p. 976. See also Joseph W. Mountin, "A Plan for Training County Health Officers," *J. AMA* 91 (1928): 717–20, for more on practical training available in Nashville.

66. Ida M. Cannon, *Social Work in Hospitals: A Contribution to Progressive Medicine* (New York: Russell Sage Foundation, 1913), pp. 208–11. I am grateful to Patricia Spain Ward for this reference.

voted to prevention; in fact, it may have decreased them.[67] Burying prevention in the clinical teaching experience reflected a popular belief that preventive medicine was "not so much a subject as it is a state of mind."[68] To many it was merely "common sense,"[69] and as such unworthy of curriculum time. Despite the positive efforts of some of medicine's most prestigious and active men, sanitarians accused the medical schools of being "extremely deficient" in the teaching of hygiene. "Instead of decreasing the number of hours given to preventive medicine . . . they should be increased and the importance of prevention should be magnified rather than subordinated to treatment and cure."[70]

It is ironic that in spite of the positive influence of the First World War on the status of preventive medicine, its actual place in the curriculum diminished during the following decade. Clinical training absorbed its practical side; bacteriology swallowed its scientific side. Preventive medicine and public health, as subjects in their own right, received little attention. The AAMC continued to recommend that 3 to 4 percent of curriculum time be devoted to hygiene and sanitation, but few schools complied.[71]

An alternate interpretation of the postwar experience is that it reflected a recognition of the importance of preventive medicine. Denied its rightful place for many years, public health at last permeated the daily activities of the student just as it would later permeate the daily activities of the practitioner. The use of clinical case studies at the Yale University School of Medicine reflected this optimism about the importance of public health. There students worked from a specific disease in a specific person back to its underlying causes in the community. They also were encouraged to seek out community resources for prevention and cure. It was hoped that in this way students would "approach patients in their private practice more constructively and humanely and that they will participate far more effectively and sympathetically in the public health programs of the community."[72] In

67. In an AAMC curriculum proposal of 1927, hygiene, sanitation and public health were allotted 128 hours, still far above actual practice in most medical schools (Fred C. Zapffe, "A Proposed New Curriculum," *Bull. AAMC* 2 [1927]: 324–26). See also "Inadequate Instruction in Public Health," *J. AMA* 89 (1927): 1655; and "Johns Hopkins University School of Medicine," *Bull. AAMC* 2 (1927): 341.

68. John M. Dodson, "Periodic Health Examinations," *Bull. AAMC* 2 (1927): 126.

69. Wendell C. Phillips, "The Physicians and the Patient of the Future," *J. AMA* 86 (1926): 1259–64.

70. "Hygiene in Medical Schools," *Am. J. Public Health* 19 (1929): 302. See also W. F. Draper, "The Unexplored Field of Preventive Medicine in Private Practice," *J. AMA* 89 (1927): 491–93.

71. "The Association of American Medical Colleges," *J. AMA* 97 (1931): 645.

72. Ira V. Hiscock, "Clinical Case Studies as Instruments in the Teaching of Public Health," *J. AMA* 96 (1931): 970–72.

a sense, the clinical teaching of preventive medicine freed the field to emphasize its practical and humane side, to teach students about the social implications of disease, to push them out into the community and force their interaction with social service and health agencies. No longer having to justify itself solely in scientific terms, preventive medicine was able to broaden its base and incorporate some of the "boundlessness" that Victor Vaughan had foreseen for it.

The Tufts College Medical School in Boston also attempted to "color the teaching of the practice of medicine with a preventive tinge." There students engaged in the home care of patients, emphasizing the social aspects of disease and the possibilities for prevention in the community.[73] The University of Illinois College of Medicine sent its students to a tuberculosis sanitorium for field clinical experience with one of the more pressing public health problems.[74]

The integration of preventive and clinical cases became fairly common practice during the 1930s. The medical student interacted with social service, public health and community agencies, and learned that the social environment was as important to disease prevention and cure as scientific processes. Family, economic, and medical problems were united, and students were expected to confront all aspects of diseases in their treatment syntheses.[75]

In these and other ways the teaching of public health and preventive medicine became more relevant to students' practice experiences. Many schools offered field work in the community, including visits to farms (to learn details of vaccine and antitoxin preparations) and department of health projects, and inspections of sewage disposal plants.[76] The University of California, for example, sent students on several field trips to a dairy, a slaughterhouse, a sewage purification plant, and required them to observe personally the routine operation of the city health office.[77] Some medical

73. Dwight O'Hara, "The Clinical Teaching of Preventive Medicine," *J. AMA* 99 (1932): 717–20. Tufts developed this program in 1928 for fourth-year students.
74. Benjamin Goldberg and Jessamine S. Whitney, "Medical Teaching in Tuberculosis," *J. AMA* 99 (1932): 707–10. See also James Alexander Miller, "The Undergraduate Teaching of Tuberculosis," *J. AMA* 104 (1935): 1336–39.
75. For more on the case study approach, see Henry E. Meleney, "Environmental Case Studies in the Teaching of Preventive Medicine," *South. Med. J.* 27 (1934): 167–70; Wilson G. Smillie, "The Incorporation of the Principles of Preventive Medicine in Clinical Teaching," *J. AMA* 102 (1934): 1232–34; Ida M. Cannon, "Social Case Teaching of Medical Students," *Bull. AAMC* 8 (1933): 139–46; Lyman Wilbur, "Report of the Council on Medical Education and Hospitals," *J. AMA* 104 (1935): 1064–65; R. H. Riley, "The Public Health Aspect of the Teaching of Obstetrics," *J. AMA* 106 (1936): 1438–40.
76. J. G. FitzGerald, "Undergraduate Instruction in Hygiene and Preventive Medicine," *Bull. AAMC* 11 (1936): 240–46.
77. Edward L. Munson and L. S. Schmitt, "On the Training of Medical Students in

schools also added new subjects like industrial hygiene,[78] vital statistics,[79] mental health and medical economics[80] to existing courses in public health and preventive medicine.

A study of Stanford University School of Medicine alumni in 1936 illustrated the extent to which efforts to upgrade the teaching of preventive medicine and public health contributed to preparing students for the practice of medicine. Fifty-eight percent of the graduates indicated that they "are or have been engaged in some form of organized public health work or in industrial medicine." The range of their activities included serving as health officer or assistant health officer; member of a board of health; and city, county, or school physician.[81]

Despite efforts in the 1930s to improve the teaching of preventive medicine, the length and content of courses throughout the country continued to vary greatly. The AMA's Council of Medical Education observed in 1937 that "preventive medicine, although of undoubted importance, has not yet developed a clear cut and generally accepted objective, so far as the teaching of undergraduate medical students is concerned."[82] J. G. FitzGerald, who conducted a survey of the teaching of preventive medicine in medical schools in the United States, Canada and Europe in 1936/37, agreed that the variation in America was enormous.[83] W. S. Leathers of Vanderbilt similarly lamented the haphazard instructional patterns. "The chief difficulty, as I understand the problem," he

Preventive Medicine," *J. AAMC* 12–13 (1930–1938): 325–30. This field work was in addition to class exercises and clinical and laboratory experiences over a three-year period. See also Leverett D. Bristol, "Preventive and Industrial Medicine and Public Health," *J. AMA* 109 (1937): 245–47.

78. Leverett D. Bristol, "The Teaching of Industrial Hygiene," *J. AMA* 102 (1934): 990–95; T. Lyle Hazlett, "Fundamentals of Industrial Hygiene," *J. AMA* 112 (1939): 1287.

79. Thomas J. LeBlanc, "What the Medical Student Should Be Taught About Vital Statistics," *Am. J. Public Health* 27 (1937): 1273–76.

80. R. R. Spencer, "The Teaching of Hygiene in Medical Schools," *South. Med. J.* 28 (1935): 381–86; Park J. White, "New Things Which Should Be Taught in a Course on Professional Conduct and Medical Economics," *Bull. AAMC* 11 (1936): 366–76.

81. Ernest C. Dickson, "On the Practical Value of Instruction of Undergraduate Medical Students in Public Health and Industrial Medicine," *Bull. AAMC* 11 (1936): 308–9.

82. "Report of the Council on Medical Education and Hospitals," *J. AMA* 108 (1937): 2136. See also Ralph M. F. Picken, "Public Health in the United States of America: The Teaching of Preventive Medicine," *Brit. Med. J.* 31 (1936): 869–70; J. N. Baker, "The Oneness of Objectives of the Association of American Medical Colleges, of the Council on Medical Education and Hospitals of the American Association and of the Federation of State Medical Boards," *J. AAMC* 12 (1937): 25–26; and H. R. Wahl, "Community Aspects of Medicine," *J. AAMC* 13 (1938): 14–18.

83. J. G. FitzGerald, "Undergraduate Instruction in Preventive Medicine," *J. AMA* 110 (1938): 1321–26. See also the discussion of FitzGerald's paper, ibid., p. 1214.

wrote, "is . . . lack of available funds and the barrier afforded too often by the conservatism of medical faculties."[84] Leathers felt reasonably optimistic that the situation would improve with additional money, like that provided by the Social Security Act of 1935, and with expanded public health knowledge. An increased sense of social responsibility by practicing physicians, evident in the 1930s, aided the cause of preventive medicine. As the president of the AMA noted in 1938, "The physician in practice has come to a realization that his obligation to society demands an extension of activity beyond the intimate personal relationship between the individual patient and himself to the broader field of preventive medicine."[85]

At least part of the failure of American medical schools to respond vigorously to the need for preventive medicine might be attributable to the growth of professional schools of public health in the twentieth century. With the burden of educating health officers transferred to the postgraduate years, medical schools could emphasize other subjects. After all, only 836 out of over 50,000 American physicians listed public health as their sole concern in 1934.[86] Deans and curriculum committees felt their responsibility was to the greater number of physicians involved in private practice.

During the 1940s attempts to upgrade the teaching of public health and preventive medicine continued to follow existing patterns. The popularity of the clinical case method increased, especially among health educators who believed that "the principles of prevention are better taught and integrated with the general curriculum of the school."[87] At Yale curriculum

84. W. S. Leathers, "Preventive Medicine: Its Outlook in Medical Education," *J. AMA* 111 (1938): 1520.

85. Irvin Abell, "The Aims of the Medical Profession as They Relate to the Public," *J. AMA* 110 (1938): 2042. Duke University inaugurated its course in public health and preventive medicine in 1939, perhaps reflecting this increase of social awareness. See James F. Gifford, Jr., *The Evolution of a Medical Center* (Durham: Duke University Press, 1972), pp. 121–22. Duke apparently ignored the AAMC guidelines until 1939.

86. The figures are from the *American Medical Directory*, as presented in *J. AMA* 103 (1934): 578. On graduate and postgraduate public health training, see Leroy E. Parkins, "The Relation of Post Graduate Medical Instruction to Public Health," *J. AMA* 103 (1934): 545–47; Thomas Parran, Jr., and Don M. Griswold, "Qualifications and Training of Local Health Officers," *Am. J. Public Health* 24 (1934): 887–91; John A. Ferrell, "Professionalization in Public Health Service," *J. AMA* 100 (1933): 1379–82; Edward S. Godfrey, Jr., "Education and Training of the Physician for a Public Health Career," *Am. J. Public Health* 39 (1940): 1447–51; and E. R. Correy, "Training for Public Health: A Review and a Forecast," *Am. J. Public Health* 30 (1940): 743–48; Mayhew Derryberry and George Caswell, "Qualifications of Professional Public Health Personnel," *U.S. Public Health Reports* 55 (1940): 2377–96.

87. S. P. Lucia, "The Integration of Preventive Medicine in the Education of the Physician," *J. AMA* 114 (1940): 1485. See also Leopold M. Rohr, "Undergraduate Medical Instruction in Public Health at the Long Island College of Medicine," *J. AAMC* 15 (1940): 189–91; Stuart P. Cromer, "The Role of Medical Schools in Public Health Education," *The Mississippi Doctor* 18 (1940): 68–73; Eleanor Cockerill, "The Preparation of the

planners found that "medical students are more interested in sick people than in preventive medicine as an abstract subject." They accordingly organized seminars around patients and then led "the discussion gradually away from the bedside" to the preventive and social aspects of the disease in question.[88] Students responded positively to this clinical approach, and numerous medical schools were soon imitating the Yale plan.

The scope of preventive medicine courses continued to expand in the 1940s,[89] embracing such topics as industrial hygiene,[90] the social and economic aspects of medicine, and the emotional concerns of patients. A more humanistic approach allowed the student "to widen his horizon from a fine, narrow focus on diseased cells or organs or organ systems to a broader view of the impact of disease upon people as individuals—upon their families and upon society; to teach an appreciation of the effects of social, economic, and emotional stresses upon the production or maintenance of symptoms or signs of disease."[91] As one professor of preventive medicine put it, "We must not permit the brilliant accomplishments of the natural sciences to overshadow the fact that social conditions under which human beings live may contribute to the causation of disease."[92]

Medical Student in the Recognition of the Social Component of Disease," *Hospital Progress* 22 (1941): 361–64.

88. John R. Paul, "Preventive Medicine at the Yale University School of Medicine, 1940–1949," *Yale J. Biol. Med.* 22 (1949–1950): 207. See also Paul's earlier article, ibid. 13 (1940): 253–58. For similar activity at the University of Illinois College of Medicine, see Henry G. Poncher and Julius B. Richmond, "The Teaching of Social Medicine on the Clinical Clerkship," *J. AAMC* 24 (1949): 97–99. See also William W. Beckman, "Some Aspects of the Clinical Teaching of the Social and Environmental Factors in Medicine," *J. AAMC* 22 (1947): 149–54. For a thorough discussion of the clinical approach, see Perrin H. Long, "The Philosophy of the Clinical Approach to Teaching in Preventive Medicine," *Proceedings of the Conference of Preventive Medicine and Health Economics* (Ann Arbor: University of Michigan School of Public Health, 1947), pp. 43–51; and W. G. Smillie, "The Integration of Teaching Content and Methods," ibid., pp. 117–25. See also William Harvey Perkins, "The Place of Preventive Medicine in the Curriculum," *J. AAMC* 22 (1947): 160–63.

89. Haven Emerson, "Purpose, Content and Methods of Teaching Public Health to Medical Students," *J. AMA* 116 (1941): 1040–44. For a sample description of students' experiences at the University of Washington School of Medicine, see Lee Powers, "Public Health and Preventive Medicine for Medical Students," *J. AAMC* 24 (1949): 344–50.

90. Donald E. Cummings, "Industrial Hygiene Instruction for Medical Students," *J. AAMC* 16–17 (1941–1942): 24–49, offers a sample lecture schedule; Dwight O'Hara, "Teaching Industrial Hygiene in the Department of Public Health and Preventive Medicine," *J. AAMC* 20 (1945): 314–16.

91. S. R. Warson, Mary M. Lewis, and G. M. Saunders, "A Method for Teaching the Emotional and Social Aspects of Preventive Medicine," *J. AAMC* 23 (1948): 135–36. See also Franz Goldmann, "Instruction in Social and Economic Aspects of Medicine," *J. AAMC* 16–17 (1941–1942): 299–307.

92. Thomas D. Dublin, "The Basis for Teaching Social and Environmental Factors in Medicine in the Undergraduate Medical Curriculum," *J. AAMC* 22 (1947): 144. Dublin

Despite all the attempts to broaden the content of public health courses, it was evident in the 1940s that sanitation frequently formed the bulk of what was actually taught. Efforts to get students out into the field increased; yet the focus remained on environmental factors such as water supply, waste disposal and food controls—the old mainstays of the nineteenth-century hygiene courses. The University of Texas Medical Branch in Galveston, for example, offered a sixty-hour public health course that stressed environmental sanitation.[93]

In general, the teaching in preventive medicine courses failed to excite large numbers of students. In fact, most did not seem to care whether it was in the curriculum or not.[94] Lectures were unpopular, especially those on environmental sanitation. Students seemed to respond favorably to preventive medicine only when it was presented in conjunction with clinical cases. There were, of course, many reasons for the students' negative attitude, as an AAMC committee investigating the teaching of preventive medicine discovered in the early 1940s. The hours allotted to preventive medicine courses were usually the ones no one else wanted and were inconvenient for students and staff. Didactic lectures given during clinical years were not well received because students wanted to see patients. Most importantly, the AAMC investigating committee perceived that "deans and faculties of medical schools, though in general professing to consider it essential to provide sound instruction in preventive medicine and public health, *do not actually regard this subject as important.*"[95]

This basic lack of commitment on the part of medical school administrators and faculty plagued preventive medicine throughout its history. The people who taught the subject and the ones who had experience in public health endeavors in the community were always dedicated to having it included in the medical curriculum. Most others gave lip service to its importance, but assigned higher priorities to other fields. Students generally shared the attitude of the faculty, either as a reflection of what their teachers felt or because instruction in public health was irrelevant or bad. This fundamental negativism was difficult to overcome.[96]

taught at Long Island College of Medicine. Health economics was also stressed as a new content area. See *Proceedings of the Conference on Preventive Medicine and Health Economics*, especially pp. 173–76, 182–84.

93. Frank M. Stead and Carl A. Nau, "A Practical Course in Environmental Sanitation for Medical Students," *J. AAMC* 18–19 (1943–1944): 173–76.

94. Hugh Leavell, "The Teaching of Preventive Medicine," *Proceedings of the Conference on Preventive Medicine and Health Economics*, pp. 23–40.

95. "Preliminary Report of the Committee on the Teaching of Public Health and Preventive Medicine Association of AMC," *J. AAMC* 17 (1942): 82 (emphasis added). See also "Final Report," *J. AAMC* 20 (1945): 152–65.

96. The attitude was prevalent throughout the medical profession. Public health officials

The AAMC committee's recommendations for improving the situation, endorsed by the Conference on Preventive Medicine and Health Economics held at the University of Michigan School of Public Health in 1946, called for more time to be allotted to preventive medicine and separate departments, staffed by full-time people, to coordinate the didactic, field and clinical teaching. The committee also pointed out the importance of distinguishing between public health and preventive medicine, terms often used interchangeably:

> Public health encompasses those activities that are undertaken for the prevention of disease and the promotion of health *that are a community-wide responsibility*. . . . Preventive medicine . . . comprises those activities that are the direct responsibility of the individual in the prevention of disease, and in the promotion of the health of himself and his family.[97]

The semantic division made during the 1940s helped lessen the confusion about what should be taught in medical school courses. Increasingly, preventive medicine became the responsibility of medical schools while postgraduate schools adopted public health.[98] This division belatedly reflected the admonition of William Sedgwick to separate the concerns of engineers from those of physicians.

The 1940s were a time of great interest in the subject of preventive medicine. It is probable that the Second World War, like earlier conflicts, stimulated some of this concern within the medical profession. But what did preventive medicine really gain? Much effort went into defining the field, clarifying department jurisdictions and integrating preventive medicine with clinical teaching. The result was a small, perhaps secure place in the curriculum for a subject that was largely diffused over the clinical years and frequently buried in other medical school concerns.

Throughout the 1950s, 1960s, and into the 1970s public health educators continued to seek "new orientations." The thrust in recent years, while

---

thought it was due to the fee-for-service economic system. A physician's income was dependent on the treatment of disease, not on its prevention. Only in a prepayment system would doctors give prevention their full commitment. See this argument in an editorial, "The Place of Preventive Medicine in the Medical Curriculum," *Am. J. Public Health* 34 (1944): 1286.

97. W. G. Smillie, "Objectives in the Teaching of Preventive Medicine and Public Health," *J. AAMC* 18 (1943): 281. The distinction is made frequently in the 1940s. See, for example, S. P. Lucia, "The Integration of Preventive Medicine in the Education of the Physician," p. 1485.

98. "The Place of Preventive Medicine in the Medical Curriculum," *Am. J. Public Health* 34 (1944): 1285–86. At a conference of professors of preventive medicine in New York this undergraduate-graduate distinction was agreed upon (W. G. Smillie, "Education of Medical Students in Preventive Medicine," *Am. J. Public Health* 36 [1946]: 855–58).

following patterns developed earlier, has been based on a new premise. Medical gains and successes have been so extraordinary that the physician today has a "new type of job. . . . It is no longer enough to describe him as a healer of the sick; he is to an increasing degree the protector of the well."[99] Physicians today actively promote health in their patients. Using periodic health examinations, medical practitioners are in the business of preventive medicine. Earlier the emphasis was on the use of public health measures to improve the health of the population; the second half of the twentieth century is using similar measures for the maintenance of a healthy population. The clinical teaching of preventive medicine, developed earlier, is also central to this modern conception.[100] The difference is that instead of teaching disease, the trend now is to teach health.[101]

One popular way of teaching health has been to assign medical students families to follow throughout their medical school years. The student follows a small group of people to observe the home environment, to assess the complexity of medical needs, and to understand the broad ramifications of health maintenance. At Vanderbilt, which introduced the family focus in 1951, students developed "a growing realization . . . of the various facets of health and normal development and of the effect of forces such as economic and emotional stresses, illness and cultural factors on individuals and families."[102] This kind of teaching allows students to look at the whole person and to appreciate "the practice of medicine as a social responsibility."[103] It aims at producing physicians who hold a broad conception both of medicine and of their own role in health maintenance, who look beyond the

99. John P. Hubbard, "Training the General Practitioner for His Job in Public Health," *Pennsylvania Medical Journal* 54 (1951): 1139.

100. David P. Barr, "The Teaching of Preventive Medicine," *J. Med. Educ.* 28 (1953): 49–56; Leonard A. Scheele, "Opportunities in the Teaching of Preventive Medicine," *J. AAMC* 25 (1950): 241–47; C. B. Stewart, "The Teaching of Clinical Preventive Medicine," *Canad. J. Public Health* 41 (1950): 157–63; Alan M. Chesney, "A Plan for the Instruction of Medical Students in Preventive Medicine and Public Health," *J. Med. Educ.* 27 (1952): 387–93; W. Palmer Dearing, "New Orientation in the Teaching of Preventive Medicine and Public Health," *J. Med. Educ.* 27 (1952): 387–93; W. Palmer Dearing, "New Orientation in the Teaching of Preventive Medicine and Public Health," *J. Med. Educ.* 27 (1952): 287–392; W. Palmer Dearing, "New Orientation in the Teaching of Preventive Medicine," *U.S. Public Health Reports* 68 (1953): 1147–55.

101. John Perry Hubbard, "Integrating Preventive and Social Medicine in the Medical Curriculum," *N. Eng. J. Med.* 351 (1954): 513–19.

102. John B. Youmans and Marian E. Russell, "Teaching Social Aspects of Medicine in the Medical School," *J. Med. Educ.* 29 (1954): 9–16. See also William W. Schottstaedt and Stewart Wolf, "Collaboration of the Medical School and the Health Department in Teaching Medical Students," *Am. J. Public Health* 45 (1955): 1097–1100, and Donald G. Anderson, "Medical Education: A Look Ahead," *J. AMA* 145 (1951): 478–80. In 1949 the University of Pennsylvania assigned families for students to follow through their medical school years.

103. John P. Hubbard and Katharine G. Clark, "Conference on Preventive Medicine in Medical Schools," *J. Med. Educ.* 28 (1953): 48. For greater detail about the conference

test tube and the virus to see a complex matrix of the social and physical aspects of health and sickness.

This conception reflects current practices. Preventive medicine is included in the medical curriculum and is considered a necessary, if small, part of the education of physicians. Its position, however, is probably as tenuous today as it has always been. Based on the rather amorphous notions of the whole man, social responsibility and humanistic medicine, its foundations could crumble in the days of nuclear medicine. Yet history is reassuring on this point. Preventive medicine has hung on, adapting itself to existing situations, through adverse times and in spite of severe curriculum pressures. It may yet lose the stigma of "softness" and become as important to the medical curriculum as the basic sciences and curative medicine.[104]

---

proceedings, see Katherine G. Clark, et al., *Preventive Medicine in Medical Schools: Report of Colorado Springs Conference, November 1952* (Baltimore: Waverly Press, 1953).

104. See Thomas Francis, Jr., "Research in Preventive Medicine," *J. AMA* 172 (1960): 993–99, for a discussion of the broad areas of prevention pertinent to physicians.

Medical Ethics and Jurisprudence

CHESTER R. BURNS

THE formal teaching of medical jurisprudence in Great Britain and the United States occurred in markedly reciprocal patterns after 1790.[1] At the University of Edinburgh, Andrew Duncan, Sr., began lecturing on the subject in 1791. In 1807 the same university established a professorship in medical jurisprudence and Andrew Duncan, Jr., was appointed to that chair.[2] The first American lectures had been given three years earlier by Dr. James S. Stringham, who was a graduate of the medical school at Edinburgh and had probably heard the lectures given by the elder Duncan. Stringham's initial lectures were delivered at Columbia College in New York City, where he had been appointed professor of chemistry. In 1813 the College of Physicians and Surgeons in New York City was reor-

---

1. For background information, see the articles by Erwin H. Ackerknecht in *Ciba Symposia* 11 (1950–1951): 1286–1304. Also see Chester R. Burns, "Thomas Percival: Medical Ethics or Medical Jurisprudence?" in Thomas Percival, *Medical Ethics* (1803; reprint ed., Huntington, New York: Robert E. Krieger, 1975), pp. xiii–xxviii.
2. Henry Harvey Littlejohn, "Department of Forensic Medicine, University of Edinburgh," in *Methods and Problems of Medical Education*, 9th ser. (New York: Rockefeller Foundation, 1928), pp. 186–88. For a list of other chairs established in European universities at the turn of the nineteenth century, see Jaroslav Nemec, *Highlights in Medico-Legal Relations* (Bethesda, Md.: National Library of Medicine, n.d.), p. 25.

ganized, becoming a division of Columbia College. Stringham was appointed professor of medical jurisprudence.

Three years previously, Benjamin Rush, who had also studied at Edinburgh, delivered a lecture on medical jurisprudence at the University of
Pennsylvania School of Medicine. The early part of the formative period
for the teaching of medical jurisprudence in the United States revolves
around Rush and his pupils at Philadelphia and those faculty and students
who sustained Stringham's legacy in New York City. Rush divided the
subject into forensic medicine and public health. The former category
included criminal injuries, poisons, accidental deaths, aberrant sexual
situations, feigned diseases, and the jurisprudence of insanity. The latter
included epidemic diseases, problems of water and food supplies, and
sources of "putrid exhalations." Rush thought that Thomas Percival had
only glanced at the subject of medical jurisprudence in his *Medical
Ethics*.[3] A syllabus of Stringham's lectures indicates that he emphasized
forensic problems associated with parturition, virginity, pregnancy, abortion, impotence and sterility, infanticide, feigned diseases, poisons, and
wounds. But Stringham also dealt with industrial nuisances, sources of
water supply, and medical etiquette, a phrase that was, for nineteenth-
century physicians, often synonymous with medical ethics.[4]

Thus, at the very birth of American concerns about medical jurisprudence, interested physicians sustained the ambiguities of definition that
had bothered their British and Continental predecessors. These ambiguities had allowed the authors of texts on medical jurisprudence to
emphasize, in varying ways, forensic medicine or medical ethics or medical police (public health). After 1800 this problem of determining the
scope of medical jurisprudence affected those Americans who developed
an interest in medical jurisprudence, including certain pupils of Rush:
Charles Caldwell, T. D. Mitchell, Reuben Mussey, and Walter Channing. Caldwell gave some lectures at Philadelphia in 1812 and 1813;
Caldwell and Mitchell intermittently taught the subject at the Transylvania Medical School in Lexington, Kentucky. Between 1814 and 1837,
Mussey was professor of surgery, obstetrics, and medical jurisprudence at
Dartmouth. Channing, a classmate of Mussey's at Pennsylvania, became
the first professor of obstetrics and medical jurisprudence at Harvard in
1815 and held that position for almost forty years.[5]

3. Benjamin Rush, *Sixteen Introductory Lectures Upon the Institutes and Practice of
Medicine, with a Syllabus of the Latter* (Philadelphia: Bradford and Innskeep, 1811), pp.
363–95.
4. The syllabus was reprinted in the *American Medical and Philosophical Register* 4
(1814): 614–15.
5. Others whose interest in medical jurisprudence was associated with Philadelphia or

Three years after his appointment to the College of Physicians and Surgeons, James Stringham died prematurely. He was succeeded by J. W. Francis, a graduate of that school who had become a professor of the institutes of medicine in 1815. With Stringham's death, medical jurisprudence was added to Francis's professorial tasks.

Another early pioneer of medical jurisprudence was Theodric Romeyn Beck, who had been a close friend and medical school classmate of Francis. After graduation in 1811, Beck began medical practice in Albany. Four years later, he was appointed professor of the institutes of medicine and lecturer in medical jurisprudence at the new College of Physicians and Surgeons of the Western District of New York founded at Fairfield. During the following year, Beck gave his first course of lectures. Seven years later, in March of 1823, Francis published a letter to Beck in which he expressed anticipation for the book on medical jurisprudence that Beck was about to publish.[6] In the fall of 1823, Beck's two volumes, *Elements of Medical Jurisprudence*, were issued in Albany. After some ten years of study, Beck had integrated the European legacies and the early American experiences. Seven chapters dealt with legal aspects of sexual and reproductive circumstances, including impotence, rape, pregnancy, legitimacy, and infanticide. Poisons were discussed in five chapters; personal identity and survivorship in two; and one chapter was devoted to each of the following: feigned diseases, mental diseases, diseases disqualifying for civic obligations, persons found dead, and wounds. Beck's two volumes were hailed as classic and they were translated into German, a remarkable honor indeed.

Theodric Beck's brother, John Brodhead Beck, had graduated from the College of Physicians and Surgeons in 1817. His graduation thesis on infanticide became the chapter on that topic in T. R. Beck's first edition. This chapter was revised for the edition of 1835 and J. B. Beck's name was added to the title page of that edition. J. B. Beck also taught medical jurisprudence at the College of Physicians and Surgeons.

T. R. Beck's only American competitor was Stephen W. Williams, who had been a student at the medical school in New York City during its reorganization, and had attended Stringham's lectures. Williams practiced medicine in Deerfield, Massachusetts, for forty years. In 1823, the year of Beck's first edition, the Berkshire Medical Institution of Massachusetts began operating in Pittsfield. Williams taught medical jurisprudence at this school for eight years. In 1835 he published a synopsis,

---

Rush included Thomas Cooper, Joseph Nancréde, and James Webster.

6. J. W. Francis, "Facts and Inferences Chiefly Relating to Medical Jurisprudence," *N.Y. Med. & Phys. J.* 2 (1823): 9–10.

undoubtedly representing lecture notes that he had used during those years.[7] Williams claimed that he had been a professor of the subject before Beck had published his treatise. However, Williams's synopsis could not compare with Beck's two volumes, which in 1835 were issued in a fifth edition.

During the third and fourth decades of the nineteenth century, the teaching of medical jurisprudence spread to other states. In 1827 Robley Dunglison, who had been brought to Virginia by Thomas Jefferson, published a syllabus of his lectures on medical jurisprudence.[8] In 1833 Dunglison lectured at the University of Maryland, and in 1836 he continued his teaching career at the Jefferson Medical College. When he left Maryland, Dunglison was succeeded by R. E. Griffith. In 1835 Griffith taught obstetrics and medical jurisprudence at the University of Virginia for one year. Later at Virginia Henry Howard was another important teacher of medical jurisprudence.[9]

In 1825, the publication year of Beck's first British edition, Griffith had published an important essay on medical jurisprudence.[10] Considering the subject "so imperfectly appreciated, and indeed almost utterly neglected," he offered a fine sample of the rhetoric of insecurity that characterized so many American analyses of medical jurisprudence during the nineteenth century. Griffith gave certain reasons for the neglect, reasons that would recur in the comments of American physicians about law and medicine. He acknowledged the general resistance of Americans to legal authority and emphasized physicians' distrust of legal and judicial inquiry, a distrust that was reciprocated by suspicious lawyers who marveled at the widespread scientific and civic controversies of medical practitioners. Griffith believed that Beck's work would generate proper attention to the subject of medical jurisprudence, and more than any other physician of this early period, he attempted to sustain a relationship between medical ethics and medical jurisprudence.

Stephen Williams had hoped that more gentlemen of the bar would investigate the subject of medical jurisprudence. Of those connected with the birth of the subject in the United States, only Thomas Cooper had had legal training. Curiously, when Beck became a professor at Albany Medi-

7. Stephen W. Williams, *A Catechism of Medical Jurisprudence* (North Hampton, Mass., 1825).

8. Robley Dunglison, *Syllabus of the Lectures on Medical Jurisprudence and on the Treatment of Poisoning and Suspended Animation* (University of Virginia, 1827).

9. Henry Howard, *Outlines of Medical Jurisprudence*, 3rd ed. (Charlottesville, Va., 1845).

10. R. E. Griffith, "On Medical Jurisprudence," *Phila. J. Med. & Phys. Sci.* 10 (1825): 36–46.

cal College in 1840, after the school at Fairfield had closed, he ceased formal teaching of medical jurisprudence in deference to Amos Dean, a lawyer who had been teaching the subject at Albany for eleven years. In 1840 Dean published a *Manual of Medical Jurisprudence*, probably the first treatise on the subject written by an American lawyer.

What William Cummin had said about Great Britain in 1834—"the teaching of state and forensic medicine is, at the present moment, only in its infancy in this country"—was also true of the United States during the first half of the nineteenth century.[11] The infant was thriving so well, though, that medical jurisprudence was among the required subjects recommended by the first committee on medical education established by the American Medical Association in 1847.

A number of American medical schools had someone labeled as a professor of medical jurisprudence, although, in many instances, the professor taught other subjects, including surgery, obstetrics, materia medica, chemistry, and institutes of medicine. For the period before 1860, William Frederick Norwood identified some forty-eight individuals as teachers of the subject at thirty-seven medical schools, scattered from Maine to California and from Wisconsin to Louisiana.[12] In addition to those previously mentioned, others who at one time or another probably gave lectures on medical jurisprudence included Nicholas Romayne, Benjamin Rush Rhees, Selah Gridley, William Tulley, David Palmer, Samuel K. Jennings, Charles B. Coventry, Levens Jaynes, John Searle Tenny, James Bryan, William Russel, Solomon Foote, William C. Kittridge, John J. H. Straith, I. J. Allen, J. Adams Allen, S. G. Armor, R. S. Holmes, Joshua Riley, Joel Parker, Charles A. Lee, John C. Dalton, R. O. Doremus, Orrin Smith, John B. Lansing, James E. Morgan, Henry Archer Mettauer, J. J. Roberts, John A. Murphy, Robert L. Rea, Ephraim Ingals, Henry G. Spofford, A. B. Smith, Isaac L. Crawcour, George Barstow, Charles Edward Brown-Séquard, H. J. Anthon, James Wynne, and James S. Harrison. From the available information it appears that most were physicians, although a few were lawyers (Parker, Spofford, Anthon). We have relatively little information about what they taught (most likely they adopted the forensic medicine emphasis of Beck and Dean), or how much they taught (treatment of the subject probably ranged from an annual lecture to a series of twenty or more). Still, medical jurisprudence received a remarkable amount of attention in nineteenth-

11. W. Cummin, "Practice of Forensic Medicine, As Conducted in This and Other Countries," *Lond. Med. Gaz.* 13 (1834): 952.

12. William Frederick Norwood, *Medical Education in the United States Before the Civil War* (Philadelphia: University of Pennsylvania Press, 1944).

century American medical schools from both physicians and lawyers, some of whom analyzed relationships between their professions.

In 1856 Chandler Gilman opened the fifty-first session of the College of Physicians and Surgeons in New York with an address on the medical and legal professions.[13] Gilman reiterated previous comments about distrust between the two professions. He emphasized the difficulties faced by physicians and thought that physicians did not understand the lawyer's obligation to argue both sides of a disputed question, nor did they understand the lawyer's desire to expose the inconsistencies of all witnesses, including medical ones. Doctors failed to appreciate that they were to provide factual information or opinions about medical evidence, and not ethical or legal opinions. Gilman believed that there was no place for a partisan spirit from either a physician or a counsellor.

Presumably, lectures and courses on medical jurisprudence provided the kind of information and understanding that would enable physicians to be effective expert witnesses. Yet we have little evidence suggesting that medical school lectures accomplished these objectives; in fact, the evidence suggests that some physicians continued to be defensive and relatively unlearned about their obligations to American courts.[14] Even so, attention to the subject did not cease.

Moreover, the need for integrating medical and legal matters was beginning to appeal to a few ambitious and talented individuals. The first treatise on medical jurisprudence written by a physician and a lawyer was published at Philadelphia in 1855.[15] Also emerging in the middle of the nineteenth century were a few outstanding individuals who had both legal and medical training: J. J. Elwell (1820–1900), Horatio Robertson Storer (1830–1922), and John Ordronaux (1830–1908).

By the time of America's centennial, regard for medical jurisprudence allowed one physician to give a major address on the subject at the International Medical Congress held at Philadelphia in September of 1876 and permitted another physician to give another major address on the history of the subject before the New York Medico-Legal Society assembled on September 6 of that same year. In the former address, Stanford Chaillé reviewed the teaching of medical jurisprudence in American medical schools.[16] Using data provided by Nathan Smith Davis, Chaillé claimed

13. Chandler Gilman, *The Relations of the Medical to the Legal Profession* (New York: Baker and Godwin, 1856).
14. Chester R. Burns, "Malpractice Suits in American Medicine Before the Civil War," *Bull. Hist. Med.* 43 (1969): 41–56.
15. Francis Wharton and Moreton Stillé, *A Treatise on Medical Jurisprudence* (Philadelphia: Kay and Brothers, 1855).
16. Stanford Emerson Chaillé, *Origin and Progress of Medical Jurisprudence, 1776–1876* (Philadelphia, 1876).

that twenty-one of forty-six regular medical schools did not teach the subject of medical jurisprudence. Of the remaining twenty-five, fourteen had professorships devoted exclusively to the subject, with five of these being held by lawyers. In the other eleven, the subject was "tacked on as a caudal appendage." Chaillé concurred with John Reese (professor of medical jurisprudence at the University of Pennsylvania), whom he quoted as follows: "There are very few of the medical colleges in which it is taught, and still fewer in which it takes rank as a distinct and independent branch along with the other departments. . . ."[17]

In the New York address, J. J. O'Dea utilized statistics provided by the Bureau of Education at Washington.[18] Data from fifty-four medical schools indicated that forty gave some instruction in medical jurisprudence. "Of this 40, no more than 9 provide instruction by full and regular courses of lectures, the remaining 31 contenting themselves with occasional lectures only, numbering from 4 to 20 in the year."[19]

It is difficult to interpret such grossly contradictory statistics. One might think that a series of twenty lectures would constitute a full and regular course. And, for some species, a caudal appendage is an important asset. If correct, it is highly remarkable that in 1876 fourteen American medical schools had professorships devoted exclusively to medical jurisprudence. On the other hand, the available evidence does not tell us if these professors gave four or ten or twenty lectures in a given year, nor if the lectures improved the responsiveness of American physicians to the legal needs of the American public.

The sparse evidence about the nature of these lectures indicates that, unlike those of Stringham, none were devoted to medical ethics or etiquette. T. D. Mitchell claimed in 1839 that the ignorance and neglect of medical ethics was, in part, caused by "teachers in our schools of medicine, who seemed to have regarded the principles of Medical Ethics as too trivial to merit their attention, or so entirely self-evident, as to incorporate by necessity, with the usual teachings of the schools."[20]

Physicians of Mitchell's day assumed that it was sufficient to bear allegiance to a code of medical ethics, such as the one adopted by the Boston Medical Association in 1808, by the State Medical Society of New York in 1823, the Medico-Chirurgical Society of Baltimore in 1832, the College of Physicians of Philadelphia in 1843, or, finally, by the American

17. Ibid., p. 13.

18. James J. O'Dea, "Medico-Legal Science: A Sketch of Its Progress, Especially in the United States," *Sanitarian* 4 (1876): 449–503.

19. Ibid., p. 503.

20. Thomas D. Mitchell, *Annual Address to the College of Physicians and Surgeons of Lexington* (Lexington, 1839), p. 6.

Medical Association in 1847. In 1855 the American Medical Association required that all constituent societies accept its code as a condition of membership. Ethical problems, therefore, were matters for practitioners, not students; and medical societies were responsible for instilling and enforcing the codified principles, even though some judged these efforts to be ineffective.

In an editorial in the *American Medical Times* dated February 2, 1861, the author, probably Stephen Smith, declared that the AMA code was ignored by most physicians. Furthermore, Smith lamented the fact that there were no lectures on medical ethics in the medical colleges. Asserting that the moral aspects of a physician were as important as the intellectual aspects, the editor pleaded for a weekly lecture, or, at least, a few lectures each year at all schools. Smith did not believe that medical schools fulfilled their responsibilities if they failed to give instruction in medical ethics.[21]

This did not mean, however, that nineteenth-century American medical practitioners were uninterested in ethical problems. In addition to the widespread concern with codification, there were many speeches about ethical issues, especially at commencements and meetings of medical societies. By 1876, though, there is no evidence that an American physician or professor had ever taught a formal course in medical ethics.

Yet lectures on law and medicine continued to be given to medical students, as some practitioners and professors heeded the call of the AMA code for doctors to attend to forensic medicine as part of their responsibilities to the American public. In 1876 Stephen Smith lectured about the legal responsibilities of physicians to students attending the University Medical College in New York City. In response to the rising number of malpractice suits, Smith was eager to inform his students that they would be responsible for appropriate knowledge and skills including the "latest improvements" and that their knowledge would have to be applied "diligently and skillfully."[22] After 1876 conscientious surgeons and physicians like Smith continued to give lectures on various aspects of law as applied to medicine.

There is no evidence that many formal courses in medical jurisprudence were established during the last quarter of the nineteenth century. There is abundant evidence that the subject continued to appear in medical school catalogues, suggesting that the medical school policies of the early part of the century were continued throughout the century. In a

21. "The Study of Medical Ethics," *Am. Med. Times* 2 (1861): 82–83.
22. Stephen Smith, "On the Legal Responsibilities of Medical Men," *Ohio Med. & Surg. J.* 1 (1876): 46–50, 148–52; ibid. 2 (1877): 63–67.

survey of catalogues in 1890, seventy-five orthodox schools and twenty-seven sectarian schools indicated that medical jurisprudence was a subject taught in their institutions.[23]

Some of these teachers also wrote important monographs and textbooks. John James Reese, professor of medical jurisprudence and toxicology at the University of Pennsylvania Medical School, prepared a popular textbook that was issued in seven editions.[24] Tracy C. Becker, a professor of medical jurisprudence at the University of Buffalo, co-authored an important text with Rudolph A. Witthaus. Ralph W. Webster, clinical professor of medicine at Rush Medical College, prepared several new editions of Frederick Peterson and Walter S. Haines's *A Textbook of Legal Medicine and Toxicology*. A lecturer on jurisprudence in the medical and dental schools of the University of Illinois, Elmer DeWitt Brothers, a lawyer, published a second edition of his *Medical Jurisprudence* in 1925.[25]

These and other physicians and lawyers were members of medico-legal societies established in the latter decades of the nineteenth century. These societies were very active. The Medico-Legal Society of New York sponsored numerous publications, including the *Medico-Legal Journal*, edited by Clark Bell for many years, and then by Alfred Herzog until his death in 1933. This society held many meetings and sponsored the first International Congress of Medical Jurisprudence held in New York City in June of 1889. The members of that congress passed a resolution which urged all medical and law schools to include a course in medical jurisprudence and require an examination in that subject for graduation.[26]

Yet the very existence of these societies indicated that American physicians and lawyers had institutionalized medical jurisprudence outside of schools of medicine and law. As with ethics, legal problems were matters for practitioners, not students. As long as these medico-legal societies responded to the needs of practitioners, there was no justification for burdening students who already had their hands filled with the more basic medical sciences. It is remarkable, indeed, that lectures on medical

23. John H. Rauch, *Report on Medical Education, Medical Colleges and the Regulation of the Practice of Medicine in the United States and Canada, 1765–1890* (Springfield: Illinois State Board of Health, 1890). In this survey, one orthodox institution (University of Missouri Medical School) and one sectarian school (Boston University School of Medicine) indicated that ethics was taught at their schools.

24. Reese occupied a professorship that had been established by Dr. George B. Wood in 1865 (J. J. Reese, "An Address before the Medico-Legal Society of Philadelphia," *Phila. Med. Times* 14 [1883–1884]: 157–61).

25. For additional information, see Frank L. Kozelka, "Legal Medicine in the United States," *Ciba Symposia* 11 (1950–1951): 1309–10.

26. Editorial, *Medico-Legal Journal* 8 (1890): 73–74.

jurisprudence continued to be supported by the medical schools during the latter decades of the nineteenth century and the early decades of the twentieth.

These early medico-legal societies also concerned themselves with matters of public health and other aspects of health legislation, but they seldom attended to problems of professional ethics. Issues of professional ethics and etiquette were debated repeatedly and heatedly during the meetings of the American Medical Association and its constituent state medical societies. As with medical jurisprudence, the subject of professional ethics was institutionalized in medical societies and thereby segregated from the institutional roles of the medical schools.

At the turn of the twentieth century, the hegemony of the AMA code of ethics was striking. Most physicians urged medical schools to teach the subject so that all graduates would understand and accept the AMA code. There is little evidence to indicate that the schools responded to these exhortations. They were too busy with basic reforms occurring in response to the recommendations of the Association of American Medical Colleges (AAMC) and the proposals of the Council on Medical Education of the American Medical Association.

Around the turn of the century, Charles Coppens, a Jesuit priest who taught at Creighton Medical College in Omaha, Nebraska, attempted to sustain one facet of the European legacy, that of relating medical ethics and medical jurisprudence. Coppens's lectures were eventually incorporated into a book entitled *Moral Principles and Medical Practice: The Basis of Medical Jurisprudence.* Coppens claimed that the term *medical jurisprudence,* as commonly used, was a misnomer.[27] In addition to a study of law, he believed, the subject ought to include a study of the moral principles upon which laws are founded. These moral principles would be applicable even in situations not governed by specific laws. Scattered throughout Coppens's lectures are various facts that belonged to forensic medicine proper. But emphasis was placed on a consideration of ethical principles applicable to abortion, sexual behavior, a physician's professional rights and duties, and insanity. In all of these areas, Coppens attempted to demonstrate the relevance of Christian ideals to the practice of medicine. His efforts symbolized the emergence of medical ethics as a medical school subject, especially at religiously affiliated schools.[28]

Four years after Coppens's fourth edition was published, the AMA's

27. Charles Coppens, *Moral Principles and Medical Practice: The Basis of Medical Jurisprudence,* 4th ed. (New York: Benziger Brothers, 1905), p. 5.
28. Someone, for example, might study the history of the teaching of medical ethics at Georgetown University School of Medicine.

Council on Medical Education asked a committee of one hundred medical school professors to prepare a comprehensive statement about the curricula of medical schools. Their report was given at a meeting of the council in April of 1909. The committee recommended that 305 hours be devoted to hygiene, medical jurisprudence, and medical ethics (including economics). Yet the committee reported a list of reduced hours under more realistic conditions. Reduced more than any other was the above category—from 305 to 120 hours.[29] Clearly, these subjects received the lowest priority.

In 1910, the year of the Flexner Report, the AAMC surveyed the curricula of fifty medical schools. The surveyor averaged the total number of hours reported by the schools and stated that thirty-seven hours were devoted to hygiene, twenty-one to medical jurisprudence, and nine to medical economics.[30] Ethics was not mentioned.

Until 1925 the Council on Medical Education continued to recommend medical jurisprudence as a curricular subject. In that year the Council omitted medical jurisprudence from its recommendations, but included hygiene and sanitation, a change that had been initiated by the AAMC in 1924.[31]

During the first quarter of the twentieth century, American medical schools, agitated with the turmoils of reform, permitted the constituent societies of the American Medical Association to remain responsible primarily for matters of professional ethics. With the exception of a few lectures, the schools also permitted these same societies and the previously mentioned medico-legal ones to attend to legal affairs. This situation began to change for medical ethics during the late 1920s and for medical jurisprudence during the early 1930s. Codified ideals were no longer sufficient and decisions of governmental agencies and legal institutions were beginning to influence the medical schools in unprecedented fashion.

In 1926 Richard Clarke Cabot, professor of medicine and professor of social ethics at Harvard, claimed that he knew of no medical school in which professional ethics was systematically taught.[32] At their November meeting that same year, the board of trustees of the American Medical Association recommended that the subject of medical ethics be a part of

29. "Report of the Council on Medical Education of the American Medical Association," *J. AMA* 52 (1909): 1522.

30. H. D. Arnold, "Report of the Subcommittee on Curriculum for the Clinical Years," *Proc. AAMC* 20 (1910): 140.

31. "Medical Education in the United States," *J. AMA* 85 (1925): 609.

32. Richard C. Cabot, *Adventures on the Borderlands of Ethics* (New York: Harper, 1926), p. 23.

the required curriculum in every medical school.[33] Responses to this recommendation began to appear.

A. D. Bevan, in reviewing the need for teaching medical ethics, did not equate medical ethics with the AMA's code, and even urged some significant revisions in that code.[34] The House of Delegates of the Ohio State Medical Society urged all Ohio medical schools to teach courses on the social relations of the physician including medical ethics, economics, jurisprudence, and history.[35]

Park J. White, a pediatrician, published an outline of a course on medical ethics which he had been teaching for four years to senior medical students at Washington University School of Medicine in St. Louis. White's six lectures covered the following general topics: acquiring practice properly; group practice; starting as assistant to a busy practitioner; proper attitudes of a doctor toward his work; coping with success; medical finance; relationships with other physicians; attending patients of another physician; public health work; hospital staff positions; doctor and nurse; doctor and druggist; salary position; railroad, insurance, factory work; quacks and cults; eugenics; euthanasia; and birth control.[36]

At the annual meeting of the Texas State Medical Association in 1927, Marvin Graves, professor of medicine at the medical department of the University of Texas at Galveston, claimed that a course of four to six lectures on medical ethics had been given to senior medical students for twenty-one years.[37] Also in that year the AMA's Council on Medical Education recommended that the "subjects of medical economics, medical jurisprudence, and medical history, and, perhaps also in some instances, pastoral medicine, might be conveniently grouped with that of medical ethics under the general title of the 'social relations of the physician.' "[38]

But medical educators did not support this recommendation nor follow the novel suggestions about teaching medical ethics offered by Chauncey Leake.[39] Medical history began to be institutionalized as a separate sub-

33. "Medical Ethics," *J. AMA* 87 (1926): 1922.
34. A. D. Bevan, "The Need of Teaching Medical Ethics," *J. AMA* 88 (1927): 617–19.
35. *J. AMA* 88 (1927): 1912.
36. Park J. White, "A Course in Professional Conduct," *J. AMA* 88 (1927): 1751. For later revisions of this course, see Park J. White, "The Teaching of Medical Ethics and Professional Conduct," *J. AAMC* 7 (1932): 353–61; and Park J. White, "New Things Which Should Be Taught in a Course on Professional Conduct and Medical Economics," ibid. 11 (1936): 366–76.
37. M. L. Graves, "Teaching of Medical Ethics," *Tex. St. J. Med.* 23 (1927): 117–118.
38. "Report of the Council on Medical Education and Hospitals," *J. AMA* 88 (1927): 1174.
39. Chauncey D. Leake, "How is Medical Ethics To Be Taught?" *Bull. AAMC* 3 (1928): 341–43.

ject;[40] pastoral medicine and medical ethics were melded in some Catholic medical schools; and medical jurisprudence remained on the periphery, occasionally offered as lectures in departments of preventive medicine and community health or as lectures by friendly neighborhood lawyers. Medical economics for the most part was ignored.

An international survey of the teaching of medical jurisprudence was published in 1928. The research, teaching, and service activities of nineteen Continental institutes were surveyed, including the highly regarded one at Vienna. The teaching activities of the departments of forensic medicine at the University of Edinburgh and the University of Glasgow were described in some detail. The Canadian author bemoaned the absence of institutes, laboratories, and courses in his country, and Charles Norris, the chief medical examiner for the city of New York, noted that in the United States, "medico-legal pathology has not, as yet, received the recognition due a science of such great importance, and in our medical schools there has been meager, if any, undergraduate instruction in these branches."[41] The phrase *medico-legal pathology* (now *forensic pathology*) suggests a further narrowing of the scope of medical jurisprudence, a narrowing that underscores the dearth of interest in teaching medical jurisprudence during the 1920s.[42]

A new surge of interest appeared in the 1930s. Harvard Medical School established the first chair of legal medicine in the United States and appointed Dr. George B. Magrath to this chair in 1932. Magrath had served many years as one of the medical examiners for Suffolk County (Boston), Massachusetts.[43] In that same year, a course was in preparation for the New York University School of Medicine and Samuel Levinson and Clarence Muehlberger were teaching an elective for senior medical students at the University of Illinois College of Medicine.[44]

During their sixteen lectures, Levinson and Muehlberger discussed the following topics: problems of legal medicine; jurisdiction of coroner and medical examiner; cause of sudden death; literature of legal medicine;

40. Chester R. Burns, "History in Medical Education: The Development of Current Trends in the United States," *Bull. N.Y. Acad. Med.* 51 (1975): 851–69.
41. Charles Norris, "Responsibility of the Chief Medical Examiner of New York City in Relation to Medical Progress, Education, and Research," in *Methods and Problems of Medical Education*, p. 347.
42. Also see William J. Curran, "The Status of Forensic Pathology in the United States," *N. Eng. J. Med.* 283 (1970): 1033–34.
43. O. T. Schultz, "Present Status and Future Development of Legal Medicine in the United States," *Arch. Path.* 15 (1933): 564–65. See F. J. Cotton, "Medicine, Ethics and Law," *N. Eng. J. Med.* 208 (1933): 584–95, for a not very satisfactory attempt to explore the intrinsic relationship between medical jurisprudence and professional ethics.
44. Samuel A. Levinson and Clarence W. Muehlberger, "An Introductory Course in Legal Medicine for Medical Students," *J. AAMC* 9 (1934): 293–301.

laws governing the body of a dead person; personal identification; medico-legal necropsy; death from burns and electricity; traumatic injuries
and fractures; identification of guns and bullets; rape and abortion; asphyx-
ial death; homicidal and suicidal poisoning; industrial poisonings;
medico-legal aspects of alcohol; examination of blood, stains, and fibers;
psycho-physiologic methods for the detection of deception; and the medical expert in court.

In 1933 H. M. Taylor, an associate professor of biochemistry and toxicology, and J. S. Bradway, professor of law, began teaching a course of
seven lectures to medical students at Duke University. In 1934 Levinson
and Muehlberger examined catalogues of seventy-seven American medical schools and discovered that 6.5 percent of the schools gave a course in
legal medicine, 58 percent gave lectures in the subject, and 35 percent
apparently did nothing. No medical school required a course in legal
medicine for graduation. Taylor and Bradway reported that their course
had become a part of the required curriculum in 1939.[45]

Interest in teaching medical ethics also appears to have increased
significantly during the 1930s. In what was probably the first survey of the
teaching of professional ethics in American medical schools, the *Journal
of the Association of American Medical Colleges* reported, in 1931, that 43
percent of sixty-seven medical schools offered definite courses in medical
ethics, with 93 percent of those courses required. There was great variation in the courses and they were often combined with medical history,
economics, and jurisprudence. Schools attending to the subject of medical ethics in other courses amounted to 28 percent; 9 percent indicated
that the subject was considered incidentally; and 20 percent indicated
that there was no instruction in medical ethics.[46]

Another survey was conducted in 1938. Although the surveyor discovered that thirty of sixty-eight medical schools (44 percent) were giving
courses in medical ethics and twenty-two of sixty-eight schools (32 percent) were giving courses in medical economics, he concluded that "only a
few schools seem to be offering courses in medical economics and ethics
which are based on sufficiently broad perspectives to obtain the proper
objectives."[47]

The revival of interest in teaching medical jurisprudence and medical

45. H. M. Taylor and J. S. Bradway, "Teaching of Legal Medicine," *Am. J. Med. Juris.* 2
(1939): 210–13.
46. "Instruction in Professional Ethics," *J. AAMC* 6 (1931): 189–90. I question this data;
if correct they meant that the number of schools teaching medical ethics had increased from
zero to 43 percent in five years.
47. J. K. Donaldson, "Relationship of Medical Schools to Medical Ethics and Medical
Economics," *South. Med. J.* 31 (1938): 327–30. In 1937, 60 percent of the medical schools
offered medical history courses. Among other reasons, history was being used to recover and

ethics continued during the 1940s and 1950s. In 1945 another survey was reported in the *Journal of the American Medical Association*. It indicated that forty-two of seventy-seven medical schools (55 percent) had some courses in medical sociology, economics, and ethics, although there was "considerable lack of uniformity" and there were "great differences in the amount of time devoted to these subjects in these schools."[48] Both physicians and non-physicians continued to urge the inclusion of courses that would educate physicians about their social and moral responsibilities.[49]

In 1955 the American Medical Association's Department of Medical Education obtained information from the deans of eighty-one medical schools about the extent of instruction in medical jurisprudence and medical ethics.[50] Seventy of the eighty-one medical schools (86 percent) allotted a prescribed amount of time for the teaching of legal medicine. Forty-five of the schools allocated over ten hours to the subject. Forty of the eighty-one schools (49 percent) indicated that a definite amount of time was allotted for instruction in medical ethics. Clearly there was little uniformity in the teaching of either subject. The lectures were given by an array of individuals whose interests ranged from the nuances of forensic pathology to the broader implications of social and environmental medicine.

In response to the extraordinary technical advances in medicine, a marked surge of interest in teaching medical ethics occurred during the 1960s. Medical ethics began to assume its rightful place as a distinctive academic subject with intrinsic merit. Symbolic of the emerging interest of clergymen in medical education was a symposium on the place of value systems in medical education, sponsored by the Academy of Religion and Mental Health in 1960. A medical ethics essay contest was sponsored by the Department of Medical Ethics of the American Medical Association, and a section of the Sixty-fifth Annual Congress on Medical Education (1969) was devoted to the teaching of human values in the medical curriculum.[51]

---

transmit traditional values of the medical profession as well as to describe and interpret the social and scientific forces that were altering the very nature of medicine (Burns, "History in Medical Education," p. 857).

48. "Instruction in Medical Sociology, Medical Economics, and Medical Ethics," *J. AMA* 129 (1945): 464.

49. For examples, see T. K. Lewis, "Resolution on Indoctrinating Medical Students with Philosophy and Ethics of Profession," *J. AMA* 134 (1947): 717; James R. Reuling, "Resolution on Teaching of Medical Economics in Medical Schools," ibid.; and Theodore M. Greene, "The Education of the Doctor in Social and Moral Responsibility," *J. AAMC* 22 (1947): 370–72.

50. "Medical Education in the United States and Canada," *J. AMA* 159 (1955): 578–79.

51. *J. AMA* 198 (1966): 9; Casey Truett, Arthur W. Douville, Bruce Fagel, and Merle Cunningham, "The Medical Curriculum and Human Values," *J. AMA* 209 (1969): 1341–45;

Since 1971 the Society for Health and Human Values has sponsored several conferences on the teaching of the humanities in medical schools, and data collected for these conferences indicates that about forty medical schools have developed some curricular strategies for relating the humanities, including ethics, to health professional education.[52]

Under the auspices of the Institute of Society, Ethics and the Life Sciences and Columbia University College of Physicians and Surgeons, the first national conference on the teaching of medical ethics was held at Tarrytown, New York, in June of 1972.[53] Some 134 participants reviewed many important issues involved in the teaching of medical ethics. The participants also heard the results of another survey of the teaching of medical ethics, a survey which indicated that three schools had required courses, thirty-three schools offered elective medical ethics courses, seventeen schools offered special lectures or programs which dealt with ethical issues in medicine, and fifty-six schools indicated that ethical issues arise in such medical school courses as community medicine, legal medicine, and psychiatry. Fifteen schools indicated that they had no specific teaching in the field of medical ethics, although it is doubtful if ethical issues do not arise somewhere in the experiences of their medical students.[54]

The teaching of medical jurisprudence has also received remarkable attention by medical schools during the last two decades. Among the many responsible factors are the following: a rising incidence of crime and a corresponding need for forensic pathology; the trials and tribulations associated with an increased number of malpractice suits; the perplexities of handling a growing number of mentally and emotionally ill persons; the increased role of the federal government in matters medical; the emergence of several formal organizations devoted to medico-legal issues; and an increased social awareness and responsiveness of the legal and medical professions. For these and other reasons, the most recent surveys

---

Edwin F. Rosinski, "Human Values and Curriculum Design," *J. AMA* 209 (1969): 1346–48; Edmund D. Pellegrino, "Human Values and the Medical Curriculum," *J. AMA* 209 (1969): 1349–53.

52. See the following publications of the Society for Health and Human Values (Philadelphia): *Proc. First Session, Institute on Human Values in Medicine*, 1971; *Proc. Second Session, Institute on Human Values in Medicine*, 1972; *Third Proc., Southwest Regional Institute, Institute on Human Values in Medicine*, 1973; *Human Values Teaching Programs for Health Professionals, Institute on Human Values in Medicine*, 1974.

53. Robert M. Veatch, Willard Gaylin, and Councilman Morgan, eds., *The Teaching of Medical Ethics* (Hastings-On-Hudson, N.Y.: Institute of Society, Ethics and the Life Sciences, 1973).

54. Ibid., pp. 97–102.

indicate a growing interest in teaching legal medicine although, viewed nationally, the institutional efforts are still quite disproportionate.

In one survey (1970) 42 of 79 four-year medical schools offered some type of course in legal medicine. Fifteen required it for graduation and 27 offered it as an elective.[55] In another survey (1970) 47 of 85 approved medical schools offered some instruction in legal medicine. A formal course was offered in 39 of these schools.[56] Another survey conducted in 1973 indicated that 46 of 116 medical schools do *not* offer courses in forensic medicine, whereas the remaining 70 offer a total of 91 courses, with 47 required and 44 elective. The fact that almost 40 percent of the medical schools do not offer any instruction in medical jurisprudence was considered "shocking and distressing" by the author and "a dereliction of the duty of the medical schools to both the student and his future patients."[57] It is encouraging to note, though, that pedagogical innovation and experimentation is a significant part of the current revival of interest in teaching medical jurisprudence in American medical schools.[58]

During the last quarter of the twentieth century, medical ethics and medical jurisprudence will continue to gain positions of increasing prominence in American medical education. The day may come when all state, national, and specialty boards will require examinations in these subjects. Perhaps, too, some professor or group of teachers will attempt to explore the pattern of social relationships that undergirded the concepts of those physicians who, two to three centuries ago, related medical jurisprudence, medical ethics, and public health. This may happen as more and more individuals participate in the renaissance of contemporary interest in the teaching of medical jurisprudence and medical ethics in American medical schools.

55. H. Richard Beresford, "The Teaching of Legal Medicine in Medical Schools in the United States," *J. Med. Ed.* 46 (1971): 401–4.

56. William H. L. Dornette, "Interdisciplinary Education in Medicine and Law in American Medical Colleges," *J. Med. Ed.* 46 (1971): 389–400.

57. Harold Hirsh, "Educational Opportunities in Forensic or Legal Medicine in Medical Schools," *Phi Delta Epsilon News* 65 (1973): 2–6.

58. In addition to Dornette, "Interdisciplinary Education in Medicine and Law," see Morton Lloyd Norton, "Development of an Interdisciplinary Program of Instruction in Medicine and Law," *J. Med. Ed.* 46 (1971); 405–11, and George J. Annas, "Law and Medicine: Myths and Realities in the Medical School Classroom," *Third Proc., Southwest Regional Institute, Institute on Human Values in Medicine* (Philadelphia: Society for Health and Human Values, 1973), pp. 45–55. For information about the teaching of legal medicine in law schools, see the following: W. J. Curran and R. H. Hamlin, "The Medico-Legal Problems Seminar at Harvard Law School," *J. Legal Ed.* 8 (1956): 499–502; W. J. Curran, "A Nationwide Survey: Medico-Legal Instruction in Law Schools," *Am. Bar Assoc. J.* 45 (1959): 815–18; 874–76. For a penetrating analysis of the views of those who have received both medical and law degrees, see William J. Curran, "Cross-Professional Education in Law and Medicine: The Promise and the Conflict," *J. Legal Ed.* 24 (1971): 42–72.

Medical History

GENEVIEVE MILLER

Es ist eine der schlimmsten Seiten unserer gegenwärtigen
Entwickelungsperiode in der Medicin, dass die historische
Kenntniss der Dinge mit jeder Generation von Studirenden ab-
nimmt. Sogar von den selbstthätigen jüngeren Arbeitern kann man
in der Regel annehmen, dass ihr Wissen im höchsten Falle nur bis
auf 3–5 Jahre rückwärts reicht. Was vor 5 Jahren publicirt ist, exis-
tirt nicht mehr.[1]

P*LUS ça change, plus c'est la même chose!* The quotation is not from
1980, but from 1870 when Rudolph Virchow was lamenting the lack of
interest in medical history among medical students. If one were to select a
leitmotif for the history of medical history in medical education, an ever-
recurring theme would be the attempt of devotees to break down medical
students' apathy and to convince them of the value of a historical component to their professional education.

In the early nineteenth century some familiarity with medical history
by the medical profession was probably acquired without conscious effort,
since medicine was largely empirical in nature and the students read
textbooks which still discussed theories of earlier medical authors. If medical history was consciously cultivated, it was for a pragmatic reason: to
extend the experience of the individual practitioner into the past in order
to provide a wiser basis for critical judgment. It is not surprising that

---

1. "That historical information about things diminishes with each generation of students
is one of the worst sides of our present period of development in medicine. As a rule one can
assume that the knowledge of even the most spontaneous younger workers reaches
backward at best only from three to five years. Whatever was published more than five years
ago, no longer exists" (cited in Georg Fischer, *Chirurgie vor 100 Jahren: Historische Studie*
[Leipzig: F. C. W. Vogel, 1876], p. 1).

Thomas Jefferson, nurtured by Voltaire and others of the French En-
lightenment who found in history a pragmatic weapon for achieving progress, should have emulated the French in instituting a course on the
history of the various theories of medicine as an integral part of the
curriculum of the new University of Virginia medical school. It was taught
between 1825 and 1833 by Robley Dunglison, a young Englishman whom
Jefferson had brought from London to teach anatomy, physiology, materia
medica and pharmacy. His lectures, which were published forty years
later by his son, were based primarily on John Freind's *History of Physic*
(1725) and Kurt Sprengel's monumental *Versuch einer pragmatischen
Geschichte der Arzneykunde* (1792–1800).[2] There is no evidence that he
continued giving his course in either Baltimore or Philadelphia, after he
left Virginia in 1833, but his famous *Dictionary* and other publications
reflect strong historical interests. He was responsible for including John
Bostock's *Sketch of the History of Medicine* with William Pulteney Ali-
son's supplement in the revised American edition of John Forbes's *Cy-
clopaedia of Practical Medicine*, which he issued as editor in 1845, and he
recommended that medical history should be given in the second year of
the two-year medical curriculum of his day.[3]

The learned, scholarly Dunglison, however, experienced discomfort in
the American intellectual climate before the Civil War in which the chief
emphasis among most citizens was on practicality. He was conscious of
anti-intellectualism even among his colleagues: "In this country [contrary
to England] to be considered highly scientific and to have published
largely on his own profession and more especially to be eminent in general literature is positively detrimental, by encouraging the idea, that the
physician may be very learned and very scientific and literary but, for that
very reason, probably not practical."[4]

The only other formal course before the Civil War of which we have any
record was given at Penn Medical University, a short-lived school which

2. Robley Dunglison, *History of Medicine from the Earliest Ages to the Commencement
of the Nineteenth Century* (Philadelphia: Lindsay and Blakiston, 1872).
3. Samuel X. Radbill, "Robley Dunglison, M.D., 1789–1869: American Medical Educator," *J. Med. Ed.* 34 (1959): 93.
4. Samuel X. Radbill, ed., "The Autobiographical Ana of Robley Dunglison, M.D.,"
Trans. Am. Phil. Soc., n.s., 53, pt. 8 (1963): 151–52. "The general impression in this
country—erroneous as it may be—is, that high literary and scientific distinction is unnecessary and many even believe, injurious in the transaction of the business concerns of life"
(ibid., p. 37). See the superb analysis of Dunglison's scholarly life and character by his
eloquent friend, Samuel D. Gross, "Memoir of Robley Dunglison, M.D., LL.D., Read
before the College of Physicians at a Special Meeting Held on the 20th of October, 1869,"
Summary of Trans. Coll. Phys. Phila., n.s., 4 (1874): 294–313.

existed in Philadelphia from 1853 to 1881. The following statement from
the *Curriculum . . . and Announcement of the Spring Session of 1854*
explains why medical history was included:

> The *history of medicine* is another branch but rarely and fragmentar-
> ily taught in our medical schools, but which deserves an important
> rank among the medical studies, both for the great light it throws on
> our present state of science, and for the scientific dignity and self-
> possession it gives to the physician in his intercourse with the eru-
> dite portion of the community who naturally look down upon any
> physician as being an ignoramus, who does not know the history of
> his own profession. In what esteem would we hold a statesman, who
> would exhibit ignorance of the history of nations?[5]

It is noteworthy that medical history was being used to defend the medical profession from its critics and to elevate the ranks of its practitioners in
the public eye. The motivation is identical with that of the Cincinnati
physician, Cornelius George Comegys, who in 1856 published a translation of Pierre Victor Renouard's *Histoire de la médecine.* In the 1850s
American medicine was under attack because of the uncertainty of its
theories, as the numerous medical sects demonstrated, and history was
believed to provide practitioners with critical judgment for accepting or
rejecting opposing theories.[6]

In addition to the formal lectures at Penn Medical University which ran
from March through June, at least one student elected to write her required thesis on a historical topic, for Sarah A. Rice of Massachusetts
graduated around 1860 with the thesis, "The History of the Origin of
Anatomy." It was an acceptable topic for student theses in other schools
also. At Cleveland Medical College there were three student theses on
the topic between 1848 and 1855.

Another source of medico-historical information for students before the
Civil War was the annual "Introductory Lecture" given at a formal convo-
cation at the beginning of each new school year. Usually delivered by one
of the professors, they were often open to the public, and although miscel-

5. Cited in Wyndham D. Miles, "An Early American Course in History of
Medicine: The History of Medicine Course at Penn Medical University in 1854," *Bull.
Hist. Med.* 38 (1964): 276–77.
6. P. V. Renouard, *History of Medicine, from Its Origin to the Nineteenth Century,
with an Appendix, Containing a Philosophical and Historical Review of Medicine to the
Present Time,* trans. Cornelius G. Comegys, M.D. (Cincinnati: Moore, Wilstack, Keys and
Co., 1856). For a discussion of Comegys's book, see Genevieve Miller, "In Praise of
Amateurs: Medical History in America Before Garrison," *Bull. Hist. Med.* 47 (1973): 588–
90.

laneous in character, they frequently contained advice for the students in the conduct of their future professional careers, as well as information about the past history of their profession, the lives of outstanding physicians, and obituaries of recently deceased professors. After the lecture it was customary for a committee of students to invite the lecturer to permit his address to be published and distributed, presumably at the school's expense. Collections of such lectures were frequently made by literary-minded physicians for their libraries.[7]

When Richard J. Dunglison published his father's lectures on medical history in 1872, he lamented that students were "left to gather their information on the previous state of medicine in whatever manner they may find it practicable or convenient to do so, *after graduation*."[8] Claiming that little was in print in English, he stated that the lectures were being published so that a condensed history would be available which might stimulate further interest in the subject. Similarly, John Charles Reeve, a professor at the Medical College of Ohio in Cincinnati, had published an English translation of Jean-Pierre-Marie Flourens's *Histoire de la découverte de la circulation du sang* (Paris, 1854) because he believed that it was important for a medical student to understand the very gradual progress in achieving medical knowledge.[9]

In spite of the absence of formal teaching of medical history in medical schools, by the middle of the century the anti-intellectualism observed by the elder Dunglison seems to have begun to recede, and numerous physicians began to cultivate literary pursuits. A few kept in touch with European developments; others built up collections of historical books and ephemera, resurrected American medical heroes, and published historical articles and books. In the final quarter of the century many professional leaders in all parts of the country became bibliophiles, as book collecting came to be equated with gentility. While John Shaw Billings was developing the Library of the Surgeon General's Office in Washington, other major collections were being made by the New York Academy of Medicine, the Philadelphia College of Physicians, and the Boston Medical Library through the energies of interested physicians. In addition to articles and books generated by anniversaries of local medical societies

7. Genevieve Miller, "Medical Education One Hundred Years Ago: The Introductory Lecture," *Ohio St. Med. J.* 54 (1958): 1578–82; ibid. 55 (1959): 40–41, 44. Two such collections made by Dr. Jared P. Kirtland and Dr. J. M. Henderson are preserved in the Cleveland Health Sciences Library.

8. Italics mine. Preface to Dunglison, *History of Medicine*, p. iv.

9. P. Flourens, *A History of the Discovery of the Circulation of the Blood*, trans. J. C. Reeve (Cincinnati: Riokey, Mallory and Co., 1859).

and institutions, the centennial celebration of 1876 stimulated historical reviews, and medical biography filled many pages.[10] It should be noted, however, that all such activity was outside of the medical school.

Ironically, at the same time that interest in medical history was slowly incubating in the United States, the rise of modern experimental medicine abroad was gradually undermining any practical use of the subject in formal medical education. When daily new discoveries made old medical theories obsolete, the past was seen to be a record of errors to be forgotten, and while many continental European countries had formerly had chairs of medical history in their government-supported universities, after the middle of the century these positions tended to disappear as nonessential.[11] A conflict thus developed between the educational ideal of a humanistically oriented individual, versed in history and belles lettres, and the rapidly evolving new medical scientist trained in new skills designed to erase past mistakes. As a practical matter, what *could* medical history contribute?

It was just at this juncture that the "humanization" of the physician came to the forefront as an educational goal for which medical history was to be the agent. Also the subject received a strong philosophical thrust from Darwinism, which by the end of the century had begun to permeate all fields of thought. Only by studying the origin and development of things could one really comprehend them. Over and over again, apologists for medical history at the turn of the century made this point. Darwinian ideas also led to interest in the general history of culture of which medicine was one component, interacting with and being influenced by other components, just as an organism interacts with its environment.[12]

The credit for attempting to make history an integral part of the medical school curriculum in America must unquestionably be assigned to John Shaw Billings, one of the major planners of the new Johns Hopkins Hospital and Medical School in Baltimore. In 1876, the year the university opened, Billings was appointed lecturer in the history of medicine, and

10. The subject is developed in detail in G. Miller, "In Praise of Amateurs," pp. 586–615; also see Whitfield J. Bell, Jr., "The Writing of American Medical History Before Professionalization," *Trans. & Stud. Coll. Phys. Phila.*, 4th ser., 42 (1974): 49–60.

11. For an extensive review of medico-historical teaching in Europe, see George Rosen, "The Place of History in Medical Education," *Bull. Hist. Med.* 22 (1948): 594–627.

12. See Julius Pagel, "Medizinische Kulturgeschichte," *Janus* 9 (1904): 285–95. Detailed discussion in Genevieve Miller, "Influences on Medical Historiography in the Late 19th Century," *Acta Congressus Internationalis XXIV Historiae Artis Medicinae 25–31 Augusti 1974 Budapestini*, 2 vols. (Budapest: Museum, Bibliotheca et Archivum Historiae Artis Medicinae de I. Ph. Semmelweis Nominata, 1976), 2:1621–25.

during the autumn of 1877 he gave twenty lectures on the history of
medicine, medical legislation and medical education that were designed
to give the background information for the plans he proposed for the new
school, which incidentally was intended to restore the original meaning to
the term *medicinae doctor* by training teachers as well as practitioners.[13]
Acknowledging that in the average American medical school, whose function was solely to train practitioners, time spent on medical history would
be of little practical value, and that sufficient information could be obtained from historical comments of the professors and from reading after
graduation, Billings insisted, however, that *university* training should be
broader:

> It appears to me that to its students an account of the various sys-
> tems of Medicine and Medical Philosophy which have from time to
> time prevailed, of the methods in which discoveries and progress
> have been made, of the principal errors and fallacies which have
> hindered this progress, and of the lives and opinions of those who
> are recognized as leaders and authorities, cannot fail to be interest-
> ing and useful; that such a course would be a means of culture, a
> stimulus to thought, and would save much labor and research when
> the time comes for the student to attempt to teach, either from the
> Professor's chair, or through the press.[14]

However he did not want such a course to become merely medical biography and bibliography, or to plead for some particular doctrine. Nor did
he wish to lay down rules preventing teachers from selecting their own
methods and topics, although he acknowledged that "some knowledge of
the lives and opinions of the great men of his Profession should be possessed by every Physician," not for biographical reasons, but because they
had "meditated and written upon many of the questions which still are
unanswered" and because a knowledge of the older medical literature
would prevent the wasteful repetition of old theories which "re-appear
and are re-exploded with the regular periodicity of organic life."[15]

Arguing again for a course in medical history in 1883 in an address to
the Medical and Chirurgical Faculty of Maryland, Billings pointed out the
benefit to the life of a physician who had medical classics and histories

13. Sanford V. Larkey, "John Shaw Billings and the History of Medicine," *Bull. Hist.
Med.* 6 (1938): 360–76.
14. Alan M. Chesney, "Two Papers by John Shaw Billings on Medical Education," *Bull.
Hist. Med.* 6 (1938): 343.
15. Ibid., pp. 344–45. At the same time, Billings established a "Notes and Queries"
section in the early issues of *Index Medicus*, the monthly citation of current literature which
he had established in 1879. Here bibliophiles could send questions about rare books and
editions, or other queries of a medico-historical or bibliographic nature.

around him into which he could dip in leisure hours. Unlike Dunglison thirty years earlier, Billings affirmed that "it certainly does not cause a lower estimate of his ability as a practical physician and surgeon to know that he reads something else besides manuals and text-books."[16]

When the Johns Hopkins School of Medicine opened in 1893, Billings was appointed lecturer in the history and literature of medicine and retained the title until 1905. However he gave only three lectures a year, and the major medico-historical activity in the new medical school was carried on by other faculty members such as William Osler, William H. Welch and Howard A. Kelly, and through the monthly programs of the Johns Hopkins Hospital Historical Club which they had founded in 1890. Osler was most successful in infecting students with historical interests. Instead of formal lectures, he injected historical remarks while teaching medicine, required students to search the literature for the original papers in which major discoveries were first described, and brought students and interns to his home for informal evenings to examine his collection of rare books, in which he took great delight.[17] Many of his students became book collectors too, and one of them, C. N. B. Camac, who was a house officer on his staff for two years, published the first American source book in medical history in 1909, believing that such information should be "considered requisite to a proper education."[18] The later source books of Ralph Major, Logan Clendening, and E. C. Kelly were also generated by the same Oslerian ideal.

In other parts of the country, activities in medical history exploded in the medical schools during the 1890s. In 1891, the same year that Billings started lecturing to the Johns Hopkins Hospital staff, Nathan Smith Davis, the historian of the American Medical Association, began to give lectures on medical history at the Chicago Medical College. The following year Charles Winslow Dulles began a compulsory course of sixteen lectures with no examination to the fourth-year class of the University of Pennsylvania; in 1895 Roswell Park initiated an extensive course at Buffalo; at Minnesota, Burnside Foster became lecturer in the history of medicine in 1897 and gave sixteen lectures to the senior class. Other

16. *Trans. Med. & Chirur. Fac. St. Md.* (1883): 79, cited in Larkey, "John Shaw Billings," p. 362.
17. He explained his method of teaching in "A Note on the Teaching of the History of Medicine," *British Med. J.* (1902), ii:93.
18. C.N.B. Camac, *Epoch-Making Contributions to Medicine, Surgery and the Allied Sciences, Being Reprints of Those Communications Which First Conveyed Epoch-Making Observations to the Scientific World Together with Biographical Sketches of the Observers* (Philadelphia: W. B. Saunders, 1909), p. vi. He first submitted the plan for the volume to Professors Welch and Osler.

schools giving formal instruction in 1901 were Boston University and Woman's Medical School in Chicago where Sarah Hackett Stevenson taught obstetrics, ethics and history of medicine.[19]

The first decade of the twentieth century continued the trend. In the same speech in which Eugene F. Cordell of the University of Maryland, the first honorary professor of the history of medicine in the United States, reproached his colleagues of the Medical and Chirurgical Faculty for their lack of interest in medical history and harangued them about its values, he presented the results of a questionnaire which he had elicited from fourteen leading medical schools. His inquiry belied his pessimism, for of the fourteen schools half had some instruction and five had faculty titles of professor or lecturer of the history of medicine.[20] In addition, the contemporary medical journals published quite a number of articles on history, and editorials were advocating its cultivation for a variety of reasons.[21] There seems to have been a good market for medico-historical textbooks, since Roswell Park's published lectures, *An Epitome of the History of Medicine*, which first appeared in 1897, sold so well that a second corrected edition was issued in 1899 and reprinted in 1908. A 1901 editorial in the *New York Medical Journal* stated:

> There have been times when we have been tempted to deplore the decadence of scholarship in the medical profession; of literary scholarship, we mean, as distinguished from a study of medical literature merely from the standpoint of utility and for purposes of applied medical science. . . . It is with pleasure that during the last years of the century that has closed we have witnessed an unmistakable increase in the bent toward it displayed by the profession at large . . . illustrated by increasingly numerous contributions to professional journals on matters of medical history, biography, archaeology, and folklore.[22]

Erwin Ackerknecht has labelled the wave of medico-historical enthusiasm which began around 1900 the Osler-Cushing-Garrison wave, implying that these individuals were chiefly responsible.[23] Perhaps this is

19. H. F. A. Peypers, "L'avancement de l'histoire de la médecine," *Janus* 6 (1901): 492.

20. Eugene F. Cordell, "The Importance of the Study of the History of Medicine," *Med. Lib. & Hist. J.* 2 (1904): 268–82.

21. E.g., "The Study of the History of Medicine," *J. AMA* 37 (1901): 453–54; "The Value of Medical Biography to the Medical Student," ibid. 41 (1903): 426–27; H. A. Geitz, "Medical History and Its Value to Medical Students," *N.Y. Med. J.* 67 (1898): 393–95; Henry L. Ambler, "The Value of Instruction in Dental History and Literature," *Dental Items of Interest* 26 (1904): 598–617.

22. "Gynecology and Surgery Among the Ancients," *N.Y. Med. J.* 73 (1901): 770.

23. Erwin H. Ackerknecht, "On the Teaching of Medical History," in Iago Galdston, ed., *On the Utility of Medical History*, Monograph I, Institute on Social and Historical Medicine,

so, but the argument has been made elsewhere that they brought focus and direction to an interest already latent in the medical profession, and that they were outstanding among many who were pursuing medico-historical interests in the United States at the time. If they became leaders it was because there were willing followers, already absorbed in the subject and carrying on activities in many parts of the country.[24] Writing in 1903, James B. Herrick, professor of medicine at Rush Medical College in Chicago, argued for a place for medical history in the medical school as an elective or as a side activity such as a medical history club. He stated, "When men like Osler advise the young physician to buy Laennec and to read Hippocrates; when Benjamin Ward Richardson said that he read Laennec every two years, there is something more to all this than a hobby."[25]

The trend to establish courses continued. Herrick began to give a seminar course around 1901; in 1910 courses were initiated at Temple and Illinois, and at Wisconsin in 1909 William Snow Miller formed a biweekly medical history seminar for medical students which met in his library. Prerequisites were a reading knowledge of French or German, regular attendance and the presentation of one paper a year. In Cleveland Henry E. Handerson lectured at the medical department of Ohio Wesleyan University; and in Baltimore, Brooklyn, Philadelphia, St. Louis, Chicago, New York, Washington, and Boston, medical history societies helped catalyze the community.[26] In 1912 Lewis S. Pilcher, a noted surgeon and book collector, speaking on Founders' Day at the University of Michigan on the liberalizing influences of historical learning as "an antitoxin for medical commercialism," urged that systematic instruction on the subject be introduced into the curriculum.[27]

Although the leading medical educators in this period were convinced that medical history was a desirable component of the curriculum,[28] the

---

The New York Academy of Medicine (New York: International Universities Press, 1957), p. 42.

24. Miller, "In Praise of Amateurs," pp. 600–611.

25. James B. Herrick, "The Study of Older Medical Writings," *Physician and Surgeon* 25 (1903): 8.

26. Fred B. Rogers, "Dr. Jules L. Prevost and the Teaching of Medical History at Temple University School of Medicine, 1910–1965," *Trans. & Stud. Coll. Phys. Phila.* 33 (1965): 139–46; William S. Middleton, "Doctor William Snow Miller and His Seminar," *Bull. Hist. Med.* 8 (1940): 1067–72.

27. Lewis S. Pilcher, "An Antitoxin for Medical Commercialism: Being Some Consideration as to the Value and Place in Medical Undergraduate Instruction of the History and Memorials of Medicine," *Physician and Surgeon* 34 (1912): 145–58.

28. Abraham Flexner, *Medical Education in the United States and Canada* (New York: Carnegie Foundation for the Advancement of Teaching, 1910), p. 52, n. 1.

various attempts to teach it met with little success. The students found the lectures boring. An editorial in the *Journal of the American Medical Association* in 1914 reviewed the discussion at a meeting of the Königsberg Society of Scientific Medicine about the best way to teach medical history. One participant mentioned that he got students interested by bringing medical history directly into his clinical demonstrations. The American reviewer commented, "We cannot too warmly commend the foregoing as the best method. . . . The history of ancient medicine is a dull subject in itself; the modern period, from the work of Vesalius and Harvey on, is the most inspiring . . . and long-winded lectures, by no matter what authority, would only crowd the medical course still further with material which could not be assimilated."[29] He pointed out that although Billings's lectures on medical history in medical education "were the best of the kind," the fruit which they bore was the method of Osler and others at Hopkins of carrying "historical medicine" directly into the clinic.

Similarly in a lecture at the opening exercises of the Syracuse Medical College in 1915, Fielding H. Garrison, whose *Introduction to the History of Medicine* had appeared two years earlier, pointed out that set medical history lectures to medical students had "been tried and tested often enough and, in most cases, found wanting . . . unless backed up by unusual eloquence or a fascinating personality." He stated that such lectures swarm with unfamiliar names "which as Coleridge said, 'are nonconductors and stop all interest,' " so that students stay away from such lectures, just as music students avoid classes in harmony and counterpoint. He too recommended the system used by Osler and Welch at Hopkins, and Harvey Cushing at Harvard, where history was integrated with studies in the laboratory or clinic. He also indicated a need for some medical men to specialize in medical history, and noted that Cushing and some other advanced teachers were already beginning to "encourage some of their pupils to take up the literary side of medicine, as a set-off to an ordinary success as internists or surgeons exclusively."[30]

An index of the strength of medico-historical interest among physicians at this time is given by the presence of 75 members at the first meeting of the Section on Historical Medicine established at the New York Academy of Medicine in 1917, and a roster of 125 members of the Boston Medical History Club.[31] From 1915 to 1920 three periodicals devoted to literary or

29. "Medical History in the Medical Curriculum," *J. AMA* 63 (1914): 2046.
30. Fielding H. Garrison, "The Uses of Medical Bibliography and Medical History in the Medical Curriculum," *J. AMA* 66 (1916): 321, 323.
31. Philip Van Ingen, *The New York Academy of Medicine: Its First Hundred Years* (New York: Columbia University Press, 1949), p. 360.

historical medicine appeared: *The Medical Pickwick: A Monthly Literary Magazine of Wit and Wisdom* (1915), the *Annals of Medical History* (1917), and *Medical Life* (1920). In 1915 Paul B. Hoeber had reissued for an American audience the medico-historical classic, William Mac-michael's *The Gold-Headed Cane*, with an introduction by William Osler. In the preface Frances R. Packard commented on the "recent great stimulation of interest in medical history which the profession in this country has shown." Dr. John Radcliffe's comment to Dr. Richard Mead, found in the *Cane*, summarized one of the reasons for this interest: " . . . for as I have grown older, every year of my life has convinced me more and more of the value of the education of the scholar and the gentleman, to the thorough-bred physician."[32]

This ideal permeated medical education up to World War II. Physicians aspired to be gentlemen, which implied a humanistic education refining them and making them superior human beings. The sentiment was voiced by W. S. Thayer of Johns Hopkins in 1913 when he recommended a premedical training not limited solely to the natural sciences, but including also mathematics, history, philosophy, and languages, both ancient and modern. Arguing that the physician's personal influence on his patients, the power "to inspire hope and confidence and affection," was one of his most necessary attributes, Thayer stated, "That which educates, softens and refines the physician as a man gives him an immense advantage over his cruder neighbor."[33] In a similar vein Charles L. Dana in his Weir Mitchell Oration at the College of Physicians of Philadelphia in 1922 extolled Mitchell for his humanistic interests and knowledge, and urged that medical schools give courses that would bring "culture" to the students, defining it as "the study, knowledge and sympathetic appreciation of the best things thought and said and done in the history of mankind, . . . the well-written stories of the achievements and mistakes of the great periods in human progress." With "culture," Dana asserted, students would tend to possess "mental balance" and sane ideas and beliefs that would counteract the current fads and follies of their profession.[34]

Medico-historical sections began to appear as regular features in some medical journals, as seen in John Rührah's column "New Books and Old" beginning with the March 12, 1921, issue of *Medical Record*, and the

32. William Macmichael, *The Gold-Headed Cane* (New York: Paul B. Hoeber, 1915), pp. xxi–xxii, 35.

33. W. S. Thayer, "Some Questions Concerning Medical Education," *Ohio St. Med. J.* 9 (1913): 1–2.

34. Charles L. Dana, "Medicine and the Humanities," *Ann. Med. Hist.* 4 (1922): 329–30.

section "Historical Medicine" which began to appear in 1924 when the journal changed its name to the *Medical Journal and Record*.[35]

Courses in medical schools continued to multiply. Walter Libby was asked to give a series of lectures at the University of Pittsburgh beginning in 1918. The bibliophile Edward Clark Streeter was appointed lecturer on the history of medicine at Harvard in 1921, and instead of lecturing at the school brought students to his home for informal evenings with his books.[36] Two students of William Snow Miller, Olof Larsell and Chauncey D. Leake, established medical history seminars similar to his at the University of Oregon and San Francisco, where Herbert M. Evans, a disciple of Osler, was also active. Morris Fishbein began teaching medical history in Chicago. The concern in the 1920s was to make medical history palatable to students. Libby chose to discuss what had aroused his curiosity when he was a medical student; Major G. Seelig, who was asked by Washington University School of Medicine in 1924 to give a course to senior students (to which seniors of St. Louis University were also invited), tried to get students interested, as noted by Garrison, "by means of a stimulating, informing, communicative literary manner." Both published their lecture notes to serve as student textbooks.[37] Another such text, prepared especially for students and issued in 1926 by Charles L. Dana, professor of nervous diseases at Cornell University Medical College, included a diagram with an exposition of medico-historical "peaks" which the students were supposed to know. He also inserted many illustrations of medical activities and institutions, in addition to the customary portraits, stating that his intention was to make the illustrations "give social atmosphere to a text which is preponderately biographical."[38] C. N. B. Camac's *Imhotep to Harvey: Backgrounds of Medical History* (New York, 1931) consisted of notes which he had used since 1926 in seminars held in the library of the College of Physicians and Surgeons at Columbia for fourth-year medical students during their clinical clerkship. He stressed that no lectures were given, but that students gathered around books, pictures, and charts spread on a large table, while he discussed

35. *Med. Record* 99 (1921): 461; *Med. J. & Record* 119 (1924): 104.

36. Henry R. Viets, "Edward Clark Streeter (1874–1947)," *Bull. Hist. Med.* 21 (1947): 843–45.

37. Walter Libby, *The History of Medicine in Its Salient Features* (Boston and New York: Houghton Mifflin, 1922), p. v; M. G. Seelig, *Medicine: An Historical Outline* (Baltimore: Williams and Wilkins, 1925), p. xv.

38. Charles L. Dana, *The Peaks of Medical History: An Outline of the Evolution of Medicine for the Use of Medical Students and Practitioners* (New York: Paul B. Hoeber, 1926), p. 7. Elsewhere Dana suggested that medical schools should have an advisory historian to work with the various departments in preparing historical lectures (Dana, "Medicine and the Humanities," p. 335).

them. There was no time in the curriculum for the students to write historical papers, but Camac mentioned that a student medical history club was being considered.[39]

In 1927 in an address to the Piersol Anatomical Society of the University of Pennsylvania, E. B. Krumbhaar, the founder of the American Association for the History of Medicine, gave suggestions about how to acquire an interest in medical history through eliminating systematic lectures unless "the teacher has the gift of tongues" and selecting topics for individual historical research projects which relate directly with one's primary medical interest.[40] Noting the "lamentable failures" in most medical schools in teaching medical history, J. M. H. Rowland of the University of Maryland reported in 1927 to the annual meeting of the Association of American Medical Colleges of the success of John Rathbone Oliver's well-attended course which included lantern slides and book demonstrations as well as a formal lecture.[41] Victor Robinson, who became professor of the history of medicine at Temple University in 1929, used a pictorial method with over five hundred slides, and he issued a thirty-two-page "Medico-Historical Curriculum, Specimen Questions and Answers."[42]

Up to this time medical history teaching in America had been distinct from the European development, where by the 1920s departments with full-time professors had been created in a number of universities, especially in Germany and Austria.[43] The subject had become a serious academic discipline for which knowledge of ancient languages and training in philology and philosophy were prerequisites. It was removed from the realm of the hobbyist and even the bibliophile, unless collecting served serious scholarly purposes. Early in the century European reviewers had been surprised and very complimentary about the Americans' interest in medical history, and Karl Sudhoff commented happily about the new chairs which sprang up.[44] However as time went on it became obvious that medico-historical education in the United States was

39. C. N. B. Camac, *Imhotep to Harvey: Backgrounds of Medical History* (New York: Paul B. Hoeber, 1931), pp. xiii–xiv.

40. E. B. Krumbhaar, "The Lure of Medical History," *Science* 46 (1927): 1–4.

41. J. M. H. Rowland, "An Experiment in the Teaching of the History of Medicine," *Bull. AAMC* 3 (1928): 317–21.

42. *Medical Life* 37 (1930): 619–50.

43. See the survey of Henry E. Sigerist, "Die Geschichte der Medizin im akademischen Unterricht: Ergebnisse einer Rundfrage des Instituts," *Kyklos* 1 (1928): 147–56; English translation in *Medical Life* 36 (1929): 41–55.

44. See Julius Pagel's comment in *Janus* 8 (1903): 502; Karl Sudhoff's in *Mitt. z. Gesch. d. Med.* 3 (1904): 214; K. Sudhoff, "Fortschritte in der Pflege der Medizingeschichte in den Vereinigten Staaten," ibid. 20 (1921): 291–92.

a matter of chance, that courses appeared and disappeared, and that few genuinely original works were being produced by Americans. The time was ripe for American graduate education in medical history in order to supply professional leadership.

As early as 1913 Arnold C. Klebs had read a paper at the Johns Hopkins Hospital Historical Club in which he had reviewed in some detail the status of the teaching and research activities of medical history in Europe, and he reminded his audience of Billings's hope that "the scheme of higher medical education which your university is about to organize will include instruction in bibliographical and *historical methods* as well as in those of the laboratory and clinic."[45] Klebs gave Sudhoff's Institute for the History of Medicine at Leipzig as a model for an ideal teaching center, where students could be instructed, not by didactic lectures, but by objective demonstration of research methods and practical bibliographical work. "Such instruction," he concluded, "will best be given in separate premises easily accessible to all departments, where the objects for demonstration should be collected and classified and where special research can be carried on." Sixteen years later, the Johns Hopkins University opened the Institute of the History of Medicine at the School of Medicine with William H. Welch as its first director.[46] Welch summoned Garrison, who had been appointed librarian of the Welch Medical Library, as lecturer in the history of medicine, and John Rathbone Oliver, whose successful lectures at the University of Maryland have already been noted. Welch had no intention of remaining long as professor, and in 1932 he was succeeded by Henry E. Sigerist, a Swiss medical historian who had been Sudhoff's successor at Leipzig. Sigerist's dynamic leadership began a new medico-historical era in the United States.

The immediate goal of the new institute was to provide leadership and to help to set standards for medico-historical teaching and research. In the thirties, although there was considerable activity, especially in popularizing medical history, the quality of many books being published was very low, "some in coarse vernacular or even doggerel," according to Garrison,[47] and Sigerist and his staff—which included his Leipzig assistant,

45. Italics mine. Arnold C. Klebs, "The History of Medicine as a Subject of Teaching and Research," *Bull. Johns Hopkins Hosp.* 25 (1914): 1, 10.

46. A detailed account of Dr. Welch's activities in founding the Johns Hopkins Institute is given by Simon Flexner and James Thomas Flexner, *William Henry Welch and the Heroic Age of American Medicine* (New York: Viking, 1941), pp. 416–43. Garrison described the possibilities of the new program in "Developmental Possibilities in Medical History as a Branch of the Medical Curriculum," *Bull. N.Y. Acad. Med.*, 2nd ser., 5 (1929): 741–56.

47. Fielding H. Garrison, "Transvaluations and Deflations in the History of Medicine and Its Teaching," *Bull. N.Y. Acad. Med.* 10 (1934): 589. An editorial in *Medical Record*

Owsei Temkin, and Ludwig Edelstein, a classicist from Berlin—undertook to introduce standards of professional historiography to the field. In 1933 Sigerist founded the *Bulletin of the Institute of the History of Medicine* (the name changed in 1939 to *Bulletin of the History of Medicine*) as a house organ for scholarly publications by the institute staff as well as articles by outsiders. One of his first publications in America was a syllabus, "On the Teaching of Medical History," containing lecture outlines and a bibliography of current books and articles designed to help lecturers in medical schools throughout the country.[48] The one thousand reprints of this syllabus disappeared within the year because of the huge demand.[49]

In addition to lecture courses and advanced seminars for students in the Hopkins medical institutions and graduate school, beginning in 1938 the institute also sponsored so-called graduate weeks in medical history, which were intended essentially to be training experiences for physicians and others who were either teaching the subject elsewhere or were engaged in medico-historical writing and research. The institute staff tactfully presented modern historiographic methods and research materials in a setting where the attendees were introduced to appropriate research tools, as well as entertained at concerts or dramatic productions relating to the theme of the graduate week. Exhibitions were also prepared to illustrate the visual techniques of education in medical history.[50]

In the spring of 1937 Sigerist sent a questionnaire to the deans of the seventy-seven grade A medical schools. He was surprised to learn that forty-six, or 70 percent of the schools, gave instruction in medical history; 60 percent of these had regular courses given by one or more instructors. Even the schools without regular courses tried to interest the students with occasional lectures or collateral reading. In the forty-six schools with instruction, thirty had required courses. Although seven professors of the

---

criticized Garrison: "But interest in medical history cannot be considered sacrosanct. It cannot be a question of all or none, of the doctor wrapping himself up in its folds in a serious and well nigh exclusive fashion, or else touching it not at all. For the doctor need not necessarily drink deep; what trickles over through popular books and articles and advertisements seems sufficient to slake the thirst of those who are not too avid in the pursuit of culture or of a liberal education. Who would deny these some taste of the history of medicine?" ("Popularization of Medical History," *Medical Record* 142 [1935]: 2).

48. *Bull. Hist. Med.* 2 (1934): 123–39.

49. See Emerson Crosby Kelly, "A Modern Method of Teaching Medical History," *J. AAMC* 12 (1937): 393–95; William G. Leaman, "Some Observations of the Teaching of Medical History," ibid. 14 (1939): 386–90.

50. See the various reports in *Bull. Hist. Med.* 6 (1938): 864–71; 7 (1939): 856–865; 12 (1942): 451–57.

history of medicine were reported, six were honorary and without stipend. Only Johns Hopkins had a full-time salaried professor.[51]

In spite of the rather optimistic picture given by the questionnaire, Sigerist was not satisfied with the quality of much of the instruction, and he noted three major difficulties: lack of time, personnel, and money. Dismissing lack of time as easily solved, he stressed the great need for training teachers to be able to present medical history effectively. He noted that most of the instructors were specialists in fields other than history and suggested that they receive postgraduate training. Sigerist also recommended that some of the other major universities establish chairs of medical history, suggesting "one university in New York, Yale, Harvard, Chicago, California or Stanford, and one southern university such as Tulane."

Sigerist's program for postgraduate training did not really materialize until after World War II and after he had left Hopkins. He could not encourage men to enter a field for which there were no openings, and although he was able to obtain Carnegie fellowships for two classics students to spend two years in the institute working on ancient medicine, no physician at that time could afford to obtain an advanced degree in a field with such an uncertain future. Only two students received degrees under Sigerist, one an M.A. in 1939 and the other a Ph.D. in 1947. Both were women who were not inhibited by the job situation.[52]

After the war other full-time chairs began to appear, led by the University of Wisconsin where in 1947 Erwin H. Ackerknecht was appointed the first professor and in 1950 a department of the history of medicine was created. A former student of Sigerist at Leipzig, Ackerknecht had been on the staff of the Johns Hopkins Institute for several years during the war. Wisconsin was followed in 1951 by Yale, where John F. Fulton was appointed Sterling Professor of the History of Medicine. In 1952 Ilza Veith developed a graduate program at the University of Chicago.

Simultaneously the American Association for the History of Medicine began to concern itself with educational problems. In 1950 the Committee on the Teaching of Medical History, composed of Richard H. Shryock (chairman), Iago Galdston, and Owsei Temkin, drew up a report analyzing the current state of the field and making recommendations to medical schools. The committee had met in the Johns Hopkins Institute on December 1, 1950, together with twenty-five others active in teaching. The

51. Henry E. Sigerist, "Medical History in the Medical Schools of the United States," *Bull. Hist. Med.* 7 (1939): 627–62.
52. Genevieve Miller and Ilza Veith. The two Carnegie fellows in 1941–1943 were Israel E. Drabkin and G. Raynor Thompson.

seven-page published report, which was distributed to the deans of all the medical schools in the United States and Canada, stressed the necessity for the inclusion of medical history in the medical school curriculum, and recommended that "some minimum work in general medical history should be required in all medical schools," giving constructive suggestions how this could be achieved. The report also stated that each school should have a full-time instructor not only to give a general course and seminars, but to serve as a historical consultant for other faculty members. For schools unable to add a full-time historian, supplementary training of instructors with avocational interests was recommended.[53]

After World War II and probably partly through Sigerist's influence, a shift in the purpose of medical history in medical education became apparent. The goal was no longer to create a humanistically oriented physician, a "cultured" man, but instead to give a physician insight into the interrelationships between medicine and society and between the various medical specialties.[54] In Raymond B. Allen's 1946 survey of American medical education he had criticized most courses in medical history because they concentrated on medical advances and great men, but failed "to bring out the broad social relations and implications of medical science and the profession in the evolution of our society."[55] Among the few schools before the war teaching "the impact of medicine and science on society" the leader was Johns Hopkins, where Sigerist's entire thrust was on the so-called social history of medicine, and where he used history to analyze contemporary events in medicine and medical care in all parts of the world.

The Committee on the Teaching of Medical History had recommended that a new survey be made, and another committee led by David A. Tucker, Jr., between 1952 and 1957 reported annually in the *Bulletin of the History of Medicine* on information which they found in medical school catalogues.[56] They reported that thirty-seven out of seventy-nine medical schools surveyed, or 47 percent of American medical schools in 1952, had organized courses in medical history, over half of which were

53. Committee on the Teaching of Medical History, "Statement of the Editorial Sub-Committee," *Bull. Hist. Med.* 25 (1951): 571–77.

54. "In the wide expanse of the present medical curriculum there are few if any areas, other than that of medical history, in which students are encouraged to step back from the technical specialties and view their science and their profession in terms of larger interrelationships—of both those within medicine and with society as a whole" (ibid., p. 573).

55. Raymond B. Allen, *Medical Education and the Changing Order* (New York: Commonwealth Fund, 1946), p. 78.

56. *Bull. Hist. Med.* 26 (1952): 562–78; 27 (1953): 358; 28 (1954): 354–58; 29 (1955): 535–44; 30 (1956): 365–69; 31 (1957): 358.

required. Three years later the total had increased to forty-two. An American Medical Association survey of the same year reported that only ten of the eighty-one medical schools in the United States reported no activity whatsoever.[57]

In the 1950s and 1960s thirteen additional schools added a full-time medical historian to their faculty, and by 1969 graduate degrees were obtainable in nine American universities: University of California at Los Angeles, University of California at San Francisco, Duke, Johns Hopkins, Minnesota, Tulane, University of Washington, Wisconsin, and Yale. A parallel development after World War II was the emergence of the history of science as an academic discipline, and in some universities like Harvard, Yale, and the University of Chicago the two subjects were included in the same department.

By the mid-1960s professional activity in medical history had been greatly stimulated by the research grant program of the National Institutes of Health, which had created a History of the Life Sciences Study Section to referee the awarding of grants in medical and related history. In order to assess the impact that this program was having on American medical education, the study section initiated a new survey based on site visits, and data was collected for ninety-five American schools. Of these, forty-three schools, or 45 percent, were found to offer regular instruction; fourteen schools, or 15 percent, had obligatory courses.[58] This represented a decline from the high point of the mid-fifties. A sampling of recent medical school catalogues indicates that formal course offerings have declined even further. However, new courses with titles such as "Medical Practice and Society" or "Society and Health Care in History" have begun to appear. Today historical data tend to merge with data from sociology and the behavioral sciences in new course formats.

The formation of the Society for Health and Human Values in 1969 brought to a focus attempts to counteract the impersonal, dehumanizing character of current medical education. In 1964 a pioneering step was taken by the new Milton S. Hershey Medical Center College of Medicine, which created a department of humanities to bring the accumulated experience of Western culture into medical education through courses in ethics, religion, and the philosophy of science. At Wisconsin the major emphasis is upon using history to elucidate current medical problems.[59]

57. Edward L. Turner, Walter S. Wiggins, and Anne Tipner, "Medical Education in the United States and Canada," *J. AMA* 159 (1955): 579.

58. Genevieve Miller, "The Teaching of Medical History in the United States and Canada: Report of a Field Survey," *Bull. Hist. Med.* 43 (1969): 259–67, 344–75, 444–72, 553–86.

59. See Guenter B. Risse, "The Role of Medical History in the Education of the

A recent study by Chester R. Burns gives a penetrating analysis of some of the reasons why past efforts to include medical history in the medical curriculum have failed. Stressing "relevance," he suggests that "too many scholars have been unwilling to adapt their scholarship to the emotional, cognitive, and vocational needs of learners at the various stages of professional development and with various images of the past" and "too many teachers have been unwilling to acquire the knowledge generated by important advances in medico-historical scholarship."[60] Unlike 1937, when Sigerist and his colleagues were the only professional medical historians in the United States, today medical history is promoted by a number of highly trained experts whose objective of making the subject a meaningful part of medical and even general education is being carried out on many different levels, including medical history museums for the general public, undergraduate premedical courses in the university, general courses in the medical schools presented topically and related to current problems, seminars devoted to medical specialties for house officers and staff, and continuing education courses for the hobbyist or bibliophile.

'Humanist' Physician: A Reevaluation," *J. Med. Educ.* 50 (1975): 458–65.

60. Chester R. Burns, "History in Medical Education: The Development of Current Trends in the United States," *Bull. N.Y. Acad. Med.*, 2nd ser., 51 (1975): 866. Burns continues the exploratory trend exemplified by the 1966 Macy Conference on Education in the History of Medicine. John B. Blake, ed., *Education in the History of Medicine*, Report of a Macy Conference sponsored by the Josiah Macy, Jr., Foundation in cooperation with the National Library of Medicine, Bethesda, Maryland, June 22–24, 1966 (New York, 1968).

Contributors

EDWARD C. ATWATER, M.D., is Associate Professor of Medicine and the History of Medicine at the University of Rochester School of Medicine and Dentistry. He has written extensively on the medical history of Rochester and on American medical education.

JOHN B. BLAKE, Ph.D., is Chief of the History of Medicine Division at the National Library of Medicine. In addition to numerous articles, he has published *Public Health in the Town of Boston, 1630–1822* (1959), *Benjamin Waterhouse and the Introduction of Vaccination: A Reappraisal* (1957), and (with Charles Roos) *Medical Reference Works, 1679–1966: A Selected Bibliography* (1967). From 1972 to 1974 he served as president of the American Association for the History of Medicine.

JEANNE L. BRAND, Ph.D., is Chief of the International Programs Division, Extramural Programs, National Library of Medicine. She is the author of *Doctors and the State: The British Medical Profession and Government Action in Public Health, 1870–1912* (1965) and editor (with George Mora) of *Psychiatry and Its History* (1970).

GERT H. BRIEGER, M.D., Ph.D., is Professor and Chairman, Department of the History of Health Sciences, University of California, San Francisco. He is editor of *Medical America in the Nineteenth Century* (1972) and *Theory and Practice in American Medicine* (1976) and author of the historical introduction to the tenth (1972) and eleventh (1977) editions of *Christopher's Textbook of Surgery*. He is presently completing a biography of the American surgeon Stephen Smith.

CHESTER R. BURNS, M.D., Ph.D., is James Wade Rockwell Associate Professor of Medical History and Associate Director of the Institute for the Medical Humanities at the University of Texas Medical Branch at Galveston. He has written widely on medical ethics and edited several anthologies, including (with John P. McGovern) *Humanism in Medicine* (1973), *Legacies in Ethics and Medicine* (1977), and *Legacies in Law and Medicine* (1977). He is past president of the Society for Health and Human Values.

DAVID L. COWEN, M.A., is Professor of History, Emeritus, Rutgers University, and Lecturer in the History of Pharmacy, Rutgers University

309

College of Pharmacy. He is the author of *America's Pre-Pharmacopoeial Literature* (1961), *Medicine and Health in New Jersey: A History* (1964), *Medical Education: The Queen's-Rutgers Experience, 1792–1830* (1966), *The New Jersey Pharmaceutical Association, 1870–1970* (1970), and *The Spread and Influence of British Pharmacopoeial and Related Literature* (1974), as well as many articles in the history of medicine and pharmacy.

MARTIN KAUFMAN, Ph.D., is Professor of History at Westfield State College in Massachusetts. His publications include *Homeopathy in America: The Rise and Fall of a Medical Heresy* (1971), *American Medical Education: The Formative Years* (1976), and *The University of Vermont College of Medicine* (1979).

JUDITH WALZER LEAVITT, Ph.D., is Assistant Professor of the History of Medicine at the University of Wisconsin, Madison. She has coedited *Medicine Without Doctors: Home Health Care in American History* (1977) and *Sickness and Health in America: Readings in the History of Medicine and Public Health* (1978), and is completing a historical study of public health in urban America.

LAWRENCE D. LONGO, M.D., is Professor of Physiology and Obstetrics and Gynecology, School of Medicine, Loma Linda University. In addition to scores of scientific articles, he has written *Oxygenation of the Fetus-in-Utero* (1978) and edited *Respiratory Gas Exchange and Blood Flow in the Placenta* (1972), *Fetal and Newborn Cardiovascular Physiology* (1978), and, since 1970, "Classic Pages in Obstetrics and Gynecology" in the *American Journal of Obstetrics and Gynecology*.

RUSSELL C. MAULITZ, M.D., Ph.D., is Assistant Professor of Medicine and of the History and Sociology of Science at the University of Pennsylvania, where he teaches medical history and practices internal medicine. He has written a number of articles on the history of nineteenth and twentieth-century scientific medicine and is currently preparing a monograph on early nineteenth-century pathology.

GENEVIEVE MILLER, Ph.D., is Associate Professor of the History of Science, Case Western Reserve University School of Medicine, and Director of the Howard Dittrick Museum of Historical Medicine in Cleveland, Ohio. Her publications include *William Beaumont's Formative Years: Two Early Notebooks, 1811–1821* (1946), *The Adoption of Inoculation for Smallpox in England and France* (1957), *Bibliography of the History of Medicine of the U.S. and Canada, 1939–1960* (1964), and *Bibliography of the Writings of Henry E. Sigerist* (1966). She is currently president of the American Association for the History of Medicine.

RONALD L. NUMBERS, Ph.D., is Professor of the History of Medicine and the History of Science, and Chairman of the Department of the History of Medicine, University of Wisconsin, Madison. He is the author of *Prophetess of Health: A Study of Ellen G. White* (1976), *Creation by Natural Law: Laplace's Nebular Hypothesis in American Thought* (1977), and *Almost Persuaded: American Physicians and Compulsory Health Insurance, 1912–1920* (1978).

LLOYD G. STEVENSON, M.D., Ph.D., is William H. Welch Professor of the History of Medicine and Director of the Institute of the History of Medicine, the Johns Hopkins University. During his distinguished career as a medical historian and educator he has served as dean of the McGill University School of Medicine, as president of the American Association for the History of Medicine, and, since 1968, as editor of the *Bulletin of the History of Medicine.*

JOHN HARLEY WARNER, M.A., is a doctoral candidate in the Department of the History of Science, Harvard University, where he is studying the history of biology and medicine. He has written on " 'The Nature-Trusting Heresy': American Physicians and the Concept of the Healing Power of Nature in the 1850s and 1860s," *Perspectives in American History* 11 (1977–78).

JAMES WHORTON, Ph.D., is Associate Professor of Biomedical History at the University of Washington, Seattle. He is the author of *Before Silent Spring: Pesticides and Public Health in Pre-DDT America* (1975) and several studies of hygienic reform in America.

Abbreviations of Journal Titles

Am. Bar Assoc. J.	American Bar Association Journal
Am. Chem. J.	American Chemical Journal
Am. Heart J.	American Heart Journal
Am. Hist. Rev.	American Historical Review
Am. J. Insan.	American Journal of Insanity
Am. J. Med. Juris.	American Journal of Medical Jurisprudence
Am. J. Med. Sci.	American Journal of the Medical Sciences
Am. J. Pharm. Educ.	American Journal of Pharmaceutical Education
Am. J. Psychiatry	American Journal of Psychiatry
Am. J. Public Health	American Journal of Public Health and the Nation's Health
Am. J. Sci.	American Journal of Science and Arts
Am. J. Surg.	American Journal of Surgery
Am. Med. Record	American Medical Recorder
Am. Med. Times	American Medical Times
Anat. Record	Anatomical Record
Ann. Int. Med.	Annals of Internal Medicine
Ann. Med. Hist.	Annals of Medical History
Ann. N.Y. Acad. Sci.	Annals of the New York Academy of Sciences
Ann. Rev. Pharmacol.	Annual Review of Pharmacology
Ann. Rev. Physiol.	Annual Review of Physiology
Ann. Sci.	Annals of Science
Ann. Surg.	Annals of Surgery
Arch. Path.	Archives of Pathology
Arch. Surg.	Archives of Surgery
Beitr. Pathol.	Beiträge zur Pathologie der Verdauungsorgane
Biogr. Mem. Nat. Acad. Sci.	National Academy of Sciences. Biographical Memoirs
Boston Med. Q.	Boston Medical Quarterly
Boston Med. & Surg. J.	Boston Medical and Surgical Journal
Brit. J. Med. Educ.	British Journal of Medical Education

313

Brit. Med. J.	British Medical Journal
Buffalo Med. J.	Buffalo Medical Journal
Bull. AMA	American Medical Association. Bulletin
Bull. Acad. Med. Cleveland	Academy of Medicine of Cleveland. Bulletin
Bull. Am. Acad. Med.	American Academy of Medicine. Bulletin
Bull. Am. Coll. Surg.	American College of Surgeons. Bulletin
Bull. AAMC	Association of American Medical Colleges. Bulletin
Bull. Hist. Med.	Bulletin of the History of Medicine
Bull. Med. Libr. Assoc.	Medical Library Association. Bulletin
Bull. Johns Hopkins Hosp.	Johns Hopkins Hospital. Bulletin
Bull. Menninger Clinic	Menninger Clinic. Bulletin
Bull. N.Y. Acad. Med.	New York Academy of Medicine. Bulletin
Bull. Wayne Univ. Col. Med.	Wayne University College of Medicine. Bulletin
Calif. Med.	California Medicine
Canad. Med. Assoc. J.	Canadian Medical Association Journal
Canad. J. Public Health	Canadian Journal of Public Health
Clin. Pharmacol. Ther.	Clinical Pharmacology and Therapeutics
Conn. Med.	Connecticut Medicine
D. S. B.	Dictionary of Scientific Biography
Eclectic Med. J.	Eclectic Medical Journal
Edinburgh Med. J.	Edinburgh Medical Journal
Federation Proc.	Federation Proceedings
Gen. Prac.	General Practitioner
Harvard Med. Alumni Bull.	Harvard Medical Alumni Bulletin
Internat. Clinics	International Clinics
J. AMA	Journal of American Medical Association
J. Am. Chem. Soc.	American Chemical Society. Journal
J. AAMC	Association of American Medical Colleges. Journal
J. Chem. Educ.	Journal of Chemical Education
J. Clin. Pharmacol.	Journal of Clinical Pharmacology
J. Hist. Med.	Journal of the History of Medicine and Allied Sciences
J. Iowa St. Med. Soc.	Iowa State Medical Society. Journal

J. Legal Ed.	Journal of Legal Education
J. Med. Educ.	Journal of Medical Education
J. Med. & Phil.	The Journal of Medicine and Philosophy
J. Mich. St. Med. Soc.	Michigan State Medical Society. Journal
J. Mt. Sinai Hosp.	Journal of the Mount Sinai Hospital
J. Nerv. Ment. Dis.	Journal of Nervous and Mental Disease
J. Soc. Hist.	Journal of Social History
Lib. Chron.	Library Chronicle
Lond. Med. Gaz.	London Medical Gazette
Long Island Med. J.	Long Island Medical Journal
Med. Ann. D.C.	Medical Annals of the District of Columbia
Med. & Biol. Ill.	Medical and Biological Illustration
Med. Comm. Mass. Med. Soc.	Massachusetts Medical Society. Medical Communications
Med. Hist.	Medical History
Med. J. & Record	Medical Journal and Record
Med. Lib. & Hist. J.	Medical Library and Historical Journal
Med. Record	Medical Record
Med. Recorder	Medical Recorder. Medicine, Surgery and Allied Sciences
Mitt. z. Gesch. d. Med.	Mittheilungen zur Geschichte der Medizin, der Naturwissenschaften und der Technik
Mt. Sinai J. Med.	Mount Sinai Journal of Medicine
N. Eng. J. Med.	New England Journal of Medicine
N. Eng. J. Med. & Surg.	New England Journal of Medicine and Surgery and Collateral Branches of Science
New Orleans Med. News & Hosp. Gaz.	New Orleans Medical News and Hospital Gazette
N.Y. Med. J.	New York Medical Journal
N.Y. Med. & Phys. J.	New York Medical and Physical Journal
N.Y. St. J. Med.	New York State Journal of Medicine
Obst. & Gynec.	Obstetrics and Gynecology
Ohio Med. & Surg. J.	Ohio Medical and Surgical Journal
Ohio St. Arch. & Hist. Q.	Ohio State Archaeological and Historical Quarterly
Ohio St. Med. J.	Ohio State Medical Journal

Peninsular J. of Med. & Col. Sci.	Peninsular Journal of Medicine and the Collateral Sciences
Perspect. Biol. & Med.	Perspectives in Biology and Medicine
Phila. J. Med. & Phys. Sci.	Philadelphia Journal of the Medical and Physical Sciences
Phila. Med. J.	Philadelphia Medical Journal
Phila. Med. Times	Philadelphia Medical Times
Proc. Am. Inst. Homeo.	American Institute of Homeopathy. Proceedings
Proc. Am. Phil. Soc.	American Philosophical Society. Proceedings
Proc. Assoc. Am. Anat.	Association of American Anatomists. Proceedings
Proc. AAMC	Association of American Medical Colleges. Proceedings
Proc. West. Pharmacol. Soc.	Western Pharmacology Society. Proceedings
Psychosom. Med.	Psychosomatic Medicine
Quart. Bull. Northw. Univ. Med. Sch.	Northwestern University Medical School. Quarterly Bulletin
Quart. Rev. Bio.	Quarterly Review of Biology
R.I. Med. J.	Rhode Island Medical Journal
Scottish M. & S. J.	Scottish Medical and Surgical Journal
St. Louis Med. Rev.	St. Louis Medical Review
South. Med. J.	Southern Medical Journal
Sudhoffs Arch. Gesch. Med.	Sudhoffs Archiv für Geschichte der Medizin und der Naturwissenschaften
Surg. Gynec. & Obstet.	Surgery, Gynecology and Obstetrics
Tex. St. J. Med.	Texas State Journal of Medicine
Trans. AMA	American Medical Association. Transactions
Trans. Am. Inst. Homeo.	American Institute of Homeopathy. Transactions
Trans. Am. Phil. Soc.	American Philosophical Society. Transactions
Trans. Am. Surg. Assoc.	American Surgical Association. Transactions
Trans. Coll. Phys. Phila.	College of Physicians of Philadelphia. Transactions

Trans. Congr. Am. Phys. & Surg.	Congress of American Physicians and Surgeons. Transactions
Trans. Maine Med. Soc.	Maine Medical Society. Transactions
Trans. Med. & Chirur. Fac. St. Md.	Medical and Chirurgical Faculty of the State of Maryland. Transactions
Trans. Med. Soc. St. N.Y.	Medical Society of the State of New York. Transactions
Trans. & Stud. Coll. Phys. Phila.	College of Physicians of Philadelphia. Transactions and Studies
U. Mich. Med. Bull.	University of Michigan Medical Bulletin
U. Mich. Med. Center J.	University of Michigan Medical Center Journal
U. Penn. Med. Bull.	University of Pennsylvania Medical Bulletin
U.S. Public Health Bull.	United States Public Health Service. Public Health Bulletin
Wis. Med. J.	Wisconsin Medical Journal
Yale J. Biol. Med.	Yale Journal of Biology and Medicine

Index

Designer:	Eric Jungerman
Compositor:	Lehmann Graphics
Printer:	Braun-Brumfield, Inc.
Binder:	Braun-Brumfield, Inc.
Text:	VIP Caledonia
Display:	Cheltenham Bold Condensed
Paper:	50 lb. P&S Offset Vellum